Your *Clinics* subscription just got better!

You can now access the FULL TEXT of this publication online at no additional cost! Activate your online subscription today and receive...

- Full text of all issues from 2002 to the present
- Photographs, tables, illustrations, and references
- Comprehensive search capabilities
- Links to MEDLINE and Elsevier journals

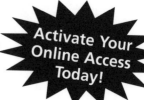

Activate Your Online Access Today!

Plus, you can also sign up for E-alerts of upcoming issues or articles that interest you, and take advantage of exclusive access to bonus features!

To activate your individual online subscription:

1. Visit our website at **www.TheClinics.com**.

2. Click on "Register" at the top of the page, and follow the instructions.

3. To activate your account, you will need your subscriber account number, which you can find on your mailing label (note: the number of digits in your subscriber account number varies from six to ten digits). See the sample below where the subscriber account number has been circled.

This is your subscriber account number

```
*****************************************3-DIGIT 001
FEB00   J0167   C7   ( 123456-89 )  10/00   Q: 1

J.H. DOE, MD
531 MAIN ST
CENTER CITY, NY  10001-001
```

4. That's it! Your online access to the most trusted source for clinical reviews is now available.

P9-ELW-477

the**clinics**.com

ELSEVIER

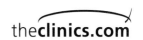
the**clinics**.com

VETERINARY CLINICS
OF NORTH AMERICA

Small Animal Practice

Emergency Medicine

GUEST EDITOR
Kenneth J. Drobatz, DVM, MSCE

March 2005 • Volume 35 • Number 2

SAUNDERS

An Imprint of Elsevier, Inc.
PHILADELPHIA   LONDON   TORONTO   MONTREAL   SYDNEY   TOKYO

W.B. SAUNDERS COMPANY

A Division of Elsevier Inc.

The Curtis Center • Independence Square West • Philadelphia, Pennsylvania 19106

http://www.vetsmall.theclinics.com

THE VETERINARY CLINICS OF NORTH AMERICA: Volume 35, Numbe
SMALL ANIMAL PRACTICE ISSN 0195-5∈
March 2005 ISBN 1-4160-284
Editor: John Vassallo

The ideas and opinions expressed in *The Veterinary Clinics of North America: Small Animal Practice* do not necessarily
flect those of the Publisher. The Publisher does not assume any responsibility for any injury and/or damage to person.
property arising out of or related to any use of the material contained in this periodical. The reader is advised to check
appropriate medical literature and the product information currently provided by the manufacturer of each drug tc
administered to verify the dosage, the method and duration of administration, or contraindications. It is the respo
bility of the treating physician or other health care professional, relying on independent experience and knowledge of
patient, to determine drug dosages and the best treatment for the patient. Mention of any product in this issue should
be construed as endorsement by the contributors, editors, or the Publisher of the product or manufacturers' claims

The Veterinary Clinics of North America: Small Animal Practice (ISSN 0195-5616) is published bimonthly (For Post Of
use only: volume 35 issue 2 of 6) by W.B. Saunders Company. Corporate and editorial offices: The Curtis Cen
Independence Square West, Philadelphia, PA 19106-3399. Accounting and circulation offices: 6277 Sea Harbor Dri
Orlando, FL 32887-4800. Periodicals postage paid at Orlando, FL 32862, and additional mailing offices. Subscript
prices are $170.00 per year for US individuals, $260.00 per year for US institutions, $85.00 per year for US stude
and residents, $215.00 per year for Canadian individuals, $325.00 per year for Canadian institutions, $225.00 per y
for international individuals, $325.00 per year for international institutions and $113.00 per year for Canadian a
foreign students/residents. To receive student/resident rate, orders must be accompanied by name of affiliated ir
tution, date of term, and the *signature* of program/residency coordinator on institution letterhead. Orders will
billed at individual rate until proof of status is received. Foreign air speed delivery is included in all *Clinics* subsc
tion prices. All prices are subject to change without notice. POSTMASTER: Send address changes to *The Veterin
Clinics of North America: Small Animal Practice*, Elsevier, Customer Service Department, 6277 Sea Harbor Drive, Orlan
FL 32887-4800, USA; phone: (+1)(877) 8397126 [toll free number for US customers], or (+1)(407) 3454020 [custom
outside US]; fax: (+1)(407) 3631354; email: usjcs@elsevier.com

The Veterinary Clinics of North America: Small Animal Practice is also published in Japanese by Gakusosha Comp⊾
Ltd., 2-16-28 Nishikata, Bunkyo-ku, Tokyo 113, Japan.

Reprints. For copies of 100 or more, of articles in this publication, please contact the Commercial Reprints Dep
ment, Elsevier Inc., 360 Park Avenue South, New York, New York 10010-1710. Tel. (212) 633-3813 Fax: (212) 4
1935, email: reprints@elsevier.com

The Veterinary Clinics of North America: Small Animal Practice is covered in *Current Contents/Agriculture, Biology*
Environmental Sciences, Science Citation Index, ASCA, Index Medicus, Excerpta Medica, and BIOSIS.

Printed in the United States of America.

GUEST EDITOR

KENNETH J. DROBATZ, DVM, MSCE, Diplomate, American College of Veterinary Internal Medicine; Diplomate, American College of Veterinary Emergency and Critical Care; Professor, Section of Critical Care; Director, Emergency Service, Department of Clinical Studies, Ryan Veterinary Hospital, University of Pennsylvania, Philadelphia, Pennsylvania

CONTRIBUTORS

JANET ALDRICH, DVM, Staff Veterinarian, Veterinary Medical Teaching Hospital, School of Veterinary Medicine, University of California-Davis, Davis, California

MATTHEW W. BEAL, DVM, Diplomate, American College of Veterinary Emergency and Critical Care; Assistant Professor, Emergency and Critical Care Medicine, College of Veterinary Medicine, Michigan State University, East Lansing, Michigan

AMANDA K. BOAG, MA, VetMB, MRCVS, Diplomate, American College of Veterinary Internal Medicine; Lecturer in Emergency and Critical Care/Internal Medicine, Queen Mother Hospital, Royal Veterinary College, North Mymms, Hertfordshire, United Kingdom

VICKI L. CAMPBELL, DVM, Diplomate, American College of Veterinary Anesthesiologists; Diplomate, American College of Veterinary and Emergency Critical Care; Assistant Professor of Emergency and Critical Care, James L. Voss Veterinary Teaching Hospital, Colorado State University, Fort Collins, Colorado

DANIEL L. CHAN, DVM, Diplomate, American College of Veterinary Emergency and Critical Care; Research Assistant Professor, Section of Emergency and Critical Care, Department of Clinical Sciences, Cummings School of Veterinary Medicine, Tufts University, North Grafton, Massachusetts

DORIS H. DYSON, DVM, DVSc, Diplomate, American College of Veterinary Anesthesiologists; Associate Professor, Anesthesiology, Department of Clinical Studies, Ontario Veterinary College, University of Guelph, Guelph, Ontario, Canada

TIM B. HACKETT, DVM, MS, Diplomate, American College of Veterinary Emergency and Critical Care; Associate Professor of Emergency and Critical Care Medicine, Department of Clinical Sciences; Director, Critical Care Unit, Veterinary Teaching Hospital, Colorado State University, Fort Collins, Colorado

ELAINE HOLT, DVM, MRCVS, Diplomate, American College of Veterinary Ophthalmologists; Staff Veterinarian, Ophthalmology Service, Department of Clinical Studies, Ryan Veterinary Hospital of the University of Pennsylvania, Philadelphia, Pennsylvania

DEZ HUGHES, BVSc, MRCVS, Diplomate, American College of Veterinary Emergency and Critical Care; Senior Lecturer in Emergency and Critical Care, Queen Mother Hospital, Royal Veterinary College, North Mymms, Hertfordshire, United Kingdom

L. ARI JUTKOWITZ, VMD, Diplomate, American College of Veterinary Emergency and Critical Care; Assistant Professor, Emergency Medicine, Department of Small Animal Clinical Sciences, College of Veterinary Medicine, Michigan State University, East Lansing, Michigan

TRACY L. LEHMAN, DVM, National Institutes of Health National Research Service Award Research Fellow, Department of Microbiology, Immunology and Pathology, Colorado State University, Fort Collins, Colorado

DEBORAH C. MANDELL, VMD, Diplomate, American College of Veterinary Emergency and Critical Care; Staff Veterinarian, Emergency Service, Department of Clinical Studies, Ryan Veterinary Hospital of the University of Pennsylvania, Philadelphia, Pennsylvania

KAROL A. MATHEWS, DVM, DVSc, Diplomate, American College of Veterinary Emergency and Critical Care; Professor, Emergency and Critical Care Medicine, Department of Clinical Studies, Ontario Veterinary College, University of Guelph, Guelph, Ontario, Canada

MAUREEN McMICHAEL, DVM, Diplomate, American College of Veterinary and Emergency Critical Care; Assistant Professor, Department of Small Animal Medicine and Surgery, College of Veterinary Medicine, Texas A&M University, College Station, Texas

TERESA M. RIESER, VMD, Diplomate, American College of Veterinary Emergency and Critical Care; VCA Newark Animal Hospital, Newark, Delaware

ELIZABETH ROZANSKI, DVM, Diplomate, American College of Veterinary Emergency and Critical Care; Diplomate, American College of Veterinary Internal Medicine (Internal Medicine); Assistant Professor, Section of Emergency and Critical Care, Department of Clinical Sciences, Cummings School of Veterinary Medicine, Tufts University, North Grafton, Massachusetts

REBECCA S. SYRING, DVM, Diplomate, American College of Veterinary Emergency and Critical Care; Assistant Professor, Section of Critical Care, Department of Clinical Studies–Philadelphia, School of Veterinary Medicine, University of Pennsylvania, Philadelphia, Pennsylvania

CONTENTS

The ability to recognize and effectively treat hypoperfusion forms the cornerstone of the emergency management of many of these patients. Global or systemic hypoperfusion can occur secondary to a reduction in the effective circulating intravascular volume (hypovolemic shock) or reduced ability of the heart to pump blood around the body secondary to reduced cardiac function (cardiogenic shock), obstruction to blood flow (obstructive shock), or maldistribution of the circulating intravascular volume (distributive shock). Global tissue hypoperfusion is initially assessed by a careful physical examination supplemented by measurement of hemodynamic and metabolic parameters. When treating hypoperfusion, the goal is to restore blood flow and oxygen delivery to the tissues rapidly, and the precise treatment used depends on the underlying cause and severity of the perfusion abnormality.

Disease of or injury to the central nervous system is a common reason for hospital admission on an emergency basis in veterinary medicine. Head injuries, seizures, and diseases that lead to intracranial hypertension frequently result in significant alteration of neurologic function. A thorough understanding of the pathophysiologic disturbances that occur during these conditions is paramount for providing stabilizing emergent care. A detailed approach that focuses on meticulous physical evaluation, provision of timely and optimal stabilizing treatment, and continued monitoring can aid in improving outcomes in animals with signs and symptoms of neurologic disease or injury.

A review of common emergencies of the urinary system is presented, with a focus on initial stabilization and treatment. Urethral obstruction, uroperitoneum, and acute renal failure are discussed.

Acute abdomen refers to the acute onset of abdominal pain. The underlying etiology of acute abdomen in the small animal patient may be minor and transient or an immediately life-threatening process. This article focuses on the approach to the patient with acute abdomen, including triage, history, physical examination, an emphasis on the diagnostic workup for these patients, and various aspects of acute management. Successful management of the patient with acute abdomen results from a proactive approach to management, including the rapid stabilization of major body systems, early identification of inciting problem(s), attention to comorbid conditions, and timely definitive therapy.

emergencies involve loss of vision, compromised globe integrity, or severe ocular pain. Delay in treating true emergencies may result in a blind eye or loss of an eye. This article discusses the clinical signs, diagnosis, and treatment as well as the prognosis of some of the more common ophthalmic emergencies.

This article discusses analgesia and chemical restraint for the emergency patient. As illness or injury affect all organ systems, specific recommendations and considerations of analgesic, anesthetic, and restraining regimens are presented. As animals of all ages, from neonates to geriatric and those that are pregnant or lactating, may require management of their illness or injury, recommendations for these patients are also presented.

Drug therapy is integral to emergency and critical care medicine but can also be the source of serious medical errors. There are important considerations with regard to drug, route, and interactions that require close attention in critical patients. The continuous development of new therapeutics and new information concerning current therapies requires practitioners to continually review drug therapies. This article addresses general guidelines, routes of administration, dosage calculations, interactions, monitoring recommendations, and resources available to help clinicians improve their drug therapy practices.

GOAL STATEMENT

The goal of the *Veterinary Clinics of North America: Small Animal Practice* is to keep practicing veterinarians up-to-date with current clinical practice in small animal medicine by providing timely articles reviewing the state of the art in small animal care.

ACCREDITATION

The *Veterinary Clinics of North America: Small Animal Practice* will be offering continuing education credits, to be awarded by a school of veterinary medicine, contract pending.

The aforementioned school of veterinary medicine is a designated provider of continuing veterinary education. Veterinarians participating in this learning activity may earn up to 6 credits per issue up to a maximum of 36 credits per year. Credits awarded may not apply toward license renewal in all states. It is the responsibility of each participant to verify the requirements of their state licensing board.

Credit can be earned by reading the text material, taking the examination online at *http:// www.theclinics.com/home/cme*, and completing the program evaluation. Each test question must be answered correctly; you will have the opportunity to retake any questions answered incorrectly. Following successful completion of the test and the program evaluation, you may print your certificate.

TO ENROLL

To enroll in the *Veterinary Clinics of North America: Small Animal Practice* Continuing Education program, call customer service at 1-800-654-2452 or sign up online at http://www. theclinics.com/home/cme. The CME program is available to subscribers for an additional annual fee of $99.95.

FORTHCOMING ISSUES

RECENT ISSUES

ELSEVIER
SAUNDERS

Vet Clin Small Anim
35 (2005) xi–xii

VETERINARY
CLINICS
Small Animal Practice

Preface

Emergency Medicine

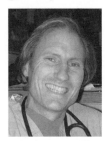

Kenneth J. Drobatz, DVM, MSCE
Guest Editor

This edition of *Veterinary Clinics of North America: Small Animal Practice* is primarily focused on the some of the more common and practical topics useful to clinicians who might see emergencies. Hence, I think it is helpful for any practicing small animal clinician. The authors of the various articles are experts in small animal emergency and critical care and are individuals who are on the clinic floor practicing what they preach. Other than just being experts, these are practical people who can provide information that is easily applied to the clinical patient. The first article, "Global assessment of the emergency patient," provides a comprehensive discussion on the physical assessment of the critically ill patient. Dr. Aldrich leaves no stone unturned and provides the most thorough article on this topic that I have ever read. The next four articles deal with the four major body systems that critical care clinicians initially focus on when dealing with unstable animals. Drs. Rozanski and Chan provide an excellent overview of how to assess and treat respiratory distress in the dog or cat. The third article by Drs. Boag and Hughes from the Royal Veterinary College is on perfusion abnormalities and is one of the most insightful reviews that I have read on this topic. Dr. Syring's article on central nervous system abnormalities follows, and her expertise and interest in this topic are clearly reflected in her presentation. To round out these articles, Dr. Rieser's review of urinary tract emergencies is extremely beneficial to any practitioner.

These first articles are followed by others on specific topics that are quite pertinent to the practicing clinician. The articles on acute abdomen and reproductive emergencies by Drs. Beal and Jukowitz, respectively, are extremely useful and thoroughly referenced. Dr. McMichael provides extremely useful information on the rarely covered topic of pediatric emergencies. Providing anesthesia is generally quite stressful for any practitioner, but giving anesthesia to the emergency patient is "giving insult to injury," so to speak. Dr. Campbell's presentation on anesthesia is a great reference for common anesthetic protocols used in emergency practice. Most people do not feel comfortable dealing with ophthalmic problems, but Drs. Mandell and Holt provide information that should alleviate some of that discomfort in handling ophthalmic emergencies. These days, any text regarding clinical veterinary medicine needs to include information on relieving pain in animals. Such needs are essential in traumatized patients. I was extremely lucky to have Drs. Mathews and Dyson provide an article on pain management in the emergency patient. Finally, but certainly not least, Drs. Hackett and Lehman give us a practical and philosophic discussion on the complexity of emergency drug therapy in critically ill animals.

I am extremely pleased with all the articles in this issue. I believe these individuals hit the mark in providing useful state-of-the-art information on common issues in emergency medicine. I hope you will enjoy it as well and that it never gathers dust on your bookshelf.

Kenneth J. Drobatz, DVM, MSCE
Department of Clinical Studies
Ryan Veterinary Hospital
University of Pennsylvania
3900 Delancey Street
Philadelphia, PA 19104–6010, USA

E-mail address: drobatz@mail.vet.upenn.edu

ELSEVIER
SAUNDERS

Vet Clin Small Anim
35 (2005) 281–305

VETERINARY
CLINICS
Small Animal Practice

Global Assessment of the Emergency Patient

Janet Aldrich, DVM

Veterinary Medical Teaching Hospital, School of Veterinary Medicine, University of California, Davis, One Garrod Drive, Davis, CA 95616, USA

Patients with life-threatening disease or injury are surviving on their physiologic reserves, which are limited. Timely therapy can be life saving, and delayed therapy can be futile. The patient's problems must be identified promptly in order of their importance to survival so that action is taken at crucial points. This is the goal of global assessment of the emergency patient.

Triage

Patients presented for emergency care have a broad spectrum of disease or injury ranging from life threatening to minor. These patients must be sorted (triaged) to determine the best order of treatment so that the sickest patients are treated first. In the emergency setting, resources like people, equipment, space, and, especially, time are limited. When emergencies occur simultaneously, prioritization by triage is essential.

Emergency team

Global assessment is a team effort, and the primary clinician is the team leader. The team goal is to achieve the best possible outcome for the patient. Tasks must be appropriately assigned so that each team member has, and can demonstrate, the knowledge, skill, and ability to fulfill his or her role. This competence should be demonstrated in practice sessions addressing issues like first contact with the owner, notification of the emergency team, transport of the patient to and within the hospital, initial triage, equipment and procedures in the emergency area, and communication with the owner.

E-mail address: jaldrich@ucdavis.edu

doi:10.1016/j.cvsm.2004.10.013
                                    vetsmall.theclinics.com

Coordination among team members is essential to ensure that streams of information flow to the team leader.

Critical thinking

Global assessment of the emergency patient should be based on principles of critical thinking, because this is the best format we know of to guide us to the truth. Critical thinking means gathering, understanding, and drawing reasonable conclusions about data so as to plan action. This is the most important activity of a clinician: to name a problem correctly; consider likely causes; and make appropriate plans for therapy, diagnosis, and client communication. In veterinary school, many of us learned a system of critical thinking called the problem-oriented approach (not to be confused with problem-based learning, which is an entirely different matter) and the accompanying problem-oriented medical record. We continue to use this system in our daily clinical practice, because the orderly and logical format helps us to avoid mistakes.

Database

Despite its importance, skill in critical thinking cannot overcome in-adequacies in the patient's database or in the clinician's database of medical information. Problems not identified because the physical examination or history is incomplete are not considered. Hypotheses about the cause of a problem cannot be generated if the clinician has insufficient knowledge about the problem. Put another way, questions not asked are not answered.

Making decisions

Emergency practice calls for willingness to make therapeutic decisions based on incomplete information. This is the nature of the emergency setting; hypotheses are generated early when little information is available. There must always be a willingness to consider new information and to reconsider previous information. Expert clinicians often consult with other team members to review and reconsider their decisions.

Clarity

Novices in emergency practice often feel pressured to act before they have clearly identified the problem. Compared with experts, novices tend to spend more time working on a solution and less time on clearly identifying the problem. Compared with novices, experts spend more time assessing the problem for the sake of clarity before they try to solve it.

Initial and comprehensive assessments

Presented next is a format for global assessment of the emergency patient using the problem-oriented approach. It is in two sections: the initial assessment and the comprehensive assessment. Both sections use the same four steps: database, problem list, assessment, and plans. Examples are provided to enhance understanding of the format. Other articles in this issue provide detailed information on the identification, assessment, and management of common problems encountered in emergency practice. The goal of this section is to provide a format to guide identification of all the patient's problems in order of their importance to survival.

Initial assessment

Initial history

Why is the patient being presented today? One member of the emergency team can briefly interview the owner while the team attends to the patient. History is important even if time is limited. For example, if the patient was hit by a car, was there loss of consciousness and was the patient observed to walk after the accident? For suspected poisoning, does the owner have information about the suspected poison, such as the package label, or knowledge of what was possibly available to the patient? This information should be promptly passed to the team leader. More information can be obtained later when more human resources are available.

The client should be asked about his or her wishes for cardiopulmonary cerebral resuscitation (CPCR) if appropriate to the situation.

Initial physical examination

Evaluate airway, breathing, and circulation to identify immediate life-threatening abnormalities of these systems. Be alert for disabling conditions, such as exsanguinating external bleeding or neurologic injury, because these might also need immediate management.

Problem list

A problem is an abnormality that interferes with the patient's well-being. In this context, we are looking for problems that immediately threaten the patient's life. Those of most concern are airway obstruction; respiratory arrest; cardiac arrest; or disabling conditions, such as exsanguinating external bleeding or neurologic (brain or spinal cord) injury.

Assessment

Assessment is how the clinician understands the problem. Assessment means understanding those associated data, identifying relations between them, and drawing reasonable conclusions. It includes whether immediate action is needed, the likely causes, and the prognosis.

For example, for the problem of severe dyspnea with stridor, immediate action is needed because oxygen delivery to the cells is likely to be at a critically low level. Tissue hypoxia depletes energy stores (ATP) needed for the processes of life. Also, the patient probably cannot tolerate any increase in oxygen demand, such as that associated with restraint.

Hypotheses about the causes of the problem are generated. For the problem of severe dyspnea with stridor, the primary hypothesis is upper airway obstruction. Causes include foreign bodies, masses (tissue or fluid), airway collapse, and laryngeal paralysis. These hypotheses are the basis for the diagnostic plan.

The prognosis is often difficult to establish in the early stages of global assessment because there is not enough information. Lack of certainty about the patient's likely response to therapy does not necessarily warrant a poor prognosis.

Plans

Therapeutic

This is the action to be taken to treat the problem. For the hypothesis of upper airway obstruction, the therapeutic plan is to provide oxygen at as high a concentration as possible, to limit manipulation of the patient, and to relieve the obstruction.

Diagnostic

This is the action to be taken to diagnose the problem. For the hypothesis of upper airway obstruction, the diagnostic plan is to choose among the various means of identifying the obstruction (direct visualization, endoscopy, or imaging), with consideration of the risks and benefits of each.

Client communication

The client must be informed of the patient's condition and the actions being taken. Risks and benefits must be explained so that the client can give informed consent for procedures. A definitive prognosis is usually not possible at this stage, but the client should be informed of the most likely hypotheses about the cause of the problem.

Comprehensive assessment

History

Complete the history of the presenting complaint. Get the past history, including the important medical and surgical events in the patient's life, immunizations, environmental history, diet, and systems review.

Although other emergency team members can help with the initial history, the veterinarian primarily responsible for the patient should get the complete history, which is essential to patient management. For example, failure to elicit the history of polyuria and polydipsia in a patient with a presenting complaint of vomiting might have disastrous consequences if the patient has diabetes insipidus and is denied free access to water while the vomiting is being managed. The resultant hypernatremia could be fatal.

Complete physical examination

Perform a rapid but complete physical examination. The importance of a complete physical examination cannot be overemphasized. Not only must problems be recognized before they can be treated, but concurrent disease can substantially affect prognosis and plans. Examples include the trauma patient with generalized lymphadenopathy that represents a previously unrecognized lymphoma; the puppy that has swallowed a fishhook and has a continuous murmur of a patent ductus arteriosus; or the cat with urethral obstruction that has a thyroid nodule representing its undiagnosed hyperthyroidism.

Problem list

All problems must be identified, but the clinician must be alert to identifying the most important first. Some examples include shock, respiratory distress, bleeding, acute abdomen, brain or spinal trauma, seizures, urethral obstruction, and dystocia. As in the initial assessment, the clinician should immediately divert to assessing and treating life-threatening problems as soon as they are identified.

Assessment

Assessment is essential; it provides the context for plans. For example, categories of shock are hypovolemic, distributive, cardiogenic, and hypoxic (hypoxemic or anemic). These categories are sufficient to guide therapy until more specific hypotheses can be investigated.

Plans

Therapeutic
Use the hypotheses to guide therapy. For example, if the problem is shock and the primary hypothesis is hypovolemia, the therapy is intravenous fluids. If the primary hypothesis is hypoxia, the therapy is oxygen, red cells, or both.
Select therapy partly on a risk/benefit basis. When the risk is low and the benefit is high, such as providing oxygen, the likelihood of need can be low.

Diagnostic
Pursue the hypothesis for the most urgent probable condition first. For example, if a surgically correctable cause of vomiting is being considered, use abdominal imaging to rule this out before pursuing metabolic causes.

Client communication

Stress prognosis, risks, benefits, and costs because these are most important to the client. Make sure your plans are acceptable to the client and in line with his or her goals for the patient.

Problem-oriented medical record

More than just fulfilling an obligation, keeping a medical record in the problem-oriented format is an excellent way to organize data and to clarify one's thoughts. The medical record should contain everything that is important and nothing that is not.

Initial and comprehensive physical examinations of the emergency patient

The physical examination is the core of emergency practice. Experienced clinicians remember many patients with normal and abnormal physical examination results and their accompanying histories. They can compare new instances with these stored data, quickly recognize patterns of disease, and use this information to establish a problem list. If they possess a good medical database about the categories of pathophysiology underlying common problems, they can quickly generate reasonable hypotheses about the cause. For example, a young cat is presented for acute respiratory distress. There is a history of intermittent cough, but the patient is otherwise healthy. On physical examination, observation shows that cat that is working hard to breathe; auscultation of the thorax reveals respiratory wheezes and no heart murmur or gallop rhythm. The problem is acute respiratory distress, and the most likely hypothesis is feline asthma. In another example, a 10-year-old, 10-lb Poodle is presented for acute respiratory distress. It has a history of coughing at night, which is increasing in frequency, but is otherwise healthy. Physical examination shows a dog that is working hard to breathe and is cyanotic, auscultation of the thorax reveals respiratory crackles, and a loud systolic murmur is heard at the left apex. The problem is acute respiratory distress, and the most likely hypothesis is pulmonary edema caused by left heart failure. Both patients have acute respiratory distress. The hypotheses generated are not the only ones possible, but they are the most likely given the pattern of the history and physical examination results of each patient. It is these mental processes that allow experienced clinicians to generate a plan quickly based on a series of rapidly made observations.

The physical examination of the emergency patient is a cycle of examinations. One must keep reviewing essential systems to verify their function and stability while moving forward to finish the examination. The physical examination is fallible; findings must be confirmed and new abnormalities sought. Following is a description of two cycles of physical examination. The first is the initial physical examination to evaluate airway, breathing, circulation, and disability. It is part of the initial assessment. The second is the complete physical examination. It is part of the comprehensive assessment. It is also focused on identifying the most life-threatening problems first but also stresses completeness so that problems are not missed.

Initial physical examination: airway, breathing, circulation, and disability

This is an initial physical examination of airway, breathing circulation, and disability. It is directed at recognizing severe respiratory distress or respiratory or cardiac arrest so that appropriate therapy can be immediately provided. There is also alertness to concurrent problems, such as exsanguinating external bleeding or neurologic injury, because these call for special management.

Is the patient conscious?

Observe the patient's mental state. Conscious patients do not need CPCR, at least not at this time. Acute deterioration in mental state can signal an impending arrest.

Airway and breathing

Is the patient trying to breathe?
Observe the movement of the chest wall and abdomen. If the patient is not trying to breathe, intubate and ventilate.

If the patient is trying to breathe, is air moving in and out of the lungs?
Listen for stridor suggesting upper airway obstruction, and auscult over the lungs for breath sounds. Be alert for sucking chest wounds, large flail segments, or decreased expansion of the chest wall suggesting pleural space disease. If air is not moving in and out of the lungs, the patient must be ventilated.

Circulation

Is the heart beating effectively? Palpate for pulses. If pulses are palpable, the heart is beating at least effectively enough to produce a pulse. If pulses are not felt, listen over the heart for heart sounds or palpate the chest wall for the precordial impulse at the left intercostal fourth to fifth space at the costochondral junction. If the patient is in lateral recumbency, the heart sounds are loudest on the side next to table. A palpable impulse means that the heart is contracting but does not equate to the strength of contraction. What is felt through the chest wall is the tension generated by the myocardium. If you cannot determine that the heart is beating and the patient is unconscious, start CPCR.

Disability

Be alert for disabling conditions that can materially affect short- or long-term outcome. Control exsanguinating external bleeding. Observe for signs of brain or spinal cord injury, such as external signs of head trauma, altered mental state, abnormal posturing, or absence of voluntary limb motion. If neurologic injury is likely, take immediate steps to protect the animal from further injury. Secure the patient to a firm supporting surface, such as a backboard. If intubation is needed, do it with the patient in lateral recumbency and without moving the neck more than is absolutely needed. Continue protective measures until the integrity of the spinal column is verified. If brain injury is likely, keep the head level with the heart. Avoid compressing the jugular veins or inducing sneezing or coughing.

Comprehensive physical examination

The order of examination continues to be directed toward identification of life-threatening problems first but without compromising the goal of performing a complete examination.

Is the patient in shock?

- Mental state
- Mucous membrane color
- Capillary refill time (CRT)
- Pulse quality
- Pulse rate
- Extremity-central temperature difference

These six parameters are often abnormal in specific patterns in patients suffering from shock. For example, in hypovolemic shock, the pattern is decreased mental state; pale, white, or cyanotic mucous membranes; slow CRT; poor pulse quality; fast pulse rate (cats in shock may have rates <180 beats per minute [bpm]); and cool extremities. In cardiogenic shock, the pattern is the same except that there may be distended jugular veins and cyanosis. In septic shock, the pattern is decreased mental state, dark red mucous membranes, fast CRT, bounding pulse quality, fast pulse rate, and warm extremities. Taken individually, the causes of any one of these variations from normal are many. It is the pattern of abnormalities in the appropriate clinical setting that should be recognized as indicative of decreased tissue perfusion. When the deviations from normal are sufficiently severe, it is appropriate to refer to this pattern of signs as a problem called shock.

Mental state

Mental state is the observer's evaluation of the patient's responsiveness to the environment. Mental state is an important physical evaluation, because the brain is an obligate user of oxygen and glucose and has few energy stores. Inadequate delivery of oxygen and glucose to the brain results in loss of the normal mental state in seconds.

Characterize the patient's mental state as alert and normally responsive, depressed or obtunded, stuporous or semicomatose, or comatose. The last two categories suggest abnormal brain function; the former are often caused by extracranial disease, such as decreased tissue perfusion, pain, or metabolic disease.

Mucous membrane color

The determinants of the color of unpigmented mucosa are volume (controlled by precapillary sphincter tone) and composition (hemoglobin concentration and hemoglobin saturation with oxygen) of blood in the underlying capillary bed. The normal color is light to dark pink. A pale to white color is caused by a deficit of volume or of hemoglobin. A red color suggests an increased volume of blood in the capillary bed because of vasodilation, as in sepsis. Cyanosis, which is represented by a blue-gray color, is caused by the presence of deoxygenated hemoglobin at a rate of at least 5 mg/dL. Its absence is not a reliable indicator that deoxygenated hemoglobin is not present. Methemoglobinemia, associated with acetaminophen poisoning (cats), can cause mucous membranes to be pale, cyanotic, and muddy or brown in color. Sulfhemoglobinemia can also cause cyanosis. Carbon monoxide poisoning can cause the mucous membranes to be cherry red. Icterus is indicated by a yellow color, which is caused by the presence of bilirubin at a rate greater than 2 mg/dL.

Lift the lip, and observe the color of the nonpigmented areas of the gingiva or buccal mucosa or of the tongue. Avoid using areas of noticeable gingivitis for this evaluation. If the oral mucosa is pigmented, one can observe the mucosa of the vulva or penis. Ambient light, pigment, and interobserver variation affect the repeatability of evaluation of mucous membrane color.

Capillary refill time

The time it takes, in seconds, for the blood to return to the capillary bed after one compresses it with a fingertip is the CRT. It is normally 1 to 2 seconds, with buccal mucosa refilling slightly slower than gingival mucosa. CRT is determined by precapillary sphincter tone, with increases in tone lengthening the CRT and decreases in tone shortening the CRT. Vasoconstriction caused by an increase in sympathetic tone, such as in response to a decrease in circulating blood volume in shock, can cause the CRT to be greater than 2 seconds. Vasodilation is characteristic of sepsis and can result in a CRT that is shorter than normal (ie, <1 second).

Pulse quality

A complete description of the assessment of pulse quality is provided in the cardiovascular section.

Find the femoral artery in the femoral triangle, and compress it with the fingertips until no pulsations are felt. Release the pressure gradually until pulsations are maximal. The digital pressure at this point is equal to mean arterial pressure.

Weak pulses are of small amplitude because of a decrease in stroke volume or an increase in peripheral resistance. Bounding pulses are caused by a large stroke volume or peripheral vasodilation.

Pulse rate

Palpate the pulse while simultaneously ausculting the heart. Determine the pulse rate, and verify that it is the same as the ausculted rate. Tachycardia (>180 bpm) is expected in seriously ill or injured patients, although cats in shock commonly have lower heart rates. Pulse deficits are usually caused by tachyarrhythmias that do not allow enough time for ventricular filling. Bradyarrhythmias may occur with diseases of the sinoatrial node.

Extremity-central temperature difference

There is normally a temperature difference between central temperature and that of the extremities of less than 8°F or 4°C. Peripheral vasoconstriction causes the temperature in the extremities to approach an ambient level.

Feel the toes, and note if they are cold. One can measure the extremity temperature in the toe web by placing a thermometer or temperature probe there and compressing the tissue over it. Compare this with the temperature obtained from a central location (usually rectal). Be alert for the presence of cold pelvic limbs in cats associated with peripheral cyanosis of the footpads, suggesting saddle thrombus.

What is the hydration state?

Dehydration is the condition resulting from loss of water from the body, but the term is usually taken to mean a loss of salt and water in an approximately isotonic concentration. Losses from the body, except for whole blood loss, come from the interstitium. Common sources of these losses are gastrointestinal and renal. Losses in the body into a third space occur with losses into the gastrointestinal tract, pleural and peritoneal spaces, and interstitium. The interstitial and intravascular volumes are normally in equilibrium across the capillary bed, such that losses from one compartment result in a decrease in volume in the other. In theory, all patients suffering an isotonic salt and water loss would thus have a decrease in vascular and interstitial volume parameters at equilibrium. The pattern of physical signs consistent with a decrease in vascular volume was described in the preceding section. Because of compensation for vascular volume losses, they are often difficult to detect until they are large. The interstitial volume parameters should always be assessed in critically ill patients because these may be the only indicator of an extracellular volume loss.

Skin turgor (elasticity) depends, in part, on the amount of salt and water as well as fat in the skin and subcutaneous tissues. Normally hydrated thin patients have decreased skin turgor, and obese patients have increased skin turgor. Puppies and kittens have increased total body water, and their skin turgor is normally greater than that of an adult. All these factors contribute to the difficulty of assessing hydration by skin turgor. That said, it is still the best physical examination parameter we have to make this crucial assessment. Experience and proper technique help to improve the repeatability of this assessment.

Gently lift the skin over the back just behind the scapula, and let it return to its resting position. The slowness of return is correlated to various degrees of dehydration, expressed as percentages of body weight (BW) as follows: mild equals 5% BW, moderate equals 7% BW, and marked equals 12% BW. Take care in interpreting the skin turgor over the dorsal neck, because the skin in this area normally returns to its resting position more slowly than skin over the back does. Assess the moistness of the mucous membranes. Interpret changes in light of the effects of other conditions, such as nausea, which causes increased salivation, and azotemia, which causes dry oral mucous membranes. Observe the corneas and conjunctivae for moistness suggesting adequate tear production. A decrease in tear production may be caused by dehydration as well as by a primary disease, such as kerato-conjunctivitis sicca. Moistness or dryness of the nose is variable in health, but a markedly dry nose might suggest dehydration.

Overhydration is usually an iatrogenic condition associated with in-travenous fluid therapy, often in patients with oliguria. Signs of overhydration include increased skin turgor, which gives the skin a jelly-like consistency; pitting edema in which the tissue can be pitted by finger pressure and retains this imprint for several seconds; chemosis in which the conjunctival tissues are glistening, white, and edematous; and, eventually, pulmonary edema.

Is the patient in pain?

There is a high likelihood that an emergency patient is suffering from pain. The entire emergency team must be constantly alert to recognize and appropriately treat pain.

Observe the patient's behavior and response to stimulation. It is important to be familiar with normal behavior for that species and breed. Patients suffering from pain may vocalize but more commonly just withdraw from interaction. Observe for painful responses to manipulation or palpation. Assume that the patient is in pain if you identify a disease or injury that would be painful to you.

Pain control is an important component of stabilizing critically ill patients and should be given concurrently with instead of after other stabilization treatments. Adequate pain control also increases the likelihood that a thorough physical examination can be performed.

Is the patient actively bleeding?

Bleeding may be obvious or occult. Exsanguinating external bleeding is usually obvious, although care must be taken to examine the entire patient and to palpate with the fingertips in heavily coated patients to identify bleeding. Substantial bleeding may occur into traumatized soft tissues, such as at fracture sites. Nasal hemorrhage is usually obvious, but substantial amounts of blood can be swallowed, thus masking the severity of the hemorrhage. Abdominal organs are highly vascular and are a common source of internal bleeding. Bleeding in the thorax may involve lung parenchyma or airways, pericardial space, or pleural space.

Signs associated with bleeding include signs of blood volume loss (shock) and the space-occupying effects of blood accumulation or excretion of blood in urine or feces or from the nose. Internal bleeding is suspected in patients that respond to initial fluid resuscitation and then deteriorate. Evidence of bleeding disorders (disease affecting primary or secondary hemostasis) includes petechiation, purpura, hematoma formation in nontraumatized areas, and rebleeding or persistent bleeding from venipuncture sites.

Complete physical examination

- Head and neck
- Respiratory
- Cardiovascular
- Abdomen
- Genitourinary
- Musculoskeletal
- Integument
- Lymphatic
- Body temperature

Head and neck

The general physical examination of the head and neck is complex because it involves examination of parts of many systems (ophthalmic, neurologic, musculoskeletal, upper part of gastrointestinal, and respiratory systems).

Observe the head for symmetry, head tilt, or nasal or ocular discharge as well as for gross structural abnormalities. Note a reluctance to move the head and neck. Observe for a change in the position of the globe in the orbit (enophthalmos or exophthalmus) or enlargement of the globe (buphthalmos). Observe the eyelids; palpebral fissures; nictitating membranes; position of the eyes; moistness of the cornea; pupil size, shape, and symmetry; symmetry and movement of the lips and muscles of facial expression; position of the tongue (if visible); and position of the ears. Be alert for abnormal eye position (strabismus) or movement (spontaneous nystagmus). Examine the cornea, anterior chamber, and lens for clarity and position of the lens. Note changes in the anterior chamber, such as hyphema or aqueous flare. Examine the conjunctiva for hyperemia or discoloration. Elicit a menace. Using the strongest possible light and the darkest possible room, elicit a pupillary light response (PLR). Palpate the face and skull for anatomic abnormalities. Examine the pinnae for discoloration and the ear canals for hemorrhage. Palpate the salivary glands, mandibular and superficial cervical lymph nodes, laryngeal cartilages, and trachea. Palpate the neck near the thoracic inlet for distention of the esophagus. In cats, palpate the ventral neck for the thyroid gland. Be alert for facial swelling in cats, which is associated with acetaminophen toxicity.

Examine the teeth, buccal and gingival mucosae, hard and soft palates, tongue, tonsillar crypts, and oropharynx for structural integrity, masses, or blood. Elicit a gag response. In cats, observe under the tongue for foreign bodies. Be alert for signs of facial fractures, such as crepitation when opening the mouth, malalignment of the mandibular teeth with the maxillary teeth, or asymmetry of the mandibular symphysis.

Respiratory

Breathing patterns are generated from the medulla and modified based on input from receptors in the airways, lungs, arterial and central chemoreceptors, muscles and tendons, and somatic pain receptors responding to stimuli, such as stretch, pressure, mechanical or chemical irritation, oxygen, carbon dioxide, hydrogen ion, exercise, and pain.

Observe the patient breathe. Note the effort, rate, and rhythm. Normal quiet breathing is nearly effortless; the chest wall and abdomen move outward on inspiration and inward on expiration, with most of the motion in the abdominal wall. No breathing sounds are heard without the stethoscope. Breathing rates are variable, and the rhythm is regular. Normal panting is open-mouthed breathing with a rapid rate and shallow respirations. Breathing sounds might be heard without the stethoscope but are not loud. The term *eupnea* is used to describe normal respiration, and *polypnea* is used to describe panting. Observe the color of the mucous membranes. Normal color is light to dark pink. Observe the neck and thorax for anatomic integrity.

Increased breathing effort. The patient with increased breathing effort seems to be working hard to breathe, with increased chest wall and abdominal movement. Breathing is often described as dyspneic, meaning difficult or labored respiration. The animal may adopt postures to ease breathing (orthopnea). These include extension of the head and neck, a preference for a standing or sitting position rather than lying down, and abduction of the elbows. Nasal flaring on inspiration may be observed. Open-mouthed breathing in cats is often a sign of severe respiratory distress. Any attempt to move the patient from the desired position causes anxiety. If a severely dyspneic patient chooses lateral recumbency, it is usually a sign of impending arrest, especially in a cat. There usually are large excursions of the chest wall and diaphragm unless the patient cannot move air into the lungs, such as with airway obstruction, or the lungs cannot be expanded, such as with pleural space (pneumothorax) or chest wall (eg, flail, sucking chest wound) disease. In paradoxic respiration, the chest wall and abdomen move in different directions. During inspiration, the chest moves outward as the intercostal muscles contract and the diaphragm and abdomen are drawn inward. Causes include obstructed upper airway, decreased lung compliance, diaphragmatic rupture, or diaphragmatic paralysis. Paradoxic respiration is also used to describe the motion of a flail segment that moves in the opposite direction as the intact chest.

The breathing rate is variable, because patients usually adopt the breathing strategy that best eases their breathing. For example, patients with extrathoracic upper airway obstruction might have long and slow inspirations, and those with intrathoracic airway collapse might have long and slow expirations. The term *tachypnea* is used to describe an excessively fast rate, and *bradypnea* is used to describe an abnormally slow rate.

Decreased breathing effort. In a patient with decreased breathing effort, the excursions of the chest wall and diaphragm are small and the rate is usually decreased. Causes include depression or injury to the respiratory center in the brain and spinal cord or neuromuscular injury causing failure of respiratory muscular function.

Abnormal breathing patterns. The following breathing patterns indicate a brain stem abnormality, but care must be taken in interpreting them because breathing patterns may also be changed by metabolic disease:

- Cheyne-Stokes: regular phases of hyperpnea and then apnea in a smooth crescendo/decrescendo pattern
- Central neurogenic hyperventilation: sustained rapid deep breathing
- Apneustic: end-inspiratory pause lasting 2 to 3 seconds
- Ataxic: disorganized irregular pattern with random deep and shallow breaths, indicating a critical state
- Apnea: complete cessation of breathing
- Agonal gasping: a gaping motion of the mouth with spasmodic contraction of the diaphragm but without significant air movement, which occurs some time after an arrest

Auscultation. Turbulent airflow in airways from the trachea to the lobar and segmental bronchi induces wall vibrations that produce sounds. Air moving through terminal bronchioles and alveoli does not produce significant sound. Loud blowing sounds are heard over the trachea during inspiration and expiration. Quieter sounds of similar character are heard over the hilar region during inspiration and the early phase of expiration. Soft rustling sounds are heard over the lung periphery during inspiration, although these may be difficult to hear during quiet breathing or in obese patients. All these are normal breath sounds whose character is modified as sounds pass from the airways through the overlying tissues.

Be alert for breath sounds heard without the aid of a stethoscope. These usually come from the extrathoracic airways. They radiate into the chest, and if they are not recognized, the sound can be inaccurately ascribed to an intrathoracic origin.

Auscult the trachea and lungs. Divide the thorax into three segments cranial to caudal and dorsal to ventral. Listen over all these areas for breath sounds as described previously. Compare the tracheal to thoracic auscultation to identify referred breath sounds. Listen for loudness of breath sounds, when they occur in the respiratory cycle (inspiration or expiration), and where they occur on the patient. The quality and loudness of normal breath sounds vary over the thorax, with louder blowing sounds heard cranioventrally and softer rustling sounds heard dorsocaudally. Breath sounds should be symmetric from one side to the other, except for a decrease in sounds on the left side over the heart.

Abnormal breath sounds. Abnormal breath sounds are wheezes and crackles. Wheezes are continuous musical (whistling) sounds caused by airway narrowing. Stridor is a wheeze usually heard without the aid of a stethoscope because it is a loud sound that occurs in the upper airways (larynx, trachea, and mainstem bronchi). Because stridorous sounds originating in the extrathoracic airways are referred into the thorax, it is important to identify their location by listening with the unaided ear and ausculting the larynx and trachea. Otherwise, the sounds may be incorrectly localized to the intrathoracic airways. Crackles are discontinuous non-musical (crackling of cellophane) sounds caused by sudden opening of airways that collapsed during a previous expiration. Wheezes and crackles originate in the intrathoracic airways (distal to the mainstem bronchi). (Note that *stertor* is a term with inconsistent definition and application, which is sometimes used to describe a snoring sound, such as that produced by soft palate entrapment. In that case, it would be another form of extrathoracic airway narrowing.)

Narrowing of the airway lumen, which causes wheeze or stridor (depending on location), has luminal or extraluminal causes. Luminal obstruction might be caused by intrusion into the airway by adjacent or associated structures (arytenoids, laryngeal saccules, soft palate, pharyngeal masses, or tracheal membrane) or by intraluminal accumulation of secretions, thickening of airway mucosa, or masses or foreign bodies. Extraluminal compression might be caused by enlargement of surrounding tissue (lymphadenopathy and tissue or fluid masses) or disruption of anatomic integrity (collapse of airway cartilage [strangulation, malacia] or stenosis).

Sudden opening of collapsed airways, which causes crackles, is associated with disease causing decreased lung volumes and a resultant predisposition to airway collapse. Causes include interstitial or obstructive lung disease; atelectasis; pulmonary edema; or masses in the lung, pleura, or chest wall. Crackles that have more of a bubbling quality can be caused by air moving through accumulated fluid in the upper airways and might be heard without the aid of a stethoscope.

Loudness of breath sounds is affected by changes in sound transmission, sound production, or both, with the former having the most effect on the loudness heard with the stethoscope on the chest wall. Sound transmission is increased by atelectasis, consolidation, or lung masses and is decreased by hyperinflation or pleural space disease (air, fluid, or tissue). Sound production is increased by increased airflow or by airway narrowing and is decreased by decreased airflow in the affected area. Causes of decreased airflow include pleural space disease (fluid, air, and tissue), chest wall disease, lung consolidation, or abdominal enlargement preventing caudal movement of the diaphragm. Because the forces affecting sound transmission and production may have opposing effects on what is heard with the stethoscope, assessment by auscultation of airflow in a specific region of the lung can be poorly correlated with the pathologic findings. The exception is with pleural space disease, where it is often possible to identify a marked decrease in or absence of breath sounds. With pleural effusion, the breath sounds are decreased ventrally; with pneumothorax, they are decreased dorsally.

Mucous membrane color. The color of unpigmented mucous membranes is a result of the volume and composition of blood in the underlying capillary bed. Cyanosis, which is characterized by a blue-gray discoloration, is caused by the presence of deoxygenated hemoglobin at a rate of at least 5 mg/dL. Give the confounding effects of ambient light, interobserver variation, and the requirement for a rather large volume of deoxygenated hemoglobin, cyanosis is not reliably identified in patients suffering from hypoxemia. Cherry-red mucous membranes can be associated with carbon monoxide poisoning.

Palpation. Palpate the neck and thorax. Evaluate the skin, subcutaneous tissues, larynx, trachea, ribs, spinous processes, sternum, and intercostal spaces for anatomic integrity. Palpate the anterior thorax of the cat to confirm its normally high compressibility. Be alert for penetrating wounds of the thorax allowing entry of room air into the pleural space, rib fractures that can lacerate the lung, segmental fractures of consecutive ribs creating a flail chest that disrupts thoracic wall integrity, subcutaneous emphysema caused by air leak from the airways and lungs, and anatomic disruption of vertebrae suggesting spinal trauma.

Percussion. Percussion produces audible vibrations, because the chest wall vibrates (like a drumhead) when it is struck. The sound from the normal thorax is resonant with a dull quality. It is hyperresonant over pneumothorax and dull over pleural effusion, pneumonia, or masses.

Place a finger in the intercostal space and tap its first phalanx briskly with the flexed finger of the opposite hand. Percuss systematically over the lung fields.

Cardiovascular

The organization of control of cardiovascular function is that intrinsic heart rate, rhythm, force of contraction, and vascular tone are influenced by neuroendocrine output from the cardioregulatory center in the medulla. This center gets neuroendocrine input from baro-, volu-, and mechano-receptors in the heart and great vessels. Output from the cardioregulatory center influences heart rate, stroke volume, cardiac output, vascular tone, and blood volume (through thirst and renal handling of salt and water).

Observation. Be aware of abnormalities of the respiratory system just examined that might be of cardiac origin, such as increased respiratory rate or effort, or pulmonary crackles. Observe for jugular vein distention, ascites, or peripheral edema. Jugular vein distention is assessed with the patient standing or in a sternal position. First, observe the vein for distention or pulsation. Next, occlude the jugular vein at the thoracic inlet to distend it, release the pressure, and observe the rate of collapse of the vein. Jugular vein distention occurs in some but not all patients with congestive right heart failure. Jugular vein pulsations occur in some patients with decreased right ventricular compliance, atrioventricular dissociation (third degree atrioventricular block), and tricuspid regurgitation. If ascites is suspected, try to elicit a fluid wave by ballottement. Right heart failure may cause ascites and, less commonly, peripheral edema.

Palpation. Pulse quality is the subjective assessment of the pulse pressure wave felt by palpation of an artery. Pulse pressure is the difference between systolic and diastolic blood pressure; it is normally in the range of 40 to 80 mm Hg. Systolic blood pressure is mainly dependent on stroke volume and arterial compliance. The components of stroke volume are preload, myocardial contractility, and afterload. Diastolic blood pressure is mainly dependent on the rate of diastolic runoff.

Palpate pulses, usually in the femoral triangle. Find the arterial pulse and apply digital pressure until the pulsations disappear. Gradually release the pressure until the pulse is palpable (digital pressure is now equal to systolic blood pressure), and continue until the pulsations are maximal (digital pressure is now equal to mean arterial blood pressure). If more or less digital pressure (than that needed to feel maximum pulsations) is applied, the pulse quality is likely to be assessed as poor when it is not. Assess rate, rhythm, amplitude, and waveform. Palpate bilateral pulses to determine symmetry. Palpate pulses in the distal extremities, note the surface temperature of feet, and inspect footpads for cyanosis.

The pulse pressure wave is a summation of many pressure waves occurring in the pulsatile arterial system; its contour is in the shape of a triangle. Variations in the height, width, or both of this contour create changes in pulse quality. The normal waveform has a smooth sharp upstroke, a momentary pause, and a fast downstroke. Common descriptions for pulses are as follows:

- Weak: small amplitude caused by decrease in stroke volume
- Bounding: abrupt upstroke and rapid downstroke with an abnormally wide amplitude commonly caused by a large stroke volume or peripheral vasodilation
- Collapsing: rapid descending limb of the pulse pressure wave caused by rapid runoff as in vasodilation
- Waterhammer: rapid ascending limb of the pulse pressure wave caused by forceful ventricular contraction as in anemia
- Pulsus paradoxus: inspiratory decrease in pulse pressure during a normal quiet inspiration, which is a normal finding that is exaggerated in pericardial tamponade
- Pulsus alternans: alternating strong and weak pulses associated with decreases in stroke volume, premature contractions, or myocardial contractile dysfunction
- Pulse deficits: during tachyarrhythmias, inadequate filling time may cause the ventricle not to eject enough blood to create a palpable pulse

Auscultation. The heart is best ausculted with the patient standing, but emergency circumstances often do not allow this. If the patient is in lateral recumbency, the heart is louder on the side next to the table, but in this position, abnormal rubbing sounds may be heard as the heart contacts the chest wall. Find the left apex, which is the point of maximal intensity, usually at fourth to fifth intercostal space at the costochondral junction. The fifth rib is normally at the level of the olecranon when the thoracic limb is in the standing position.

With the stethoscope, auscult for the first (closure of the mitral and tricuspid valves) and second (closure of the pulmonic and aortic valves) heart sounds. Listen at the apex (mitral valve area) and base (pulmonic and aortic valve area) on the left side. Listen on the right side at the third through fifth intercostal spaces at the costochondral junction (tricuspid valve area). Note whether the rhythm is regular, regularly irregular, or irregular. Characterize murmurs by location, loudness, and whether they occur during systole, diastole, or both. Simultaneously palpate the femoral pulse while ausculting the heart to identify pulse deficits.

Murmurs are caused by prolonged vibrations of the heart or great vessels. They are usually caused by valvular insufficiency or anemia, where the combination of decreased viscosity and compensatory increased stroke volume creates turbulence. Gallops are auscultable third or fourth heart sounds caused by vibration of ventricular walls and are associated with stiff walls because of cardiomyopathy or a large volume of blood entering the ventricle. In patients with extremely compressible chest walls (cats), abnormal heart sounds can be created by excess compression of the chest wall by the stethoscope.

Heart rate is normally controlled by the rate of diastolic depolarization and the threshold potential of the sinoatrial node. Heart rate is modified by the balance between sympathetic and parasympathetic tone. Normal heart rates for dogs are 60 to 80 bpm at rest and 140 to 180 bpm during excitement (up to 220 bpm in puppies); in cats, normal rates are 100 bpm at rest and 240 during excitement. Seriously ill or injured patients are expected to have heart rates higher than 180 bpm, although cats may have lower rates.

The normal heart rhythm is regular or regularly irregular (varying with respiration). Tachyarrhythmias in emergency patients are often caused by premature depolarizations of cells before they have received a depolarization wave originating in the sinoatrial node. These ectopic pacemakers develop because of the effects of hypoxia, trauma, stretch, or drugs. Bradyarrhythmias are less common in emergency patients but may occur because of diseases of the sinoatrial node (sick sinus syndrome). Arrhythmias can interfere with cardiac output by adversely affecting stroke volume or heart rate. If an apparent arrhythmia is detected, an electrocardiogram is called for to define it and to help distinguish life-threatening from non–life-threatening arrhythmias. Tachyarrhythmias with the potential to be life threatening include supraventricular tachycardia, fast ventricular tachycardia, ventricular flutter, and fibrillation. Bradyarrhythmias with this potential include third degree atrioventricular block and sinus arrest.

Abdomen

The term *acute abdomen* refers to the sudden onset of clinical signs caused by disease in the abdominal cavity. Causes of acute abdomen are inflammation, distention, traction, or ischemia of abdominal structures. Care must be taken in localizing pain to the abdomen based on the patient's response, because extra-abdominal causes of apparent abdominal pain, such as back pain, are common.

Abdominal distention is common in emergency patients and may be caused by accumulation of gas, blood, pus, or salt and water in the organ lumens or in the peritoneal or retroperitoneal spaces. Frequent re-evaluation of the abdomen for progressive distention is important.

Observation. Observe for visible injury to the abdomen and for abdominal distention. Observe the patient's posture for signs of abdominal pain, such as arching the back, guarding the abdomen, and adopting the praying position (crouching with the forelegs and standing with the rear legs). Observe the skin over the abdomen for signs of trauma.

Palpation. Abdominal palpation should start with gentle pressure to assess for a painful response. Adequate pain control allows a more complete examination. Palpate the abdomen using an organized format of the examiner's choice. If ascites is suspected, try to elicit a fluid wave by ballottement. Try to palpate the liver (caudal border), spleen, kidneys, intestines, and bladder. The stomach may be palpable if distended. A rectal examination is part of the complete physical examination in dogs, except for extremely small dogs. It is not usually done in cats without a specific indication. On rectal examination, one can assess anal sphincter tone, the pelvis (for symmetry), the ventral sacrum, ventral coccygeal vertebrae and adjacent muscles, the neck of the bladder, the prostate in male dogs, the cervix and body of the uterus in female animals, the urethra, the rectum, the anus, and anal sacs. Sublumbar lymph nodes are not usually palpable per rectum unless they are massively enlarged because they are in the sublumbar area at the level of the fifth to seventh lumbar vertebrae rather than in the pelvis. Hypogastric lymph nodes are in the pelvis. Note the character of the feces in the rectum, and observe the color and consistency of feces on the glove. Visually inspect the anus and surrounding skin. Palpate the body wall, inguinal rings, and scrotum for hernias.

Other structures in the abdomen that are not usually palpable are the ureters, pancreas, adrenals, ovaries and nondistended uterus in female animals, and lymph nodes.

Percussion. Perform percussion by placing a finger on the abdominal wall and tapping the first digit briskly with the flexed finger of the other hand. Percuss over several areas on both sides. Tympany suggests gas, whereas fluid produces a dull sound.

Auscultation. Listen over the abdomen for the sound of borborygmus, which is a rumbling sound of gas moving through the intestines. Several cycles of borborygmus per minute suggests adequate gut motility. Absence of sounds for several minutes suggests ileus, and increased frequency of sounds may occur with enteritis.

Genitourinary
Female animals. Examine the mammary glands for discharge or discoloration, and palpate for swelling or masses. Examine the vulva for discharge,

discoloration, swelling, or masses. The uterine horns may be palpable abdominally if they are distended. A vaginal examination should be performed if clinically indicated. The external vulva should be cleaned, and the examiner should use a sterile glove.

Male animals. Examine the scrotum for swelling, redness, ulceration, or masses. Palpate the testes to assess symmetry, prominence of epididymis, and for masses. Extrude the tip of the penis to examine for discoloration, masses, or mineral material (cats). Examination of the bladder and urethra has been described in the section on the abdomen.

Musculoskeletal

If the patient sustained trauma severe enough to disrupt bones or joints, it is likely that there are internal injuries. Respiratory, cardiac, vascular, urinary, and neurologic injuries are common and have priority for treatment.

Observe the patient for gross anatomic disruption and for symmetry. Characterize the body condition, usually with a scoring system ranging from 1 to 9, with 1 being emaciated and 9 being morbidly obese. There is no corresponding system for rating muscle mass, but a decrease in muscle mass, whether generalized or local, should be noted. If the patient is able to walk, observe the gait for coordination, strength, and symmetry. Palpate each limb from a distal to proximal direction. Examine the interdigital skin and foot pads. Palpate the soft tissue of the limbs, flex and extend each joint individually, and then palpate the long bones for anatomic disruption. Flex and extend the neck, and palpate the spinous processes of the cervical, thoracic, and lumbar vertebrae. Palpate the sacrum and the tail, and note tail movement and anal tone. Note painful responses, lacerations, areas of swelling, crepitus, or angular deformity. Be aware that substantial blood loss can occur into fracture sites; these areas should be continually monitored for expansion of swelling.

Injured structures should be handled gently. Motion at fracture sites and further contamination of open fractures should be minimized.

Integument

Intact skin is the major barrier to contamination of underlying tissues by environmental substances. Lacerations or abrasions compromise this barrier; severe lacerations can also allow substantial blood loss. Primary dermatologic emergencies do exist. These include drug eruptions and various immune-mediated skin diseases in which there is a risk of infection and sepsis. The marked discomfort suffered by patients with pruritic skin disease or with otic foreign bodies is often a reason for the owners to seek emergency care.

Observe the hair coat for shine and fullness, and identify alopecia and note its distribution. Examine the skin, including the otic epithelium.

Primary skin lesions include macules, papules, nodules, pustules, tumors, wheals, and vesicles. If any are present, note their size, shape, consistency, color, and location.

The skin often displays important clues to the origin of bleeding disorders. Impairment of primary hemostasis (vasoconstriction and primary platelet plug) is characterized by petechiae and purpura (confluent petechiae). Impairment of secondary hemostasis (coagulation factors and stable clot) is characterized by hematomas. Continual bleeding after venipuncture is consistent with a defect of primary hemostasis, whereas rebleeding is more consistent with a defect of secondary hemostasis.

Lymph nodes

Superficial lymph nodes commonly evaluated are mandibular, superficial cervical (prescapular), and popliteal. If generalized lymphadenopathy is present, one can also evaluate the axillary and inguinal nodes. Isolated lymphadenopathy usually suggests disease in the area drained by the affected node.

Body temperature

Body temperature is regulated around a normal setpoint by output from the anterior hypothalamus to regulate thirst, panting, other behavioral changes, and autonomic and endocrine output to conserve or lose heat. Endogenous pyrogens trigger the hypothalamus to reset the setpoint at a higher level to achieve fever, which is usually considered to be beneficial. Severe prolonged muscular activity, high environmental temperatures, or inability to ventilate adequately (brachycephalic dogs) can overwhelm the patient's ability to dissipate heat and cause life-threatening hyperthermia. Temperatures of 107°F or greater may cause increased cell membrane permeability and production of inflammatory mediators and can cause direct thermal denaturation of proteins and alterations in cell structure.

Decreases in body temperature are caused by cold environments, sedation or anesthesia and surgery, and metabolic disease. At temperatures less than 94°F, the ability to shiver is lost. Consequences of severe decreases in body temperature include decreases in heart rate, cardiac output, and blood pressure.

Get a rectal temperature as part of the complete physical examination. Consider the history and physical examination findings to differentiate fever (which usually should not be treated with active cooling) and hyperthermia because of the inability to dissipate heat, which should be treated as an emergency with active cooling.

Neurologic system and examination

A brief neurologic survey was part of the disability evaluation in the initial assessment. Many aspects of the neurologic system are evaluated in the course of performing a complete physical examination. A general screening neurologic examination is indicated if neurologic disease or injury is suspected. Problems that are of neurologic origin include seizures, altered mental state (stupor or semicoma, coma, or disorientation), paresis or paralysis, head tilt, and spontaneous nystagmus. Because the brain requires a steady supply of oxygen and glucose, abnormalities of tissue perfusion must be resolved before assigning abnormalities of mentation to primary brain disease.

Neural trauma includes the mechanical damage caused by physical forces (concussion, contusion, laceration or transection, compression, and distraction) and the subsequent processes of hemorrhage, vasospasm, ischemia, and hypoxia. The dysfunction is caused by blockage of action potential generation or conduction in damaged neurons.

Neurologic dysfunction can be immediate or delayed in onset. Prolonged seizures are associated with periods of hypoventilation and hypoxemia during the most active part of the seizure. These, combined with the intense neuronal activity, can cause brain swelling.

Spinal cord compression causes, in order of increasing severity of injury, conscious proprioceptive deficits, loss of voluntary motion, loss of superficial pain, and, finally, loss of deep pain.

This examination is to find out whether neurologic disease is present and, if so, to provide neuroanatomic localization. Anatomic divisions are the cerebrum, subcortical area, cerebellum, C1 through C5, C6 through T2, T3 through L3, L4 through S2, S1 through S3, and coccygeal.

If brain or spinal cord injury was suspected in the earlier examinations, the patient should already have been stabilized with a backboard. The cautions about manipulating the patient's position still apply.

Mental state. A normal mental state depends on the function of the ascending reticular activating system. Input along sensory pathways ascends to the reticular formation in the brain stem, which has output by way of projections to the cerebral cortex to regulate arousal.

Observe the patient's mental state, and characterize it as alert and normally responsive, depressed or obtunded, stuporous or semicomatose, or comatose. Note abnormalities of response, such as disorientation or compulsive behavior.

Examination of the head. Observe the face and head for signs of external trauma, and palpate for anatomic integrity. Note abnormal posturing, such as hyperextension of the neck with extensor rigidity of the forelegs (Schiff-Sherrington sign). Note spontaneous nystagmus, strabismus, and head tilt. Observe for scleral hemorrhage or blood in ear canals or from the nose.

Observe pupil size, symmetry, and responsiveness to light. Elicit the PLR using the brightest possible light in the darkest possible room. Note spontaneous abnormal eye movements (nystagmus). In patients suspected of having suffered brain trauma, assess brain stem reflexes of physiologic nystagmus, gag, and swallow. Assessing physiologic nystagmus involves moving the head from side to side to elicit the reflex and should be done with care or not at all if the patient is suspected of having cervical spine injury. Evaluate gag and swallow, which are also brain stem reflexes.

Signs of brain stem involvement.

- Unconsciousness
- Bilaterally unresponsive pupils
- Absent gag and swallow
- Absence of the normal vestibular reflex
- Irregular breathing patterns or apnea
- Decerebrate rigidity (extensor rigidity × 4 plus opisthotonus)

Pupils and pupillary light response in order of increasing severity.

- normal size, slow PLR
- miosis, intact PLR
- pinpoint, no PLR
- mydriasis, no PLR.

Pupils are the single most important sign differentiating metabolic from primary neurologic causes of coma. The PLR is resistant to metabolic insult but is affected by drugs like atropine and opioids.

Examination of the spine. Palpate the entire spinal column (C1 to coccygeal). Note areas of swelling, crepitation, bony deformity, or pain. Elicit spinal reflexes of panniculus, patellar, gastrocnemius, biceps and triceps, perineal, and withdrawal. Assess deep pain, remembering that withdrawal of a limb in response to a noxious stimulus shows intactness of the reflex arc but does not mean that the patient feels its toes. A purposeful response by the patient is called for to show intactness of the ascending sensory pathways. Assess anal tone and tail movement.

Gait and postural responses. Gait and postural responses are not evaluated until the patient is stable and only if it is safe to move the patient (see cautions described in the section on disability). If it is safe to do so, proceed to evaluate the ability to stand and support, voluntary motion, gait, and conscious proprioception.

Seizures and tremors. Generalized seizures are caused by paroxysmal cerebral dysrhythmia. They are characterized by loss of consciousness as well as by generalized muscle contraction (tonus) and then jerking (clonus) and are often accompanied by autonomic dysfunction (urination and defecation). In status epilepticus, seizures occur in quick succession and there is inadequate time for recovery between them. The intense neuronal activity during seizures causes metabolic derangements that can damage neurons and cause brain swelling.

Generalized tremors may be associated with poisoning by tremorogenic toxins or organophosphates. A patient history is important to elicit exposure.

The repetitive vigorous muscular activity and interference with respiratory function that occur in seizures or tremors predispose the patient to hyperthermia, hypercapnia, hypoxemia, and metabolic acidosis.

Summary

The approach to the global assessment of the emergency patient must be an organized, focused, and efficient pursuit of identification all the patient's problems in the order of their importance to survival. The format of the problem-oriented approach serves as a guide. The patient's history and physical examination results serve as the database for global assessment; they are the core of emergency practice.

Suggested reading

Crowe DT. Triage and trauma management. In: Murtaugh RJ, Kaplan PM, editors. Veterinary emergency and critical care medicine. St. Louis: Mosby-Year Book; 1992. p. 77–121.

Facione PA. Critical thinking: what it is and why it counts. Milbrae (CA): California Academic Press; 1998.

Fagella AM. First aid, transport, and triage. Vet Clin N Am Small Anim Pract 1994;24:997–1014.

Kassirer JP, Kopelman RI. Learning clinical reasoning. Baltimore: Williams & Wilkins; 1991.

Kittleson MD. Signalment, history, and physical examination. In: Kittleson MD, Kienle RD, editors. Small animal cardiovascular medicine. St. Louis: Mosby; 1998. p. 16–46.

Kotlikoff MI, Gillespie JR. Lung sounds in veterinary medicine. Part I. Terminology and mechanisms of sound production. Compend Contin Educ Pract Vet 1984;5(8):634–8.

McCurnin DM, Poffenbarger EM. Small animal physical diagnosis and clinical procedures. Philadelphia: WB Saunders; 1991.

Weed LL. Medical records, medical education and patient care. Chicago: The Press of Case Western Reserve University; 1971.

ELSEVIER
SAUNDERS

Vet Clin Small Anim
35 (2005) 307–317

VETERINARY
CLINICS
Small Animal Practice

Approach to the Patient with Respiratory Distress

Elizabeth Rozanski, DVM*, Daniel L. Chan, DVM

*Section of Emergency and Critical Care, Department of Clinical Sciences, Cummings School
of Veterinary Medicine, Tufts University,
200 Westboro Road, North Grafton, MA 01536, USA*

Respiratory distress of any origin represents a true emergency requiring rapid identification of the underlying cause, immediate alleviation of the sensation of difficulty in breathing, and provision of diagnostic and therapeutic information for the owners of affected animals. Clearly, there are a variety of potential underlying reasons for the development of respiratory distress. For the clinician in emergency practice, successful management of patients in respiratory distress revolves around developing a knowledge base of the potential causes of respiratory distress and "pattern recognition" of common emergent problems affecting dogs and cats. Prompt recognition of the underlying condition and appropriate therapeutic interventions are essential in the management of respiratory emergencies. The goals of this article are to review the function of the respiratory system, to describe pathophysiologic causes for hypoxemia, to illustrate various methods for classifying respiratory distress, to highlight common emergency conditions resulting in respiratory distress, and to provide guidelines for emergent management.

Gas exchange

As a review, the primary goal of the respiratory system is to promote gas exchange. Air enters the upper respiratory system via the nose or the mouth. The air is warmed and humidified and then passes down the respiratory tree. Larger particles of debris are filtered out. The trachea branches into the successive generation of smaller and smaller airways. Gas exchange occurs at the level of the alveoli. Although the flow of air (ventilation, termed V) is

---

* Corresponding author.
E-mail address: Elizabeth.rozanski@tufts.edu (E. Rozanski).

0195-5616/05/$ - see front matter © 2005 Elsevier Inc. All rights reserved.
doi:10.1016/j.cvsm.2004.12.003
vetsmall.theclinics.com

obviously essential, the other aspect of gas exchange involves the delivery of blood (perfusion, termed Q) to the level of the alveoli. Blood reaches the capillaries adjacent to the alveoli by way of the pulmonary vasculature. The blood exits the right heart via the pulmonary outflow tract and then flows through the pulmonary arteries. These arteries branch into smaller and smaller vessels until they reach the level of the capillary. Red cells traverse the capillaries in single file; during contact with the alveoli, the oxygen diffuses out of the alveoli and binds to the hemoglobin, because the carbon dioxide (CO_2, waste gas) diffuses off the hemoglobin molecule into the alveoli for expiration. In normal animals, the capillary endothelium is impermeable to larger molecules, such as albumin.

Causes of hypoxemia

In animals that develop hypoxemia, there are five possible broad causes. Each disease observed clinically fits into one of more of the following categories. These causes include a low inspired oxygen concentration (Fio_2), hypoventilation, shunt, ventilation-perfusion (V-Q) mismatch, and diffusion impairment [1]. Normal oxygen concentration in room air is approximately 21%, and low Fio_2 is an uncommon cause of hypoxemia. This may occur at higher altitudes or because of anesthesia machine dysfunctioning, however [1]. Low Fio_2 may be simply corrected by supplementing oxygen. Hypoventilation results from absent or ineffective (low) tidal volumes as a result of such causes as drug therapy side effects (eg, opioids, propofol) or loss of central respiratory drive [2]. Respiratory muscle fatigue in patients with prolonged and severe dyspnea can result in hypoventilation [3]. Hypoventilation is treated by mechanical ventilation or by reversing the cause that triggered the hypoventilation. It should be emphasized that hypoventilation may not be appreciated as respiratory compromise because respiratory attempts are limited or depressed.

Shunt refers to the complete bypassing of ventilated areas of the lungs by deoxygenated blood and re-entry into the circulatory system [4]. The classic example of a shunt is the right-to-left shunt that accompanies the cardiac defect of the tetralogy of Fallot (right ventricular hypertrophy, ventricular septal defect [VSD], pulmonic stenosis, and overriding aorta). In affected animals, the severity of the pulmonic stenosis results in the shunting of deoxygenated blood through the VSD into the left ventricle. Because oxygen supplementation cannot affect shunted deoxygenated blood, pure shunts are described as nonresponsive to oxygen supplementation. In certain conditions, significant alveolar pathologic changes can contribute to shunting. Alveoli filled with inflammatory exudates, edema, or blood can reduce gas exchange efficiency. Because this is not a true shunt, however, oxygen supplementation can improve oxygenation.

V-Q mismatch refers to the poor coordination of the areas of the lung that are adequately perfused versus those that are appropriately ventilated, resulting in impairment of gas exchange [4]. Normally, there is a good match between areas that are appropriately ventilated and those that are adequately perfused. In some cases, however, areas of the lungs can be perfused but are not well ventilated (low V/Q ratio), whereas in other conditions, well-ventilated areas are inadequately perfused (high V/Q ratio). Conditions associated with a low V/Q ratio include pneumonia, edema, hemorrhage, and inflammatory exudates. Pulmonary thromboembolism is an example of a condition resulting in a high V/Q ratio. This mismatching results in the development of hypoxemia but is not necessarily accompanied by hypercarbia. Diffusion of CO_2 is many times more efficient than that of oxygen, explaining the discrepancy when gas exchange is compromised. As a result of physiologic responses by the lung, V-Q mismatch generally responds to oxygen supplementation.

The final area that may result in hypoxemia is diffusion impairment. Typically, during the transition phase through the capillary bed, the oxygen diffuses within the first third of the length of the capillary. If the alveolar-capillary membrane is significantly thickened, however, there may be diffusion impairment and gas exchange can become compromised. Diseases resulting in diffusion impairment include pulmonary interstitial pathologic findings such as fibrosis, severe interstitial pneumonia, and interstitial hemorrhage. Oxygen supplementation can increase the oxygen tension within the alveoli sufficiently to overcome diffusion impairment and alleviate hypoxemia.

Oxygen therapy

Although an understanding of the potential causes of respiratory distress is indispensable, the first steps in the clinical evaluation of a patient presented with respiratory distress are to provide a supplemental source of oxygen and to obtain a brief history from the client or owner. All emergency facilities should be equipped to provide a form of supplemental oxygen. Supplemental oxygen may be provided by means of a variety of options, including flow-by oxygen, a face mask, nasal oxygen, an Elizabethan collar and cellophane wrap ("oxygen hood"), an oxygen cage, and intubation with intermittent positive-pressure ventilation (IPPV). Flow-by oxygen is provided by holding oxygen tubing near the mouth and nostrils of the affected patient. The flow rate is usually set at 100 mL/kg/min or greater. Flow-by oxygen is an easy and rapid solution; however, the actual increase over room air's 21% oxygen content may be minimal, particularly with an anxious or uncooperative animal. Oxygen may also be provided with a face mask, with the oxygen tubing attached to a cone that is placed over the nose and mouth of the patient. The Fio_2 with a face mask is also variable, although a high percentage may be reached in weak animals. Flow-by and face mask oxygen may require veterinary personnel to hold the pet and the oxygen supply.

Nasal oxygen involves placement of a flexible catheter into the nasal passages and insufflation of humidified oxygen. Nasal oxygen is particularly useful in pets that are not panting or are demonstrating open-mouthed breathing. Nasal oxygen is commonly placed after patient stabilization rather than urgently in the emergency setting. An improvised oxygen hood may be created with an Elizabethan collar and cellophane wrap or may be commercially purchased (Jorgenson Laboratories, Loveland, CO). An oxygen cage is also frequently used to provide supplemental oxygen. Oxygen cages are commonly well tolerated by cats and dogs and are also capable of achieving a high concentration of oxygen; however, if the cage door is opened for patient manipulation, the Fio_2 falls rapidly. Finally, intubation and IPPV represent the best option for providing high levels of supplemental oxygen, removing respiratory fatigue, and eliminating patient fear and anxiety.

Assessment

During the initial stabilization of the pet, a history should be obtained from the owner. In some cases, the precipitating cause of the respiratory distress is straightforward, such as with traumatic injuries, whereas in other cases, the onset may be more insidious. Animals with preexisting medical conditions, such as cardiac disease, neoplasia, or megaesophagus, may also be predisposed to the development of respiratory distress. Owners should be questioned as to past medical conditions and history of routine veterinary care, including heartworm prophylaxis; finally, progression of the signs of respiratory distress should be described. Specifically, distress may be acute in onset or may be more progressive. Particularly in cats, the development of respiratory distress may be preceded by anorexia, lethargy, or abnormal behavior.

Respiratory distress may be further characterized by the location of the lesion or the underlying pathophysiologic condition. Often, localization of the lesion can help to guide the clinician to the most likely cause. Specifically, respiratory distress may be localized to the upper airway, lower airway, parenchyma, or pleural space. Common pathophysiologic causes for respiratory distress include anatomic abnormalities, airway collapse, infection, inflammation, trauma, and pulmonary edema of cardiac and noncardiac causes. For the emergency clinician, the most appropriate first step is to localize the lesion and then to review specific differential diagnoses based on signalment, history, and other physical examination findings.

Diseases of the upper airway

Upper airway diseases may be appreciated by loud stridulous breathing with an increased inspiratory time. Many dogs are hyperthermic on initial presentation because of a decreased ability to cool. The upper airways represent the primary source of resistance to airflow. Upper airway obstructions can be dynamic or fixed. Dynamic obstructions are characterized by the paradoxic movement of tissues into the lumen of airways during inspiration. Common dynamic obstructions include laryngeal paralysis and tracheal collapse, whereas fixed obstructions include extraluminal obstructions, such as neoplasia or cellulitis, and intraluminal obstructions, such as laryngeal tumors or nasopharyngeal polyps. Dynamic and fixed severe upper airway obstructions also result in the development of airway mucosal edema and possibly everted laryngeal saccules as a result of irritation from the increased air flow rates through a narrow lumen.

Emergently, upper airway obstruction should be suspected in any dog with loud and noisy breathing. Therapy for a suspected dynamic obstruction should include sedation and supplemental oxygen. In case of dynamic obstruction, sedation is beneficial in reducing the anxiety associated with inspiration, because with increased inspiratory efforts, there is a resulting paradoxic decline in airway diameter. Low doses of acepromazine (0.03–0.05 mg/kg administered intravenously) alone or in combination with butorphanol (0.1 mg/kg administered intravenously) are often effective. Hyperthermia should be treated by active cooling with room temperature (not cold) intravenous fluids and by placing the dog in a cool area. Because of airway swelling and edema, a single dose of a short-acting anti-inflammatory glucocorticoid is advisable. If the dog has not improved within 15 to 30 minutes or the distress is worsening, more aggressive therapy is warranted. The dog should be heavily sedated or anesthetized and intubated. The emergency clinician should be competent in evaluating airway function and anatomy and in performing a tracheostomy if necessary. Additionally, because many upper airway conditions require medical or surgical interventions, the emergency clinician should fully discuss long-term outcomes and expectations with clients.

The most common causes of upper airway obstruction may vary depending on location; however, in our practice, they include laryngeal paralysis, tracheal collapse, brachycephalic airway syndrome, and severe cellulitis. A complete discussion on the management of these conditions is beyond the scope of this article; however, despite their similarities, differences among the underlying diseases do exist regarding optimal management of affected patients. Awareness of the different nuances of these conditions is critical in their successful management.

Laryngeal paralysis primarily affects older large-breed dogs, particularly retrievers. Usually, the clinical signs of noisy breathing have been present for some length of time before a crisis. Crises often occur during the first hot and humid days of the spring or summer months and may be associated with exercise. Dogs typically respond well to sedation. Dogs that do not rapidly improve should be sedated, have their laryngeal function evaluated, and be intubated. If palliative surgery is not readily available, dogs may require a tracheostomy or may be kept sedated/intubated until normothermia and eupnea are restored. In our practice, we commonly anesthetize patients with propofol for 30 to 60 minutes. If a dog cannot be safely extubated after this time, a tracheostomy may be performed rather than keeping a patient intubated and thereby raising the risk of aspiration pneumonia.

Conversely, in dogs with severe brachycephalic airway syndrome or tracheal collapse, avoidance of a tracheostomy is preferable as compared with dogs with laryngeal paralysis. The reason for this is that many of these dogs become permanently dependent on the tracheostomy tube once placed. If a tracheostomy is unavoidable, plans should be made for surgical correction of the obstruction as soon as feasible. Brachycephalic dogs may also develop laryngeal collapse, which is not amenable to laryngoplasty and may ultimately necessitate a permanent tracheostomy.

In cats, upper airway obstructions are less common but may be caused by nasopharyngeal polyps or infiltrative laryngeal diseases (neoplastic or granulomatous diseases). Nasopharyngeal polyps are a condition of young cats. Occasionally, cats with severe pleural effusion have the appearance of severe inspiratory distress. If sedation for an oral examination of a cat with a suspected upper airway obstruction is planned, supplies should be collected ahead of time for an emergency tracheostomy. The laryngeal lumen of affected cats may be only 1 or 2 mm in diameter and may require an urgent tracheostomy. If biopsy of a laryngeal mass is performed in a cat, a tracheostomy is almost always required because of subsequent airway swelling. Cats may also have a permanent tracheostomy placed, although it is less well tolerated than in dogs.

Diseases of the lower airways

Respiratory distress may also result from lower airway disease, parenchymal lung disease, or pleural space disease. Thoracic radiographs are essential to help clarify the degree of pulmonary or pleural space involvement. Nevertheless, it is important to recall that radiography can be stressful, particularly in cats that are experiencing respiratory distress. Lower airway diseases include chronic bronchitis and feline asthma. Chronic bronchitis rarely presents emergently, although flare-ups do occur in some patients. Chronic bronchitis is defined as the presence of a cough on most days for the preceding 2 months, without evidence of other underlying cause. Canine chronic bronchitis commonly affects small-breed dogs. On auscultation, a mitral murmur is commonly identified. Conversely, feline lower airway disease may present as an emergency. In cats, airway disease seems to represent a continuum, with some cats having primarily inflammatory airway disease with cough and excessive mucus production, whereas other cats are the more prototypical "asthmatics" with reversible bronchoconstriction. Cats with severe bronchoconstriction are often presented emergently. It is important to distinguish the airway disease from congestive heart failure (CHF). Cats with airway disease are typically normothermic and have had a history of cough. Heart failure and airway disease may be accompanied by crackles.

Diseases affecting the lungs

Parenchymal lung disease is often responsible for respiratory distress. Common causes of parenchymal lung disease include pulmonary edema (cardiogenic and noncardiogenic), pulmonary contusion, pneumonia, and neoplasia. Heart failure commonly manifests as respiratory distress. Heart failure in cats is usually appreciated by hypothermia combined with an increased respiratory rate and effort. Jugular venous distention may be present. A gallop or a murmur may be ausculted. Cats with CHF commonly have slow heart rates (130–140 beats per minute [bpm]). Heart disease in dogs is usually chronic valvular disease or dilated cardiomyopathy. Animals with a history of trauma or possible trauma that are presented with respiratory distress can be assumed to have some component of pulmonary contusion (or pneumothorax). Therapy for respiratory distress associated with pulmonary infiltrates includes supplemental oxygen and therapeutic agents directed toward the presumptive underlying cause. The distribution of the pulmonary infiltrates may be useful to help determine the underlying problem. Cardiogenic pulmonary infiltrates most often surround the perihilar region in dogs, whereas the distribution of pulmonary edema may vary in cats. Bacterial pneumonias typically have a cranioventral distribution. Neoplasia usually results in a nodular pattern, although metastatic disease may appear variable.

Animals with suspected cardiogenic pulmonary edema should be treated initially with diuretics (furosemide, administered intravenously or intramuscularly, either 4 mg/kg every 4–6 hours or 1–2 mg/kg every 1–2 hours), cage rest, and supplemental oxygen. If rapid improvement is not observed, additional therapy with vasodilators (nitroprusside titrated to effect) is warranted. In practice, despite published guidelines, measurement of blood pressure during infusion of nitroprusside is usually not performed so as to limit patient stress, loss of supplemental oxygen (by opening the cage door), and technical difficulties in obtaining repeatable and reliable measurements. Specifically, it may be challenging or impossible to place an arterial line for direct blood pressure determinations in an animal with CHF. Oscillometric techniques are commonly inaccurate with small dogs or cats, and Doppler techniques are time-consuming and require a patient with respiratory distress to be restrained. Dobutamine, given as a continuous rate infusion (CRI), is useful in increasing cardiac output in dogs with dilated cardiomyopathies. Intravenous fluids should not be administered to a patient with heart failure, although the patient should be permitted ad libitum access to water. Hemodynamically significant arrhythmias should be treated. Patients should be transitioned to long-term medications after stabilization. Although an echocardiogram is not considered an emergent procedure, emergency clinicians should have a basic knowledge of echocardiography, including assessment of left atrial size, contractility, and the presence or absence of pericardial effusion.

Noncardiogenic pulmonary edema may occur for a variety of reasons. In the emergency room, head trauma, upper airway obstruction, seizures, and electric cord injury are common triggers for the development of non-cardiogenic edema [5]. Noncardiogenic pulmonary edema is typically characterized by high protein; it occurs as a result of permeability shifts in the capillaries rather than hydrostatic forces, as is the case with cardiogenic edema. There is no specific therapy that has been proven beneficial for hastening recovery from noncardiogenic edema [5]. Treatment recommendations include cage rest and supplemental oxygen. More specific therapy with diuretics or colloids has been advocated by various clinicians, although no consensus statement exists. Most dogs with noncardiogenic pulmonary edema rapidly improve within 24 to 48 hours [5].

Pulmonary contusions are common after traumatic injury, particularly in dogs. Animals severely affected with pulmonary contusions are presented short of breath soon after the injury, although, radiographically, the infiltrates often worsen over the first 12 to 24 hours. Dogs with contusions commonly have small- to moderate-volume pneumothoraces as well. Contusions generally heal rapidly. One study in dogs was unable to support the use of prophylactic antibiotics or corticosteroids [6]. Diuretics are also not indicated for animals with pulmonary contusions.

Dogs with pneumonia may be presented to the emergency room with respiratory distress. Bacterial pneumonia is rare in cats. Pneumonia can be subdivided into community-acquired and hospital-acquired forms. Examples of community-acquired pneumonia include severe bronchopneumonia (eg, infectious kennel cough complex) and aspiration pneumonia in a dog with laryngeal paralysis or megaesophagus. Any dog that develops pneumonia while hospitalized for treatment of another condition is considered to have hospital-acquired pneumonia. Therapy for pneumonia includes broad-spectrum antibiotics, physiotherapy, and intravenous fluids. Ideally, a bacterial culture is performed before the institution of antibiotics.

Animals are infrequently presented on an emergent basis with dyspnea secondary to metastatic disease, although cough and lethargy are common. Spontaneous pneumothorax may occasionally develop in a patient with pulmonary neoplasia. Treatment of suspected neoplastic disease is directed at supportive care. Common metastatic tumors include hemangiosarcoma and mammary gland adenocarcinoma. Occasionally, further imaging is indicated to attempt to localize a primary tumor; however, this is generally futile. Pulmonary lymphoma may respond well to therapy. It is also important to exclude a recent travel history in dogs with a nodular pulmonary pattern, because the systemic mycoses can mimic metastatic disease. Other less common causes of pulmonary infiltrates include eosinophilic pneumonitis, smoke inhalation, and pulmonary fibrosis [7–10].

Diseases of the pleural space

Pleural space disease commonly results in marked respiratory distress. Common causes are pleural effusion, pneumothorax, and diaphragmatic hernia. Pleural space disease may often be suspected clinically based on a restrictive (short and shallow) breathing pattern. Thoracic radiographs are useful in documenting the extent of the pleural space disease but may not be safely obtained in animals with severe respiratory distress. Therapeutic thoracocentesis can remove significant volumes of effusion and results in rapid improvement in respiratory rate and effort. Effusions may be classified based on fluid characteristics (transudate, modified transudate, or exudate) or based on the underlying cause. Most effusions are modified transudates. Common causes for the development of pleural effusion include CHF and neoplasia. Other less common causes include chylothorax and pyothorax. An aliquot of fluid should be analyzed, and bacterial culture should be submitted if there is suspicion of an infectious cause. Anticoagulant rodenticides commonly result in substantial intrapleural hemorrhage. Thus, in dogs at risk of anticoagulant rodenticide intoxication, a prothrombin time should be evaluated before thoracocentesis. Pleural effusion is best treated based on the underlying cause. Pyothorax generally requires chest tube placement for drainage [11]. In dogs, chest tubes are generally inadequate; therefore, exploratory thoracotomy is indicated. Animals with long-standing effusion recognized by history or radiographically by rounding of the lung lobes may develop severe iatrogenic pneumothorax after thoracocentesis. Some pulmonary neoplasms are sensitive to chemotherapy, and this mode of therapy can improve respiratory compromise. Diuretics and vasodilators are almost always effective in relieving signs of CHF.

Pneumothorax may be classified as traumatic or spontaneous. Traumatic pneumothorax is more common. For animals with a known history of injury, needle thoracocentesis may be performed if there is clinical suspicion that pneumothorax may be the cause of dyspnea. Because of the high density of tissue thromboplastin, a previously healthy injured lung heals rapidly; thus, chest tubes are not commonly required in the trauma patient. A commonly cited guideline is that three or more thoracocenteses ("three-strike rule") within 24 hours is sufficient justification for placement of the chest tube in the traumatic pneumothorax. It is exceedingly rare to have a patient with trauma require a thoracotomy for resection of the traumatized lung. Conversely, most cases of spontaneous pneumothorax require surgical resection of the affected lobe. Spontaneous pneumothorax is defined as pneumothorax occurring without trauma [12]. Common causes include bulla/blebs and neoplasia (primary or metastatic) [12]. Additionally, cats with lower airway disease may occasionally develop spontaneous pneumothoraces [13]. For affected dogs, rapid surgical exploration and resection have been associated with decreased morbidity and expense [12].

Diaphragmatic hernia should be corrected as soon as the patient is considered stable enough for surgery [14]. In traumatic injuries, concurrent pulmonary contusions may markedly worsen gas exchange; thus, anesthesia and surgery may be postponed until clinical improvement. If significant herniation exists, however, including the presence of the stomach within the intrathoracic cavity, surgical repair is urgent. Anesthesia may still be safely performed with pulmonary contusions, although in addition to the positive-pressure ventilation required because of the loss of diaphragmatic integrity, a small amount of positive end-expiratory pressure (PEEP) may be beneficial to help recruit collapsed alveoli. In chronic hernias, re-expansion pulmonary edema may result in severe respiratory failure [15]; thus, correction of chronic hernias should be undertaken with care and gradual reinflation of the lung.

Summary

Respiratory emergencies are common presentations to emergency clinicians. Appropriate assessment and timely interventions may be crucial in the stabilization of dyspneic patients. The emergency clinician should be fully prepared and equipped to correctly ascertain and treat the most likely cause of respiratory compromise of a patient. Based on history, signalment, clinical presentation, and brief physical examination findings, the clinician should be able to formulate a plan of action to relieve respiratory distress and communicate with the owner about the diagnostic and therapeutic strategies and overall prognosis of the patient. Prompt recognition of the underlying respiratory disease and complete familiarity with emergency diagnostic and therapeutic procedures can lead to the successful management of many emergency respiratory patients.

References

[1] Lee JA, Drobatz KJ. Respiratory distress and cyanosis in dogs. In: King LG, editor. Textbook of respiratory disease in dogs and cats. St. Louis: Elsevier; 2004. p. 1–11.
[2] Rose DK, Cohen MM, Wigglesworth DF, et al. Critical respiratory events in the postanesthesia care unit. Patient, surgical, and anesthetic factors. Anesthesiology 1994; 81(2):410–8.
[3] Barton L. Respiratory muscle fatigue. Vet Clin N Am Small Anim Pract 2002;32(5):1059–71.
[4] West JB. Ventilation-perfusion relationships. In: Coryell PA, editor. Respiratory physiology—the essentials. 5th edition. Baltimore: Williams & Wilkins; 1998. p. 51–69.
[5] Drobatz KJ, Saunders HM, Pugh CR, et al. Noncardiogenic pulmonary edema in dogs and cats: 26 cases (1987–1993). J Am Vet Med Assoc 1995;206(11):1732–6.

[6] Powell L, Rozanski EA, Tidwell A, et al. A retrospective analysis of pulmonary contusion secondary to motor vehicle accidents in 143 dogs: 1994–1997. J Vet Emerg Crit Care 1999;9: 127–36.

[7] Drobatz KJ, Walker LM, Hendricks JC. Smoke exposure in cats: 22 cases (1986–1997). J Am Vet Med Assoc 1999;215(9):1312–6.

[8] Drobatz KJ, Walker LM, Hendricks JC. Smoke exposure in dogs: 27 cases (1988–1997). J Am Vet Med Assoc 1999;215(9):1306–11.

[9] Clercx C, Peeters D, Snaps F, et al. Eosinophilic bronchopneumopathy in dogs. J Vet Intern Med 2000;14(3):282–91.

[10] Corcoran BM, Cobb M, Martin MW, et al. Chronic pulmonary disease in West Highland white terriers. Vet Rec 1999;144(22):611–6.

[11] Waddell LS, Brady CA, Drobatz KJ. Risk factors, prognostic indicators, and outcome of pyothorax in cats: 80 cases (1986–1999). J Am Vet Med Assoc 2002;221(6):819–24.

[12] Puerto DA, Brockman DJ, Lindquist C, et al. Surgical and nonsurgical management of and selected risk factors for spontaneous pneumothorax in dogs: 64 cases (1986–1999). J Am Vet Med Assoc 2002;220(11):1670–4.

[13] White HL, Rozanski EA, Tidwell AS, et al. Spontaneous pneumothorax in two cats with small airway disease. J Am Vet Med Assoc 2003;222(11):1547, 1573–5.

[14] Schmiedt CW, Tobias KM, Stevenson MA. Traumatic diaphragmatic hernia in cats: 34 cases (1991–2001). J Am Vet Med Assoc 2003;222(9):1237–40.

[15] Stampley AR, Waldron DR. Reexpansion pulmonary edema after surgery to repair a diaphragmatic hernia in a cat. J Am Vet Med Assoc 1993;203(12):1699–701.

ELSEVIER
SAUNDERS

Vet Clin Small Anim
35 (2005) 319–342

VETERINARY
CLINICS
Small Animal Practice

Assessment and Treatment of Perfusion Abnormalities in the Emergency Patient

Amanda K. Boag, MA, VetMB, MRCVS*, Dez Hughes, BVSc, MRCVS

Queen Mother Hospital, Royal Veterinary College, Hawkshead Lane, North Mymms, Hertfordshire AL9 7TA, United Kingdom

The term *perfusion* refers, to the pumping of a fluid through an organ or tissue. Although, experimentally, isolated tissues may be perfused with a variety of fluids, in the living patient, perfusion refers to the pumping of blood to organs and peripheral tissues via the circulatory system. In a healthy animal, this results in the delivery of oxygen and other metabolic substrates to the tissues and the removal of byproducts of tissue metabolism, notably carbon dioxide. Failure of adequate oxygen delivery at the tissue level and, subsequently, the cellular level results in decreased oxidative metabolism, leading to decreased synthesis of high-energy phosphates and impaired cellular function. Ultimately, cellular death and organ failure may occur. When global tissue perfusion fails to the extent that cellular oxygen delivery is impaired, this is termed *shock*. Although decreased perfusion may occur primarily at a local level, for example, hind limb hypoperfusion secondary to aortic thromboembolism in cats, the emergency clinician is more often concerned with the challenging task of assessing global tissue perfusion. Some degree of global tissue hypoperfusion is common in many emergency patients because it can result from a large variety of underlying disease processes; hence, the ability to recognize and treat hypoperfusion is fundamental to the stabilization of these patients. Overperfusion (ie, increased blood flow to the tissues) may occur, especially in patients unable to excrete fluid normally (eg, patients with oliguric renal failure). Although this may have important clinical sequelae, it is unlikely to occur before veterinary intervention (especially fluid therapy), and thus is rarely a concern of the emergency clinician.

---

* Corresponding author.
E-mail address: aboag@rvc.ac.uk (A.K. Boag).

0195-5616/05/$ - see front matter © 2005 Elsevier Inc. All rights reserved.
doi:10.1016/j.cvsm.2004.10.010   *vetsmall.theclinics.com*

Classification of hypoperfusion

The criteria used to assess the presence and severity of hypoperfusion, and thus to formulate treatment plans, are dependent on the underlying cause of the perfusion abnormality. Global or systemic hypoperfusion can occur secondary to a reduction in the effective circulating intravascular volume (hypovolemic shock) or reduced ability of the heart to pump blood around the body secondary to reduced cardiac function (cardiogenic shock), obstruction to blood flow (obstructive shock), or maldistribution of the circulating intravascular volume (distributive shock). Common causes of systemic hypoperfusion in small animal patients are shown in Table 1. In the emergency patient, hypoperfusion is most commonly seen secondary to hypovolemia. More than one cause of hypoperfusion may exist in a given patient at any one time (eg, patients with severe sepsis have evidence of hypovolemic and distributive shock and may also have a component of cardiogenic shock).

Consequences of hypoperfusion

As hypoperfusion, of whatever cause, worsens, cellular hypoxia ultimately occurs. Although brief periods of cellular hypoxia may be tolerated, for example, during strenuous exercise, prolonged decreases in tissue oxygen tension result in profound disturbances in cellular metabolism. Under aerobic conditions, cellular energy is generated in the form of high-energy phosphate compounds (primarily ATP) produced via three processes: glycolysis, the citric acid cycle, and oxidative phosphorylation or the electron transport chain. Under anaerobic conditions, only the first of these

Table 1
Causes of hypoperfusion in small animal patients

Hypovolemia	Cardiogenic	Obstructive	Distributive
Hemorrhage	Cardiomyopathy	Pericardial	Systemic inflammatory
Trauma	Dilated	tamponade	response syndrome
Coagulation	Hypertrophic	Restrictive pericarditis	Pancreatitis
disorders	Valvular disease	Pulmonary	Neoplasia
Neoplasia	Severe	thromboembolism	Burns
Burns	dysrhythmias		Sepsis
Vomiting and			Severe tissue
diarrhea			trauma
Severe polyuria			
Marked internal			
fluid losses			
Pleural			
Peritoneal			
Interstitial			
Severe dehydration			

pathways, glycolysis, can function. This allows energy production to continue in the face of cellular hypoxia but generates much less energy on a molar basis. Metabolism of 1 mol of glucose leads to the generation of 38 mol of ATP under aerobic conditions but only 2 mol of ATP under anaerobic conditions, although this is somewhat offset by the fact that anaerobic energy production is more rapid than aerobic energy production. Glycolysis produces pyruvate and consumes nicotinamide adenine di-nucleotide (NAD^+). To allow anaerobic metabolism to continue, the cell must dispose of pyruvate and regenerate NAD^+, which it does by converting pyruvate to lactate. A disadvantage of lactate production is the concomitant production of hydrogen ions and the development of an organic metabolic acidosis within the cell and systemically, because lactate equilibrates rapidly across the cellular membrane. Interestingly, intracellular acidosis after ATP depletion delays cell death and may have a protective response at the cellular level [1].

Tissue hypoxia, cellular energy depletion, and acidosis lead to disturbed ionic homeostasis across cell membranes [2,3], abnormal intracellular signaling [4,5], and reduced cellular functional capacity [6]. Eventually, hypoxic cells die, and this results in further local inflammation and reduction in organ function. Ultimately, patient outcome after an episode of systemic hypoperfusion is related to the severity and duration of hypoperfusion and the degree of impairment in oxygen metabolism and resultant cellular damage. Experimental studies in animals [7,8] and clinical studies in people [9–11] have correlated decreased systemic oxygen metabolism and cumulative oxygen debt with mortality and the develop-ment of organ failure. A recent study has also shown an improved outcome in people with severe sepsis or septic shock when therapy to maximize tissue oxygen delivery was introduced at an early stage [12].

One of the challenges of assessing hypoperfusion in the emergency patient is recognition of the patient in which global indices of perfusion are adequate but in which local perfusion to certain organs may be significantly impaired. In the early stages of global hypoperfusion, such as hemorrhage, blood flow is redirected to the vital organs, such as the brain and heart [13–15]. Global indicators of tissue perfusion may be relatively normal at this stage; however, significant cellular hypoxia may be occurring in other organ systems, notably the skin and gastrointestinal tract [16]. Similarly, in distributive shock, it is recognized that occult oxygen deficits may exist despite adequate systemic perfusion parameters [17,18]. Failure to identify and treat these patients may result in subsequent organ dysfunction and increased morbidity and mortality.

Clinical assessment of perfusion status

Evaluation of any emergency patient should start with a physical exam-ination focusing on the major body systems (respiratory, cardiovascular, and neurologic). A careful evaluation of the cardiovascular system of the animal can provide a large amount of information regarding the animal's systemic perfusion. The initial assessment should encompass heart rate, cardiac auscultation, mucous membrane color, capillary refill time (CRT), and pulse quality (amplitude and duration) in the proximal and distal limbs. The initial perfusion assessment can be supplemented by evaluating jugular and peripheral venous filling, jugular pulsation, apex beat, and rectal and extremity temperature.

In uncomplicated hypovolemia, these cardiovascular parameters tend to change in a relatively predictable manner (Table 2) and provide a useful assessment of the animal's systemic perfusion. A normovolemic dog in the setting of a veterinary emergency clinic is likely to have a heart rate of 80 to 120 beats per minute (bpm) and pink mucous membranes, with a CRT of approximately 1 to 1.75 seconds. Although small-breed dogs tend to have a higher resting heart rate than the large and giant breeds, the effect of body size on heart rate tends to be overemphasized in the veterinary literature. Femoral and metatarsal pulses should be easily palpable. Careful palpation of the height (amplitude) and width (duration) of the femoral pulse should allow the astute clinician to generate a mental image of the pulse profile (Fig. 1A) that allows an estimation of pulse volume. In strict terms, the pulse palpated is representative of pressure waves in the arterial wall rather than actual flow in the vessel; however, the physical qualities of the pulse seem to equate to pulse volume.

In response to hypovolemia, a number of compensatory responses occur to maintain arterial blood pressure (ABP), which is the product of cardiac output (CO, heart rate × stroke volume) and peripheral vascular resistance. Loss of blood volume results in decreased venous return to the heart and decreased CO. Homeostatic mechanisms initiated by baroreceptors, including catecholamine release and inhibition of the vagal parasympathetic center, lead to increases in heart rate, cardiac contractility, and systemic vascular resistance that act to restore ABP toward normal. In this compensated stage of hypovolemia, heart rate and cardiac

Table 2
Physical examination parameters to assess the stages of uncomplicated hypovolemia

Clinical parameter	Mild hypovolemia	Moderate hypovolemia	Severe hypovolemia
Heart rate	130–150 bpm	150–170 bpm	170–220 bpm
Mucous membrane color	Normal to pinker than normal	Pale pink	Gray, white, or muddy
Capillary refill time	Rapid (<1 second)	Approximately normal (1–2 seconds)	Prolonged (>2 seconds) or absent
Pulse amplitude	Increased	Mild to moderate decrease	Severe decrease
Pulse duration	Mildly reduced	Moderately reduced	Severely reduced
Metatarsal pulse	Easily palpable	Just palpable	Absent

Abbreviation: bpm, beats per minute.

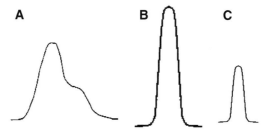

Fig. 1. (*A*) Normal pulse profile. (*B*) Tall and narrow pulse profile as palpated in compensated hypovolemia. (*C*) Short and narrow pulse profile as palpated in decompensated hypovolemia.

contractility are mildly increased and the CRT is faster than normal. Careful palpation of the pulse reveals a pulse profile that is taller and narrower than normal (see Fig. 1B), reflecting a slightly decreased pulse volume. This pulse profile is often described as being "hyperdynamic," "bounding," or "snappy"; however, these words often serve to confuse rather than to clarify.

As hypovolemia progresses, compensatory mechanisms gradually fail and the animal progresses to decompensated hypovolemic shock in which global tissue perfusion is severely compromised. These patients show markedly increased heart rates (170–220 bpm in dogs). Cardiac auscultation may reveal quiet heart sounds secondary to the decreased blood volume. Mucous membranes are pale to white, gray, or muddy (depending on background pigmentation), with a prolonged or absent CRT. The femoral pulse profile is short and narrow (see Fig. 1C), often described as weak or "thready," and metatarsal pulses are absent. CO plateau then falls at heart rates in excess of approximately 180 bpm [19]. Consequently, heart rates faster than 220 to 240 bpm are unlikely to represent a physiologic sinus tachycardia in response to hypovolemia and are more likely to be a primary tachyarrhythmia warranting urgent assessment with ECG.

The assessment of hypoperfusion secondary to hypovolemia in cats is similar but more challenging. Normal feline mucous membranes are paler than in dogs, and although possible, it is harder to appreciate a pulse profile. Resting heart rates are higher than in dogs and are usually 160 to 200 bpm in a veterinary clinic. The proportional increase in heart rate with hypovolemia is not as marked, probably because even normal cats in a veterinary clinic already have sympathetic nervous system activation.

The clinical assessment of perfusion status using the previously discussed criteria works well in dogs with hypoperfusion secondary to hypovolemia. Not all patients with significant hypoperfusion have uncomplicated hypovolemia, however. Cross-referencing the various physical parameters discussed previously should be done whenever a clinical assessment is performed, because this may provide evidence of other forms of hypoperfusion. If they still have an adequate circulating blood volume, canine patients with distributive shock secondary to sepsis or systemic inflammatory response syndrome (SIRS) exhibit classic hyperdynamic signs (tachycardia, tall and narrow pulses, and bright pink or red mucous membranes with a rapid CRT). Once these patients develop concurrent serious hypovolemia, they have more severe tachycardia, weak femoral pulses, and a prolonged CRT; however, their mucous membrane color may still be pink or indeed injected. A dog with severe hypoperfusion caused by uncomplicated hypovolemia normally has much less color in the mucous membrane than a dog with SIRS. It is this discrepancy in the mucous membrane color compared with the other perfusion parameters that should alert the clinician to the fact that the dog may have something other than uncomplicated hypovolemia. Urgent diagnostic procedures should be undertaken together with stabilization in these patients to identify the source of the inflammatory response. In some dogs with severe hypovolemia and maldistribution, the mucous membranes show cyanosis, presumably because of increased tissue transit time, resulting in more oxygen offloading from hemoglobin. An inappropriately slow heart rate for the degree of hypoperfusion can be seen in dogs with septic peritonitis, possibly because of intra-abdominal vagal stimulation.

Feline patients with conditions like severe sepsis associated with distributive shock rarely demonstrate the injected mucous membranes commonly seen in dogs. Cats with sepsis or SIRS are more commonly presented with signs of severe mental depression, poor or unpalpable femoral pulses, pale mucous membranes (often with an undetectable CRT), and inappropriate bradycardia. In a recent retrospective study of 29 cats with confirmed severe sepsis, 66% had a heart rate lower than 140 bpm on presentation [20].

Many dogs with congestive heart failure caused by valvular heart disease do not have forward failure or severe hypoperfusion. In contrast, forward failure is more common in dogs and cats with cardiomyopathy. Nevertheless, patients with hypoperfusion secondary to cardiogenic causes exhibit the same signs of hypoperfusion as those seen with hypovolemia (ie, poor pulse quality, pale mucous membranes with a prolonged CRT, tachycardia). On examination of their cardiovascular system, they often have other abnormalities that lead one to suspect a cardiogenic cause. Such abnormalities may include a heart murmur or gallop rhythm, or arrhythmia with or without pulses deficits. If the cardiac disease is significant enough to be causing global hypoperfusion, it is likely that the patient will show also some degree of respiratory compromise, with the presence of dyspnea secondary to pulmonary edema or pleural effusion. Despite arterial hypotension, many of these patients actually have increased intravascular volume secondary to chronic neurohormonal responses to impending cardiac failure.

Hemodynamic monitoring

A detailed and thorough physical examination is undoubtedly the most useful sole means of assessing global perfusion status in veterinary emergency patients. An experienced clinician can assess whether mild to severe global hypoperfusion exists within minutes of the patient arriving at the emergency clinic. A physical examination does not require expensive equipment, and it can be repeated multiple times and used to assess response to therapy. More information can be gleaned, however, when the physical examination is supplemented by hemodynamic monitoring. The most commonly measured parameters in veterinary medicine include ABP and central venous pressure (CVP). Whenever hemodynamic monitoring is used, it is incumbent on the clinician to understand the relevant technical aspects of the device used, including its accuracy and precision and the sources of spurious results. Furthermore, to be able to use the information obtained for the benefit of the patient, the mechanisms responsible for hemodynamic homeostasis must be understood.

Arterial blood pressure

ABP peaks immediately after cardiac systole and then falls to a nadir at the end of diastole (Fig. 2). The difference between systolic and diastolic blood pressure is the pulse pressure, which determines the height (amplitude) of the palpated arterial pulse. Mean arterial pressure (MAP) is calculated as the sum of the diastolic pressure and a third of the difference between systolic and diastolic pressures. Diastolic blood pressure is thus a more important determinant of tissue perfusion than systolic pressure.

ABP can be measured in a number of ways. Noninvasive methods include Doppler and oscillometric techniques. In most people's hands, the Doppler method only allows assessment of systolic pressure but is more likely to give meaningful readings than oscillometric techniques in the face of significant hypotension in small animals, especially cats [21], or when arrhythmias are

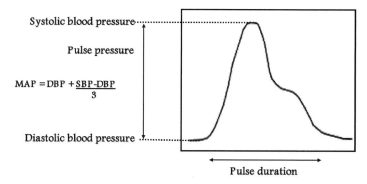

Fig. 2. Arterial pressure tracing.

present. Oscillometric methods use a cuff that is gradually inflated and deflated by a machine. Pressure changes within the cuff caused by arterial pulsations are detected and allow the machine to calculate systolic, diastolic, and mean pressures. Heart rate is also often displayed.

The placement of an arterial catheter, commonly in the dorsal pedal artery, allows direct measurement of ABP when connected to an electronic pressure transducer, which allows continuous display of arterial pressure. This provides the most accurate measurement of blood pressure but is more invasive, and placement of arterial catheters can be challenging, especially in small patients or those with severe hypoperfusion.

Although a low ABP (systolic <80 mm Hg, mean <60 mm Hg) implies severe hypoperfusion and requires urgent treatment, ABP is an insensitive indicator of mild to moderate hypoperfusion, because the body's homeostatic mechanisms act to maintain ABP within a narrow range by changing heart rate, stroke volume, and systemic vascular resistance. Furthermore, ABP is not synonymous with tissue perfusion. Patients with a low CO but intense peripheral vasoconstriction may have normal ABP yet dangerously low tissue blood flow.

Central venous pressure

CVP is measured by placement of a catheter into the central venous compartment, commonly the intrathoracic vena cava, via the jugular vein. In cats and small dogs, a long intravenous catheter can be advanced into the caudal vena cava via the saphenous or medial femoral vein. Readings can be taken intermittently, or, as with direct ABP, it is possible to connect the catheter to an electronic transducer and display a continuous output and waveform. Normal CVPs are between 0 and 5 cm H_2O. The value obtained reflects the balance between central venous blood volume, venous capacitance, and right-sided cardiac function. When the catheter tip is in the intrathoracic venous vasculature, changes in intrathoracic pressure may also affect the CVP reading; thus readings should be interpreted with caution in dyspneic patients or those on positive-pressure ventilation [22]. Because the venous circulation is a low-pressure system with minimal autoregulation, CVP is generally a better indicator of intravascular volume status than ABP. Patients with hypoperfusion secondary to hypovolemia are likely to have a low CVP, and changes in CVP can be used to help guide therapy. There is some experimental evidence that acute hypovolemia may lead to decreased ventricular distensibility and venoconstriction as well as an increase in CVP [23]; thus, it is possible that CVP could be insensitive in the acutely bleeding patient. CVP is especially useful in those patients at risk of volume overload, notably patients with anuric renal failure, heart disease, or parenchymal lung disease. Measurement of CVP can also be used in the assessment and diagnosis of patients with hypoperfusion secondary to the rare condition, restrictive pericarditis, in which CVP is elevated despite clinical evidence of systemic hypoperfusion.

Advanced hemodynamic monitoring

Measurement of more advanced cardiovascular parameters, such as CO, pulmonary artery occlusion pressure, and systemic vascular resistance, is often used to guide therapy in critically ill human patients. Measurement of these parameters has traditionally been performed using thermodilution techniques and a CO computer after placement of a pulmonary artery (Swan-Ganz) catheter; thus, these parameters are rarely measured in the veterinary emergency patient. Recently, there has been interest in less invasive methods of measuring CO, including thoracic electrical bioimpedance (TEB), the lithium dilution indicator method (LiDCO), and pulse contour analysis (PulseCO) [24,25]. TEB calculates CO by using the known changes in electrical impedance produced by blood flow through the aorta. Although initial experimental studies in dogs showed good correlation between CO measured by TEB and by thermodilution [26,27], a later study is less encouraging [28]. Human clinical studies using TEB have also shown variable results [29,30]. The LiDCO method involves the injection of a bolus of lithium chloride into a central vein, with measurement of the concentration of diluted lithium at the site of a peripheral arterial catheter. The LiDCO computer can then construct a dilution curve and determine the CO. The LiDCO method shows good correlation with thermodilution methods in horses [31], pigs [32], and dogs [33]. A recent study demonstrated good agreement between CO determined after lithium administration into a central or peripheral vein [34]. This raises the possibility that CO could be measured with a technique needing placement of only a peripheral venous catheter and an arterial catheter. This may make monitoring of CO more accessible for use in veterinary emergency patients. Further studies in clinical veterinary patients are needed before the usefulness of this technique can be evaluated. Pulse contour analysis is a more advanced technique that provides a near-continuous display of CO based on analysis of arterial waveforms. It requires calibration by thermodilution or lithium dilution on a regular basis (every 8 hours); however, results from trials in human patients show good correlation with more traditional methods of measuring CO [35–37]. Its use has not yet been reported in a veterinary clinical setting. The ability to measure CO reliably in veterinary emergency patients may help to identify patients with early global hypoperfusion and may allow better tailoring of therapy.

Lactate

The clinical value of measuring serum lactate concentrations to aid in the assessment of hypoperfusion has been recognized for more than 40 years

[38]. As hypoperfusion progresses and tissues become hypoxic, anaerobic metabolism occurs and lactate is generated from pyruvate to allow cellular energy production to continue. Lactate equilibrates rapidly across cellular membranes; thus, increased intracellular lactate results in an increased interstitial and blood lactate concentration. Hyperlactatemia occurs whenever the rate of lactate production exceeds that of lactate extraction. Brief periods of relative tissue hypoxia, such as with exercise [39] or seizures [40], can lead to dramatic increases in lactate; however, the hyperlactatemia resolves quickly as lactate is rapidly metabolized, principally by the liver. In patients with systemic hypoperfusion, the major determinant of the relative contribution to lactate production and extraction by different tissues seems to be blood flow. In mild hemorrhage in dogs, blood flow to the gastrointestinal tract is reduced, whereas blood flow to the liver is initially preserved. Although intestinal lactate production is increased, the liver is still able to extract and metabolize lactate [41]. In severe hemorrhagic shock, the liver actually becomes a net producer of lactate [41,42]. Numerous experimental studies have documented that increases in blood lactate concentration correlate well with oxygen debt and critical levels of oxygen delivery [7,43–45]. Clinical experience suggests that mild systemic hypo-perfusion is associated with a plasma lactate concentration of 3 to 5 mmol/L, moderate hypoperfusion with a lactate concentration of 5 to 7 mmol/L, and severe hypoperfusion with lactate levels exceeding 7 mmol/L. A retrospective study performed by one of the authors evaluating plasma lactate concentration in dogs with hemorrhagic shock secondary to anticoagulant rodenticide toxicity showed that lactate concentration was significantly higher as clinical perfusion parameters deteriorated. Lactate concentrations [mean (range)] in 41 dogs classified into mild, moderate, and severe hypoperfusion groups were 2.4 (1.4–3.4), 3.6 (2.3–5.5), and 7.9 (6.1–10.5) mmol/L, respectively (D. Hughes, BVSc, MRCVS, unpublished data, 2000).

High lactate concentrations have prognostic implications. An early study in people demonstrated that as lactate concentrations increased from 2.1 to 8.0 mmol/L, survival decreased from 90% to 10% [45]. Because of the extremely heterogeneous nature of causes of hyperlactatemia, however, it has proved difficult to identify a critical level of oxygen delivery associated with lactic acidosis [46,47]. A decrease in serum lactate concentration after therapy for hypoperfusion may be more useful prognostically and seems to discriminate between human survivors and nonsurvivors better than peak or admission lactate concentration [48,49]. Our clinical experience indicates that this is likely true in dogs and cats and depends on the severity and reversibility of the underlying disease. Severe hyperlactatemia after acute severe hemorrhage that is rapidly controlled and treated is not associated with high mortality, whereas it usually is in dogs with septic peritonitis. In veterinary patients, lactate concentration has been shown to be predictive of survival in dogs with heartworm caval syndrome [50,51], dogs in a veterinary intensive care unit [52], and horses with acute abdominal crises [53]. In dogs with gastric dilatation volvulus syndrome, a high serum lactate concentration has been shown to be a moderately sensitive but specific indicator of the presence of gastric necrosis [54]. Despite these studies, it is important to note that for individual patients, as opposed to groups of patients in studies, lactate concentration should not be used alone to guide therapy but used in conjunction with all other clinical features.

There are limitations to the use of lactate to assess hypoperfusion, however. First, hyperlactatemia implies that oxygen extraction has already been maximized, tissue hypoxia is present, and anaerobic metabolism is occurring to attempt to support cellular energy production [44,55]. It is thus a late marker of hypoperfusion. Second, because the liver and other tissues in the body have a large capacity to oxidize lactate, it is possible that significant regional hypoperfusion may exist with a normal serum lactate concentration. Third, hyperlactatemia may occur secondary to other causes, such as neoplasia, diabetes mellitus, and severe liver disease [56]. In the authors' experience, this is rare in the absence of concurrent hypoperfusion, although it does occur occasionally in dogs with lymphoma and hemangiosarcoma. In patients with hyperlactatemia that are not showing signs of global hypoperfusion, it is likely that they have occult regional hypoperfusion.

Hyperlactatemia seen in patients with sepsis and septic shock seems to be a much more complicated situation. Certainly, when these patients have more severe hypovolemia, lactate concentration is often increased. The hypermetabolic state seen with sepsis may result in increased glycolysis and pyruvate production at a rate faster than it can enter the citric acid cycle. Some of the pyruvate is consequently converted to lactate. In these patients, although lactate is increased, the lactate/pyruvate ratio would be expected to be normal. There is increasing evidence from experimental studies [57–59] and clinical studies in people [60,61] that the hyperlactatemia seen in volume-replete septic patients is related to hypermetabolism. In the authors' experience, patients with sepsis that are relatively volume replete have only mild hyperlactatemia and moderate to severe hyperlactatemia is usually associated with hypovolemia.

Systemic oxygenation parameters

During the development of hypoperfusion, there is a period when oxygen delivery to the tissues is decreased but tissue oxygen consumption is maintained by the tissues increasing oxygen extraction from the blood. The oxygen extraction ratio (OER) gradually increases, resulting in decreased mixed venous oxygen saturation. Thus, desaturation of mixed venous blood may be an earlier marker of tissue hypoperfusion than serum lactate. Mixed venous blood is obtained from the pulmonary artery, necessitating placement of a pulmonary artery catheter. In people with normal perfusion, central venous oxygen saturation using blood drawn from the superior vena cava tends to underestimate mixed venous oxygen saturation because of the relatively high OER of the heart and brain. Conversely, in patients with systemic hypoperfusion, redistribution of blood flow to the heart and brain leads to an overestimation of mixed venous levels [62]. Nevertheless, changes in central venous oxygen saturation tend to follow changes in mixed venous samples [63–65]. The maintenance of central venous oxygen saturation has been used as a goal in a recent human clinical study assessing the emergency fluid resuscitation of patients in septic shock [12]. The measurement of central venous oxygen saturation in veterinary emergency patients could play a role in assessing patients with early hypoperfusion; however, the technical requirements would make it difficult.

Assessment of local hypoperfusion

The assessment of hypoperfusion in the emergency patient commonly focuses on the global indicators of systemic perfusion discussed previously. Significant local hypoperfusion of certain organs, notably the gastrointestinal tract and skin, may occur before systemic hypoperfusion [15,18,66]. This has two important consequences. First, detection of hypoperfusion in these organs can provide an early indicator of impending global hypoperfusion. Second, occult hypoperfusion of individual organs may have a significant impact on morbidity and mortality.

The gastrointestinal tract is one of the first organs to suffer from decreased blood flow in hypovolemic and cardiogenic shock. Moreover, reduction in splanchnic blood flow may persist, even in the face of normal hemodynamic parameters, after resuscitation from hemorrhagic or septic shock [67,68]. Decreased gastrointestinal perfusion may contribute to increased morbidity and is implicated in the development of progressive organ dysfunction [69,70]. Gastrointestinal perfusion can be assessed using the technique of gastric tonometry [71]. A catheter equipped with a silicone balloon filled with physiologic saline and permeable to gas but not to fluid is introduced into the stomach. After a period of equilibration (usually 60–90 minutes), the saline is withdrawn from the balloon and the P_{CO_2} is measured. With knowledge of arterial bicarbonate concentration, gastric intramucosal pH can be calculated using the Henderson-Hasselbalch equation. Studies in experimental animals [72] and critically ill people [68,69] have shown gastric intramucosal pH to be a more sensitive predictor of complications and death than many of the systemic indicators of hypoperfusion. Despite the apparent sensitivity of gastric tonometry, its use is limited in emergency patients because of the need to place a nasogastric tube and to allow an equilibration period of at least 1 hour.

A new technique is measurement of sublingual P_{CO_2}. There seems to be good correlation between serum lactate and sublingual P_{CO_2} in animals with circulatory shock [73]. Sublingual P_{CO_2} has also been found to correlate well with gastric intramucosal P_{CO_2} [74,75]. When hemodynamic variables, arterial lactate, and sublingual P_{CO_2} were compared as prognostic indicators in human intensive care patients, sublingual P_{CO_2} and, more specifically, the difference between sublingual and arterial P_{CO_2} were the best predictors of mortality [76]. Although its use has not yet been evaluated in veterinary patients, sublingual capnometry may prove to be a noninvasive and inexpensive method of assessing early tissue hypoperfusion in veterinary emergency patients.

Cutaneous hypoperfusion has been assessed by various methods in experimental models of hemorrhagic shock [66] and human trauma patients [77,78]. Despite showing promising results, its use has not been evaluated in veterinary patients and may be compromised by the hair coat of veterinary patients. Urinary oxygen tension to assess renal oxygen supply has been evaluated in critically sick people [79]. In anesthetized dogs, there is good correlation between renal blood flow and urinary oxygen tension [80]. This correlation was better than that between renal blood flow and femoral arterial pressure or urinary flow rate. The use of urinary oxygen tension has not been evaluated in veterinary clinical patients.

Treatment

The ultimate goal in treating hypoperfusion is to restore blood flow, and thus oxygen delivery, to tissues, with the aim of preventing further organ damage and the risk of progression to multiorgan failure. Intuitively, one might expect that rapid normalization of perfusion would be associated with a better outcome, and this is supported by human clinical studies [12,81,82]. There is no doubt that the initial treatment of hypoperfusion varies depending on the underlying cause. At an extreme, pericardiocentesis is a specific and successful method of treating hypoperfusion secondary to pericardial effusion and obstructive shock. In many scenarios, however, debate exists regarding the most successful and appropriate methods of resuscitation and the end-points that should be achieved even for common causes of hypoperfusion such as hemorrhage.

Treatment of hypovolemia

Therapy for hypovolemia unsurprisingly revolves around replacement of the intravascular volume deficit with fluid therapy. Rational decision making on the type and rate of administration of intravenous fluid therapy most appropriate in any individual patient relies on an understanding of fluid homeostasis within the body and on the nature of the fluid loss. Patients with fluid loss solely or principally from the intravascular compartment, such as that occurring with hemorrhage, are treated differently from those patients in which there is likely to have been interstitial and intracellular fluid loss (dehydration) as well. This most commonly occurs in patients in which fluid loss exceeds fluid intake over a longer time (often days), such as with protracted vomiting and diarrhea. Consequently, there is time for fluid shifts between body compartments to occur, and the interstitial and, ultimately, intracellular compartments lose fluid as well.

Hemorrhage

Hemorrhage is one of the more common causes of severe hypoperfusion in veterinary emergency patients. A number of different fluid therapy strategies can be used in the reversal of hypoperfusion in these patients:

- Isotonic crystalloid replacement solutions at rapid rates (60–90-mL/kg bolus in dogs, 40–60-mL/kg bolus in cats)
- Hypertonic saline solution (4–7 mL/kg in dogs, 2–4 mL/kg in cats)
- Colloid administration, including hemoglobin-based oxygen-carrying solutions (10–20-mL/kg bolus)
- Blood products

A large body of experimental research and human clinical trials has addressed the issue of the optimal resuscitation strategy for hemorrhagic shock; however, there is a dearth of information specifically relating to veterinary clinical patients. Although any of these strategies may be successful in an individual patient, there is no consensus in human or veterinary medicine as to the single best method, and because of the heterogenous nature of patients with hemorrhagic shock, a strategy that works for every patient is unlikely to exist. An understanding of the controversies should help the astute clinician to make informed decisions for his or her patients.

For many years, aggressive resuscitation with large volumes of crystalloids has been the recommended treatment for patients presented with hypotension secondary to hemorrhage [83]. This recommendation was partially based on experimental animal models of controlled hemorrhage [84,85]; however, these models do not necessarily mimic the hemodynamic situation in most of our acutely bleeding patients. In more recent experimental models of severe uncontrolled hemorrhage, it has been found that aggressive fluid resuscitation may be harmful, resulting in a greater volume of blood loss and worse short-term mortality [86–88]. In animals in which ongoing bleeding is a concern, hypotensive resuscitation to a MAP of 60 mm Hg may be associated with a better outcome and may not lead to significant end organ damage [89,90].

The use of colloids for restoration of intravascular volume after hemorrhage is also controversial. Because colloids are retained within the intravascular space and exert a colloid osmotic pressure, they are more efficient in expanding plasma volume and achieve similar resuscitation end points more rapidly with smaller infused volumes compared to crystalloids

[91,92]. There are, however, a number of issues to be considered before using colloids in patients with hemorrhage. First, they are associated with coagulopathy in a proportion of people [93,94] and dogs [95,96], essentially acquired Von Willebrand's disease. Second, if the animal has active ongoing bleeding and colloids escape the intravascular space, they still exert a colloid osmotic effect. If this occurs in certain sites, such as the pulmonary parenchyma or cranium, they may worsen clinical signs associated with these organs. Third, because they are more efficient at increasing intravascular volume, there is a greater potential for intravascular volume overload if patients are not monitored carefully.

The treatment of hypoperfusion with colloid solutions in human patients has recently been questioned in several meta-analyses of human randomized clinical trials [97–101]. Although there are important limitations of the randomized controlled trials used in the studies and of the meta-analyses themselves [102], all show a trend toward increased mortality when colloids are used to resuscitate human trauma patients. The only meta-analysis designed a priori to investigate resuscitation after trauma showed a lower mortality rate associated with the use of crystalloid fluids [100]. It should be noted that the colloid used in many of the randomized controlled trials was albumin, which, until recently, has been rarely used in veterinary emergency patients.

Hypertonic saline is another option for fluid resuscitation after hemorrhagic shock. Its use is based on the principle that by injecting a hypertonic solution into the vascular space, a large (albeit temporary) osmotic gradient is created that mobilizes endogenous fluid from the interstitial and intracellular spaces to support intravascular volume. Because saline rapidly equilibrates with the interstitial space, it is commonly used in conjunction with a colloid, such as dextran 70 or hydroxyethyl starch, to prolong its effect [103]. Because of its hyperosmolar nature, it may also be beneficial in reducing organ injury by affecting neutrophil-endothelial cell interactions in postischemic tissue [104,105] and reducing endothelial cell swelling [106]. A meta-analysis of human clinical trials concluded that there were insufficient data to decide whether hypertonic crystalloids were better than isotonic crystalloids for the resuscitation of human trauma patients [107]. Clinical experience suggests that hypertonic saline can rapidly improve perfusion in patients with severe hemorrhagic hypovolemia but that its rapid effects may be deleterious in patients with ongoing bleeding, especially pulmonary contusions.

The use of crystalloid or colloid solutions to restore tissue perfusion tends to result in dilution of the red cell mass, leading to decreased oxygen-carrying capacity, although this may be somewhat offset by the decrease in blood viscosity. The decrease in hematocrit is difficult to predict, especially in canine patients, because the spleen acts as a major reservoir for red cells [108]. Although blood products may be used in the initial treatment of hypoperfusion in veterinary emergency patients, their use is often delayed until after tissue perfusion is restored using other intravenous fluid therapy. At this time, an assessment can be made of the need for increased oxygen-carrying capacity. Even in institutions with sufficient blood donors or blood products on site, the time taken to obtain or warm stored blood necessitates treatment with other fluids before blood in severely compromised patients.

Hemoglobin-based oxygen-carrying solutions (Oxyglobin; Biopure Corporation, Cambridge, MA) may provide a treatment for hemorrhagic shock that acts to restore tissue perfusion and to enhance oxygen-carrying capacity. Patient groups that may benefit from their use remain to be defined. A recent comprehensive review of clinical and experimental studies of hemoglobin-based oxygen-carrying solutions reported variable results when assessing their efficacy for the treatment of hemorrhagic shock [109]. A major concern is the potential deleterious side effect of increased pulmonary and systemic vascular resistance secondary to vasoconstriction [109].

Nonhemorrhagic hypovolemic shock

Nonhemorrhagic hypovolemic shock is most commonly seen in patients that have sustained fluid losses greater than fluid intake over a number of days. These patients commonly have a significant component of interstitial and intracellular dehydration as well as hypovolemia. As such, they are candidates for treatment with isotonic replacement crystalloid solutions. Because these solutions distribute rapidly to the interstitium, they treat hypoperfusion as well as dehydration. In patients that have also had significant and rapid loss of protein leading to decreased intravascular colloid osmotic pressure, therapy with colloids may be indicated to reduce the development of interstitial edema.

Distributive shock

A component of distributive shock is suspected when an animal is presented with evidence of peripheral vasodilation (injected mucous membranes) despite other clinical, hemodynamic, or biochemical evidence of hypoperfusion. Distributive shock is most often associated with SIRS, and an aggressive search for the underlying cause should be instituted together with initial treatment in all cases. Inadequate effective circulating intravascular volume is often a component of the tissue hypoperfusion, and treatment of patients with suspected distributive shock should always begin with aggressive volume loading using crystalloid or colloid fluids provided there are no other contraindications, such as heart or lung disease. In addition to hypovolemia, the inadequate effective circulating volume may be caused by increased microvascular permeability and peripheral vasodilation. It is especially challenging in these patients to assess the volume of intravenous fluids necessary to ensure an adequate intravascular volume.

Volume overload and the development of interstitial or pulmonary edema is a concern, especially because there is currently no way to quantitate alterations in microvascular permeability. The patient should be carefully monitored for any change in respiratory status or the development of peripheral edema. Peripheral edema is first noted by careful palpation over the gastrocnemius tendon or by the development of chemosis. The placement of a central venous line and measurement of CVP may be helpful in judging intravascular volume status.

In the absence of cardiogenic or obstructive causes or ongoing hemorrhage, hypotension in the face of aggressive volume resuscitation is often caused by septic shock. If advanced hemodynamic monitoring is available, these patients are commonly seen to have normal or increased CO, with low systemic vascular resistance [110]. Sepsis is also characterized by systolic and diastolic dysfunction, however, and cardiac contractility may be decreased [111]. In this situation, inotrope or pressor therapy is indicated, usually with catecholamines (Table 3). The choice of vasoactive agent should be based on an understanding of the goals of therapy and clinician familiarity. Generally, in vasodilatory states in which restoration of perfusion pressure is the goal, α-adrenergic agonists, such as norepinephrine or phenylephrine, should be used. If depressed cardiac function may also be contributing to hypoperfusion, however, an agent with β-adrenergic agonist properties, such as dobutamine, dopamine, or epinephrine, can be used. In veterinary emergency medicine, the hemodynamic information necessary to make such choices is not often immediately available, so it has been suggested that empiric β-agonism be tried before α-agonism.

Vasopressin is being recommended increasingly as a vasoactive agent in the treatment of refractory septic shock in people at a dose of 0.01 to 0.04 U/min [112]. It is of particular interest that, unlike the catecholamines, where vascular hyporesponsiveness commonly occurs in shock states [113], the vasoconstrictor activity of vasopressin seems to be enhanced in septic shock [114]. Doses of vasopressin that lead to significantly increased ABP in people with septic shock [115] do not seem to have pressor effects in normal people [116]. Its use in veterinary clinical patients has yet to be evaluated.

Table 3
Doses of vasoactive agents used in the treatment of distributive shock in dogs

Vasoactive agent	Recommended dose
Dopamine	3–20 µg/kg/min
Dobutamine	2–15 µg/kg/min
Norepinephrine	0.5–2 µg/kg/min
Phenylephrine	1–3 µg/kg/min
Epinephrine	0.1–1.0 µg/kg/min

It is recommended that treatment be initiated at the lower end of the dose range and titrated upward.

Decisions on vasoactive therapy should be based on all the information available to the clinician, and the patient should be carefully monitored. An increase in blood pressure per se does not always indicate improved tissue perfusion, and administration of vasoactive agents may improve blood pressure at the expense of tissue perfusion. Moreover, blood flow to some organs may improve, whereas perfusion in other tissues remains unchanged or is reduced [117–119]. The treatment and monitoring of patients with refractory hypotension and hypoperfusion secondary to distributive shock are particularly challenging. The high mortality rate associated with septic shock, even in human patients, despite advanced hemodynamic monitoring may be a partial result of occult tissue hypoperfusion.

One of the few clinical studies in people to show a significant difference in mortality in patients with septic shock showed improved survival in patients with early (within 6 hours) optimization of hemodynamic variables, emphasizing the importance of the emergency clinician in the successful management of sepsis and septic shock [12]. The hemodynamic parameters optimized in this study were ABP, CVP, and central venous oxygenation. All these parameters can be obtained with the placement of central and arterial lines, procedures that are commonly performed in veterinary emergency patients.

Cardiogenic shock

The treatment of hypoperfusion secondary to cardiogenic causes relies on diagnosis and characterization of the underlying cardiac abnormality. Many patients with cardiogenic shock also have evidence of respiratory compromise on presentation. This needs to be addressed concurrently, if not more urgently, with the hypoperfusion. Depending on the cardiac abnormality, specific treatment may be directed toward improving myocardial contractility, controlling serious arrhythmias, or reducing preload or afterload. Treatment of cardiac emergencies is covered in elsewhere in this issue.

Summary

Many patients presented to the emergency veterinarian are suffering from global or local tissue hypoperfusion. Global or systemic hypoperfusion can occur secondary to a reduction in the effective circulating intravascular volume (hypovolemic shock) or reduced ability of the heart to pump blood around the body secondary to reduced cardiac function (cardiogenic shock), obstruction to blood flow (obstructive shock), or maldistribution of the circulating intravascular volume (distributive shock). Initial assessment involving physical examination supplemented by measurement of hemodynamic and metabolic parameters allows the clinician to recognize and treat patients with severe global hypoperfusion. Use of techniques like sublingual capnometry and measurement of central venous oxygen saturation may aid recognition and evaluation of early hypoperfusion. Treatment decisions are made based on an assessment of the severity of the hypoperfusion and its probable underlying cause. Early effective treatment of hypoperfusion is likely to lead to a better outcome for the patient.

References

[1] Gores GJ, Nieminen AL, Wray BE, et al. Intracellular pH during "chemical hypoxia" in cultured rat hepatocytes. Protection by intracellular acidosis against the onset of cell death. J Clin Invest 1989;83(2):386–96.

[2] Trunkey DD, Ilner H, Wagner IY, et al. The effect of hemorrhagic shock on intracellular muscle action potentials in the primate. Surgery 1973;74(2):241–50.

[3] Trunkey DD, Ilner H, Wagner IY, et al. The effect of septic shock on skeletal muscle action potentials in the primate. Surgery 1979;85(6):638–43.

[4] West MA, Wilson C. Hypoxic alterations in cellular signal transduction in shock and sepsis. New Horiz 1996;4(2):168–78.

[5] Abraham E. Physiologic stress and cellular ischemia: relationship to immunosuppression and susceptibility to sepsis. Crit Care Med 1991;19(5):613–8.

[6] Haljamae H. The pathophysiology of shock. Acta Anaesthesiol Scand Suppl 1993;98:3–6.

[7] Dunham CM, Siegel JH, Weireter L, et al. Oxygen debt and metabolic acidemia as quantitative predictors of mortality and the severity of the ischemic insult in hemorrhagic shock. Crit Care Med 1991;19(2):231–3.

[8] Dunham CM, Fabian M, Siegel JH, et al. Hepatic insufficiency and increased proteolysis, cardiac output and oxygen consumption following hemorrhage. Circ Shock 1991;35(2): 78–86.

[9] Shoemaker WC, Czer LSC. Evaluation of the biologic importance of various hemodynamic and oxygen transport variables: which variables should be monitored in post-operative shock? Crit Care Med 1979;7:424–31.

[10] Siegel JH, Rivkind AI, Dalal S, et al. Early physiologic predictors of injury severity and death in blunt multiple trauma. Arch Surg 1990;125(4):498–508.

[11] Rixen D, Siegel JH. Metabolic correlates of oxygen debt predict posttrauma early acute respiratory distress syndrome and the related cytokine response. J Trauma 2000;49(3): 392–403.

[12] Rivers E, Nguyen B, Havstad S, et al. Early goal-directed therapy in the treatment of severe sepsis and septic shock. N Engl J Med 2001;345(19):1368–77.

[13] Bounos G, Hampson LG, Gurd FN. Regional blood flow and oxygen consumption in experimental hemorrhagic shock. Arch Surg 1963;87:340–54.

[14] Dyess D, Powell RW, Swafford AN, et al. Redistribution of organ blood flow after hemorrhage and resuscitation in full-term piglets. J Pediatr Surg 1994;29(8):1097–102.

[15] Schlichtig R, Kramer DK, Pinsky MR. Flow redistribution during progressive hemorrhage is a determinant of critical O_2 delivery. J Appl Physiol 1991;70(1):169–78.

[16] Dabrowski GP, Steinberg SM, Ferrara JJ, et al. A critical assessment of the end points of shock resuscitation. Surg Clin N Am 2000;80(3):825–44.

[17] Vallet B, Lund N, Curtis SE, et al. Gut and muscle tissue PO_2 in endotoxemic dogs during shock and resuscitation. J Appl Physiol 1994;76(2):793–800.

[18] Whitworth PW, Cryer HM, Garrison RN, et al. Hypoperfusion of the intestinal microcirculation without decreased cardiac output during live Escherichia coli sepsis in rats. Circ Shock 1989;27(2):111–22.

[19] Kumada M, Azuma T, Matsuda K. The cardiac output-heart rate relationship under different conditions. Jpn J Physiol 1967;17(5):538–55.

[20] Brady CA, Otto CM, Van Winkle TJ, et al. Severe sepsis in cats: 29 cases (1986–1998). J Am Vet Med Assoc 2000;217(4):531–5.
[21] Brown S, Haberman C, Morgan J. Evaluation of Doppler ultrasonic and oscillometric estimates of blood pressure in cats. J Vet Intern Med 2001;15(3):281.
[22] Gookin JL, Atkins CE. Evaluation of the effect of pleural effusion on central venous pressure in cats. J Vet Intern Med 1999;13(6):561–3.
[23] Walley KR, Cooper DJ. Diastolic stiffness impairs left ventricular function during hypovolemic shock in pigs. Am J Physiol 1991;260:701–12.
[24] Hirschl MM, Kittler H, Woisetschlager C, et al. Simultaneous comparison of thoracic bioimpedance and arterial waveform-derived cardiac output with thermodilution measurement. Crit Care Med 2000;28(6):1798–802.
[25] Chaney JC, Derdak S. Minimally invasive hemodynamic monitoring for the intensivist: current and emerging technology. Crit Care Med 2002;30(10):2338–45.
[26] Tremper KK, Hufstedler SM, Barker SJ, et al. Continuous non-invasive estimation of cardiac output by electrical bioimpedance: an experimental study in dogs. Crit Care Med 1986;14(3):231–3.
[27] Spinale FG, Reines HD, Crawford FA. Comparison of bioimpedance and thermodilution methods for determining cardiac output: experimental and clinical studies. Ann Thorac Surg 1988;45(4):421–5.
[28] Tibballs J, Hochmann M, Osborne A, et al. Accuracy of the BoMED NCCOM3 bioimpedance cardiac output monitor during induced hypotension: an experimental study in dogs. Anaesth Intensive Care 1992;20(3):326–31.
[29] Raaijmakers E, Faes TJ, Scholten RJ, et al. A meta-analysis of three decades of validating thoracic impedance cardiography. Crit Care Med 1999;27(6):1203–13.
[30] Shoemaker WC, Belzberg H, Wo CC, et al. Multicenter study of non-invasive monitoring as alternatives to invasive monitoring of acutely ill emergency patients. Chest 1998;114(6): 1643–52.
[31] Linton RA, Young LE, Marlin DJ, et al. Cardiac output measured by lithium dilution, thermodilution and transesophageal Doppler echocardiography in anesthetized horses. Am J Vet Res 2000;61:731–7.
[32] Kurita T, Morita K, Kato S, et al. Comparison of the accuracy of the lithium dilution technique with the thermodilution technique for measurement of cardiac output. Br J Anaesth 1997;79:770–5.
[33] Mason DJ, O'Grady M, Woods JP, et al. Assessment of lithium dilution cardiac output as a new method of cardiac output measurement in the dog. Am J Vet Res 2001;62: 1255–61.
[34] Mason DJ, O'Grady M, Woods JP, et al. Comparison of a central and a peripheral (cephalic vein) injection site for the measurement of cardiac output using the lithium-dilution cardiac output technique in anesthetized dogs. Can J Vet Res 2002;66: 207–10.
[35] Buhre W, Weyland A, Kazmaier S, et al. Comparison of cardiac output assessed by pulse contour analysis and thermodilution in patients undergoing minimally invasive direct coronary artery bypass grafting. J Cardiothorac Vasc Anesth 1999;13:437–40.
[36] Zollner C, Haller M, Weis M, et al. Beat-to-beat measurement of cardiac output by intravascular pulse contour analysis: a prospective criterion standard study in patients after cardiac surgery. J Cardiothorac Vasc Anesth 2000;14:125–9.
[37] Hamilton TT, Huber LM, Jessen ME. Pulse CO: a less invasive method to monitor cardiac output from arterial pressure after cardiac surgery. Ann Thorac Surg 2002;74(4 Suppl): S1408–12.
[38] Broder G, Weil MH. Excess lactate: an index of reversibility of shock in human patients. Science 1964;143:1457–9.
[39] Rose RJ, Bloomberg MS. Responses to sprint exercise in the greyhound: effects on hematology, serum biochemistry and muscle metabolites. Res Vet Sci 1989;47:212–8.

[40] Orringer CE, Eustace JC, Wunsch CD, et al. Natural history of lactic acidosis after grand-mal seizures. A model for the study of an anion-gap acidosis not associated with hyperkalemia. N Engl J Med 1977;297(15):796–9.
[41] Berry MN, Scheuer J. Splanchnic lactic acid metabolism in hyperventilation, metabolic alkalosis and shock. Metabolism 1967;16:537–47.
[42] Cucinell SA, O'Brien JC, Bryant GH, et al. Lactate generation by liver in hemorrhagic shock. Proc Soc Exp Biol Med 1981;168(2):222–7.
[43] Cain S. Appearance of excess lactate in anesthetized dogs during anemia and hypoxic hypoxia. Am J Physiol 1965;209:604–10.
[44] Cilley R, Scharenberg A, Bongiourno P, et al. Low oxygen delivery produced by anemia, hypoxia and low cardiac output. J Surg Res 1991;51:425–33.
[45] Weil MH, Afifi AA. Experimental and clinical studies in lactate and pyruvate as indicators of the severity of acute circulatory failure. Circulation 1970;41(6):989–1001.
[46] Astiz ME, Rackow EC, Kaufman B, et al. Relationship of oxygen delivery and mixed venous oxygenation to lactic acidosis in patients with sepsis and acute myocardial infarction. Crit Care Med 1988;16(7):655–8.
[47] Bakker J, Coffemils M, Leon M, et al. Blood lactate levels are superior to oxygen-derived variables in predicting outcome in human septic shock. Chest 1992;99(4):956–62.
[48] Tuchschmidt J, Fried J, Swinney R, et al. Early hemodynamic correlates of survival in patients with septic shock. Crit Care Med 1989;17(8):719–23.
[49] Vincent JL, Dufaye P, Berre J, et al. Serial lactate determinations during circulatory shock. Crit Care Med 1983;11(6):449–51.
[50] Kitagawa H, Yasuda K, Sasaki Y. Blood gas analysis in dogs with pulmonary heartworm disease. J Vet Med Sci 1993;55(2):275–80.
[51] Kitagawa H, Yasuda K, Kitoh K, et al. Blood gas analysis in dogs with heartworm caval syndrome. J Vet Med Sci 1994;56(5):861–7.
[52] Lagutchik MS, Ogilvie GK, Hackett TB, et al. Increased lactate concentrations in ill and injured dogs. J Vet Emerg Crit Care 1998;8:117–26.
[53] Orsini JA, Elser AH, Galligan DT, et al. Prognostic index for acute abdominal crisis (colic) in horses. Am J Vet Res 1988;49(11):1969–71.
[54] dePapp E, Drobatz KJ, Hughes D. Plasma lactate concentration as a predictor of gastric necrosis and survival among dogs with gastric dilatation-volvulus: 102 cases (1995–1998). J Am Vet Med Assoc 1999;215(1):49–52.
[55] Cain S. Oxygen delivery and uptake in dogs during anemia and hypoxic hypoxia. J Appl Physiol 1977;42:228–34.
[56] Lagutchik MS, Ogilvie GK, Wingfield WE, et al. Lactate kinetics in veterinary critical care: a review. J Vet Emerg Crit Care 1996;6(2):81–95.
[57] Hotchkiss RS, Karl IE. Reevaluation of the role of cellular hypoxia and bioenergetics failure in sepsis. JAMA 1992;267(11):1503–10.
[58] Song SK, Hotchkiss RS, Karl IE, et al. Concurrent quantification of tissue metabolism and blood flow via 2H/31P NMR in vivo: III. Alterations of muscle blood flow and metabolism in sepsis. Magn Reson Med 1992;25(1):67–77.
[59] Vary TC. Sepsis-induced alterations in pyruvate dehydrogenase complex activity in rat skeletal muscle: effect on plasma lactate. Shock 1996;6(2):89–94.
[60] Levy B, Bollaert PE, Charpentier C, et al. Comparison of norepinephrine and dobutamine to epinephrine for hemodynamics, lactate metabolism and gastric tonometric variables in septic shock: a prospective randomised study. Intensive Care Med 1997;23(3):82–7.
[61] Gore DC, Jahoor F, Hibbert JM, et al. Lactic acidosis during sepsis is related to increased pyruvate production, not deficits in tissue oxygen availability. Ann Surg 1996;224(1):97–102.
[62] Scheinman MM, Brown MA, Rapaport E. Critical assessment of the use of central venous oxygen saturation as a mirror of mixed venous oxygen in severely ill cardiac patients. Circulation 1969;40(2):165–72.

8 BOAG & HUGHES

[63] Tahvanainen J, Meretoja O, Nikki P. Can central venous blood replace mixed venous blood samples? Crit Care Med 1982;10(11):758–61.
[64] Reinhard K, Rudolph T, Bredle DL, et al. Comparison of central-venous to mixed-venous oxygen saturation during changes in oxygen supply/demand. Chest 1989;95(6):1216–21.
[65] Ladakis C, Myrianthefs P, Karabinis A, et al. Central venous and mixed venous oxygen saturation in critically ill patients. Respiration 2001;68(3):279–85.
[66] Hartmann M, Montgomery A, Jensson K, et al. Tissue oxygenation in hemorrhagic shock measured as transcutaneous oxygen tension, subcutaneous oxygen tension and gastrointestinal intramucosal pH in pigs. Crit Care Med 1991;19(2):205–10.
[67] Oud L, Kruse JA. Progressive gastric intramucosal acidosis follows resuscitation from hemorrhagic shock. Shock 1996;6(1):61–5.
[68] Oud L, Haupt M. Persistent gastric intramucosal ischemia in patients with sepsis following resuscitation from shock. Chest 1999;115:1390–6.
[69] Marik PE. Gastric intramucosal pH: a better predictor of multiorgan dysfunction syndrome and death than oxygen derived variables in patients with sepsis. Chest 1993;104:225–9.
[70] Pastores SM, Katz DP, Kvetan V. Splanchnic ischemia and gut mucosal injury in sepsis and the multiple organ dysfunction syndrome. Am J Gastroenterol 1996;91:1697–710.
[71] Groeneveld ABJ, Kolkman JJ. Splanchnic tonometry: a review of physiology, methodology, and clinical applications. J Crit Care 1994;9(3):198–210.
[72] Knudson MM, Bermudez KM, Doyle CA, et al. Use of tissue oxygen tension measurements during resuscitation from hemorrhagic shock. J Trauma 1997;42(4):608–14.
[73] Nakagawa Y, Weil MH, Tang W, et al. Sublingual capnometry for diagnosis and quantitation of circulatory shock. Am J Respir Crit Care Med 1998;157(6):1838–43.
[74] Povoas HP, Weil MH, Tang W, et al. Comparisons between sublingual and gastric tonometry during hemorrhagic shock. Chest 2000;118(4):1127–32.
[75] Marik PE. Sublingual capnography. A clinical validation study. Chest 2001;120(3):923–7.
[76] Marik PE, Bankov A. Sublingual capnometry versus traditional markers of tissue oxygenation in critically ill patients. Crit Care Med 2003;31(3):818–22.
[77] Velmahos GC, Wo CCJ, Demetriades D, et al. Early continuous noninvasive hemodynamic monitoring after severe blunt trauma. Injury 1999;30:209–14.
[78] Tatevossian RG, Wo CCJ, Velmahos GC, et al. Transcutaneous oxygen and CO_2 as early warning of tissue hypoxia and hemodynamic shock in critically ill emergency patients. Crit Care Med 2000;28:2248–53.
[79] Morelli A, Rocco M, Conti G, et al. Monitoring renal oxygen supply in critically ill patients using urinary oxygen tension. Anesth Analg 2003;97:1764–8.
[80] Kainuma M, Kimura N, Shimada Y. Effect of acute changes in renal arterial blood flow on urine oxygen tension in dogs. Crit Care Med 1990;18(3):309–12.
[81] Kern JW, Shoemaker WC. Meta-analysis of hemodynamic optimization in high-risk patients. Crit Care Med 2002;30(8):1686–92.
[82] Mock C, Visser L, Denno D, et al. Aggressive fluid resuscitation and broad spectrum antibiotics decrease mortality from typhoid ileal perforation. Trop Doct 1995;25(3):115–7.
[83] Committee on Trauma. Advanced trauma life support manual. Chicago: American College of Surgeons; 1997. p. 103–12.
[84] Shires T, Coln D, Carrico J, et al. Fluid therapy in hemorrhagic shock. Arch Surg 1964;88:688–93.
[85] Dillon J, Lynch JL, Myers R, et al. The treatment of hemorrhagic shock. Surg Gynecol Obstet 1966;122:967–77.
[86] Bickell WH, Bruttig SP, Millnamow GA, et al. The detrimental effects of intravenous crystalloid after aortotomy in swine. Surgery 1991;110(3):529–36.
[87] Kowalenko T, Stern S, Dronen S, et al. Improved outcome with hypotensive resuscitation of uncontrolled hemorrhagic shock in a swine model. J Trauma 1992;33(3):349–53.

[88] Solomonov E, Hirsh M, Yahiya A, et al. The effect of vigorous fluid resuscitation in uncontrolled hemorrhagic shock after massive splenic injury. Crit Care Med 2000;28(3): 749–54.

[89] Stern SA, Dronen SC, Birrer P, et al. Effect of blood pressure on hemorrhage volume and survival in a near-fatal hemorrhage model incorporating a vascular injury. Ann Emerg Med 1993;22(2):155–63.

[90] Stern SA, Wang X, Mertz M, et al. Under-resuscitation of near-lethal uncontrolled hemorrhage: effects on mortality and end-organ function at 72 hours. Shock 2001;15(1): 16–23.

[91] Haupt MT, Rackow EC. Colloid osmotic pressure and fluid resuscitation with hetastarch, albumin and saline solutions. Crit Care Med 1982;10(3):159–62.

[92] Boura C, Caron A, Longrois D, et al. Volume expansion with modified hemoglobin solution, colloids, or crystalloid after hemorrhagic shock in rabbits: effects in skeletal muscle oxygen pressure and use versus arterial blood velocity and resistance. Shock 2001; 19(2):176–82.

[93] Karlson KE, Garzon AA, Shaftan GW, et al. Increased blood loss with administration of certain plasma expanders: dextran 75, dextran 40 and hydroxyethyl starch. Surgery 1967; 62(4):670–8.

[94] Barron ME, Wilkes MM, Navickis RJ. A systematic review of the comparative safety of colloids. Arch Surg 2004;139(5):552–63.

[95] Glowaski MM, Moon-Massat PF, Erb HN, et al. Effects of oxypolygelatin and dextran 70 on hemostatic variables in dogs. Vet Anaesth Analg 2003;30(4):202–10.

[96] Concannon KT, Haskins SC, Feldman BF. Hemostatic defects associated with two infusion rates of dextran 70 in dogs. Am J Vet Res 1992;53(8):1369–75.

[97] Velanovich V. Crystalloid versus colloid fluid resuscitation: a meta-analysis of mortality. Surgery 1989;105(1):65–71.

[98] Bisonni RS, Holtgrave DR, Lawler F, et al. Colloids versus crystalloids in fluid resuscitation: an analysis of randomized controlled trials. J Fam Pract 1991;32(4): 387–90.

[99] Schierhout G, Roberts I. Fluid resuscitation with colloid or crystalloid solutions in critically ill patients: a systematic review of randomised trials. BMJ 1998;316:961–4.

[100] Choi PT, Yip G, Quinonez MD, et al. Crystalloids vs colloids in fluid resuscitation: a systematic review. Crit Care Med 1999;27(1):200–10.

[101] Alderson P, Schierhout G, Burns I, et al. Colloids versus crystalloids for fluid resuscitation in critically ill patients [Cochrane review]. In: The Cochrane Library. Issue 3. Chichester: John Wiley & Sons; 2004.

[102] Rizoli SB. Crystalloids and colloids in trauma resuscitation: a brief overview of the current debate. J Trauma 2003;54(Suppl):S82–8.

[103] Walsh JC, Kramer GC. Resuscitation of hypovolemic sheep with hypertonic saline/ dextran: the role of dextran. Shock 1991;34(3):336–43.

[104] Nolte D, Bayer M, Lehr MA, et al. Attenuation of postischemic microvascular disturbances in striated muscle by hyperosmolar saline dextran. Am J Physiol 1992;63:H1411–6.

[105] Rizoli SB, Kapus A, Fan J, et al. Immunomodulatory effects of hypertonic resuscitation on the development of lung inflammation following hemorrhagic shock. J Immunol 1998;161: 6288–96.

[106] Corso CO, Okamoto S, Leiderer R, et al. Resuscitation with hypertonic saline dextran reduces endothelial cell swelling and improves hepatic microvascular perfusion and function after hemorrhagic shock. J Surg Res 1998;80(2):210–20.

[107] Bunn F, Roberts I, Tasker R, et al. Hypertonic versus near isotonic crystalloid for fluid resuscitation in critically ill patients [Cochrane review]. In: The Cochrane Library. Issue 3. Chichester: John Wiley & Sons; 2004.

[108] Dillon AR, Hankes GH, Nachreiner RF, et al. Experimental hemorrhage in splenectomised and nonsplenectomised dogs. Am J Vet Res 1980;41(5):707–11.

[109] Day TK. Current development and use of hemoglobin-based oxygen-carrying (HBOC) solutions. J Vet Emerg Crit Care 2003;13(2):77–93.

[110] Parker MM, Shelhammer JH, Natanson C, et al. Serial cardiovascular variables in survivors and nonsurvivors in human septic shock: heart rate as an early predictor of prognosis. Crit Care Med 1987;15:923–9.

[111] Parrillo JE, Burch C, Shelhammer JH, et al. A circulating myocardial depressant substance in humans with septic shock: septic shock patients with a reduced ejection fraction have a circulating factor that depresses in vitro myocardial cell performance. J Clin Invest 1985; 76:1539–53.

[112] Dellinger RP, Carlet JM, Masur H, et al. Surviving sepsis campaign guidelines for management of severe sepsis and septic shock. Crit Care Med 2004;32(3):858–71.

[113] Thiemermann C, Szabo C, Mitchell JA, et al. Vascular hyporeactivity to vasoconstrictor agents and hemodynamic decompensation in hemorrhagic shock is mediated by nitric oxide. Proc Natl Acad Sci USA 1993;90:267–71.

[114] Baker CH, Sutton ET, Zhou Z, et al. Microvascular vasopressin effects during endotoxin shock in the rat. Circ Shock 1990;30:81–95.

[115] Malay MB, Ashton RC Jr, Landry DW, et al. Low-dose vasopressin in the treatment of vasodilatory septic shock. J Trauma 1999;47(4):699–703.

[116] Wagner HN Jr, Braunwald E. The pressor effect of the antidiuretic principle of the posterior pituitary in orthostatic hypotension. J Clin Invest 1956;35:1412–8.

[117] Marik PE, Mohedin M. The contrasting effects of dopamine and norepinephrine on systemic and splanchnic oxygen utilization in hyperdynamic sepsis. JAMA 1994;272(17): 1354–7.

[118] Sautner T, Wessely C, Riegler M, et al. Early effects of catecholamine therapy on mucosal integrity, intestinal blood flow and oxygen metabolism in porcine endotoxin shock. Ann Surg 1998;228(2):239–48.

[119] Malay MB, Ashton JL, Dahl K, et al. Heterogeneity of the vasoconstrictor effect of vasopressin in septic shock. Crit Care Med 2004;32(6):1327–31.

ELSEVIER
SAUNDERS

Vet Clin Small Anim
35 (2005) 343–358

VETERINARY
CLINICS
Small Animal Practice

Assessment and Treatment of Central Nervous System Abnormalities in the Emergency Patient

Rebecca S. Syring, DVM

*Section of Critical Care, Department of Clinical Studies–Philadelphia,
School of Veterinary Medicine, Ryan Veterinary Hospital, University of Pennsylvania,
3900 Delancey Street, Philadelphia, PA 19104, USA*

Disease of or injury to the central nervous system (CNS) is a common reason for hospital admission on an emergency basis in veterinary medicine. Head injuries, seizures, and diseases that lead to intracranial hypertension frequently result in significant alteration of neurologic function. A thorough understanding of the pathophysiologic disturbances that occur during these conditions is paramount for providing stabilizing emergent care. A detailed approach that focuses on meticulous physical evaluation, provision of timely and optimal stabilizing treatment, and continued monitoring can aid in improving outcomes in animals with signs and symptoms of neurologic disease or injury.

Regulation of cerebral hemodynamics

In health, cerebral blood flow is maintained within a narrow range, ensuring adequate oxygen and glucose delivery to the brain to maintain aerobic metabolism and normal neurologic function. Pressure autoregulation maintains constant cerebral blood flow, via changes in cerebral vascular resistance, over a wide range (50–150 mm Hg) of systemic mean arterial blood pressures (MAPs). Above and below this range, cerebral blood flow is directly proportional to systemic blood pressure [1]. In some disease states, such as head trauma, pressure autoregulation may be disrupted focally or globally in the brain, making cerebral blood flow entirely dependent on systemic blood pressure [2].

E-mail address: resyring@vet.upenn.edu

Intracranial pressure (ICP) is the pressure exerted between the skull and its intracranial components. It is determined by changes in volume of the three intracranial components (blood, brain, and cerebrospinal fluid volume) according to intracranial compliance. An increase in volume of any of these components can result in intracranial hypertension if compensatory decreases in the other components cannot accommodate these changes to maintain intracranial volume. Normal ICP in dogs and cats is 5 to 10 mm Hg [3]. Intracranial hypertension is harmful initially because it limits cerebral perfusion, resulting in hypoxic or ischemic injury to neurons and perpetuation of the cascade of secondary injury. As it becomes more severe, it can cause compression of the brain stem, resulting in depressed mental, cardiac, and respiratory function, ultimately culminating in brain herniation or death.

Cerebral perfusion pressure (CPP) is a clinically useful calculated value that serves as the primary determinant for blood flow, and thus nutrient delivery, to the brain. It is determined by the difference between MAP and ICP (CPP = MAP − ICP). In human medicine, physicians strive to maintain CPP greater than 70 mm Hg [4]. Although ICP is rarely measured in veterinary medicine, this concept emphasizes the importance of maintaining optimal blood pressure in the presence of intracranial hypertension. Systolic blood pressure should be maintained greater than 90 mm Hg at all times in patients with intracranial disease to increase the likelihood of adequate CPP [5].

Pathophysiology of neurologic injury

The original disturbance that occurs to the brain is referred to as primary neurologic injury. This nomenclature is widely used when referring to traumatic brain injury (TBI) because it refers to the insult that occurs at the time of trauma. The concept, however, can be extended to other disease processes that affect normal physiologic processes in the brain (eg, neoplasia, seizure activity). Although primary injury is important, in most situations, there is little that can be done to change the damage incurred as a result of the initial insult. Instead, most treatment regimens focus on limiting progression of neurologic damage.

Secondary neurologic injury refers to a series of detrimental events that can stem from the initial insult to the brain, resulting in progressive neuronal damage at the site of initial insult or extending globally to the brain as a whole. The brain, with its high metabolic rate, is sensitive to impaired oxygen or glucose delivery, the sources for ATP production under aerobic conditions. Impaired ATP production causes failure of cell membrane pumps, which can result in intracellular accumulation of water and calcium and extracellular liberation of excitatory amino acids, such as glutamate. These processes can lead to vasogenic and cytotoxic cerebral edema, excitotoxicity, oxidative injury, activation of the inflammatory and coagulation cascades, vasospasm, and cell death [6]. Although hypoglycemia is harmful, it is well documented that hyperglycemia, in the face of cerebral ischemia, promotes an intracellular acidosis that results in neuronal and glial cell death [7,8]. Two factors that have a significant impact on the perpetuation of secondary injury are systemic hypoxia and hypotension, both of which can be easily recognized and addressed clinically.

Initial evaluation

When evaluating animals with manifestations of intracranial disease, it is important to realize that extracranial disturbances, such as systemic hypotension or hypoxemia, can have a dramatic influence on outcome. For example, studies in human patients with TBI indicate that approximately 60% have concurrent injuries to other major organs [9]. In a retrospective study evaluating head injuries in dogs and cats, most dogs with TBI had sustained blunt vehicular trauma, whereas most cats were young kittens that had been stepped on accidentally [8]. In both of these situations, multisystemic injury affecting perfusion and oxygenation is likely. Patients with seizure activity can develop hypoxia secondary to noncardiogenic edema [10]. Maintenance of systemic blood pressure is essential in patients with intracranial hypertension to maintain cerebral perfusion. All these scenarios demonstrate that an initial patient assessment evaluating all major body systems (cardiovascular, respiratory, and neurologic) is mandatory to ascertain the extent of injury, address emergent needs, and optimize outcome.

Assessment of the cardiovascular system should include evaluating mucous membrane color, capillary refill time, heart rate and rhythm, and peripheral pulse quality. Evidence of pale mucous membranes, a capillary refill time exceeding 2 seconds, tachycardia, and weak pulses may indicate hypovolemia (ie, hemorrhagic shock) or altered tissue perfusion requiring immediate stabilizing treatment. Marked compression of the brain stem and medulla can result in arrhythmias and cardiac instability in the absence of significant extracranial disturbances; however, this is generally seen as a preterminal event [11].

Assessment of the respiratory system should focus on respiratory rate, effort, mucous membrane color, and thoracic auscultation. The goal in assessing the respiratory system is to ensure that adequate oxygenation and ventilation are maintained in the patient with neurologic disease. Multiple system trauma can predispose the patient to thoracic injuries, such as pulmonary contusions, pneumothorax, or pleural space disease, which may limit the ability to oxygenate. TBI can result in significant damage to the nasal and oropharyngeal regions, resulting in difficulty in ventilation, and thus carbon dioxide accumulation. Because hypoxia and hypercarbia can worsen secondary injury in the diseased brain, timely supplementation of oxygen therapy and intubation with or without positive-pressure ventilation in the hypoventilating patient can improve outcome.

Assessment of the neurologic system should initially focus on three major aspects: level of consciousness, brain stem reflexes, and motor activity/ posture. A detailed neurologic evaluation is often not performed until after the patient has been fully resuscitated and stabilized. Level of consciousness can be defined as normal, depressed/obtunded, stuporous, or comatose. An obtunded animal is arousable with noise or gentle touching but has a decreased responsiveness to its environment. Stupor describes an animal that is responsive only to noxious stimulation, whereas a comatose animal does not respond to this stimulation. Decreased mentation is a normal response to shock (decreased tissue perfusion) that should improve after resuscitation.

Initial assessment of brain stem reflexes should include evaluating pupils for size, symmetry, responsiveness to light, and the presence of physiologic nystagmus. Intracranial causes of miotic pupils include loss of cortical input or direct damage to sympathetic centers in the midbrain, allowing unopposed oculomotor pupillary constriction [12]. In the absence of ocular pathologic findings, midrange to dilated pupils that lack a pupillary light response imply injury to the oculomotor nerve in the brain stem ipsilateral to the injury as a result of compression, swelling, or hemorrhage [13]. The presence of anisocoria may indicate a lateralizing or more focal lesion within the brain. Physiologic nystagmus is a normal response that involves a tracking movement of the eyes in a horizontal direction in response to head movement. Normally, the eyes move slowly away from the direction in which the head is rotated, followed by a fast-phase motion in the direction of head movement. Lack of physiologic nystagmus often indicates brain stem injury, again as seen with compression, hemorrhage, or swelling.

Assessment of motor activity and posture may help to localize neurologic lesions. The presence of ataxia, hemiparesis, or tetraparesis may be the result of lesions affecting the cerebral cortex, brain stem, or spinal cord. The evidence of other cranial nerve abnormalities helps to differentiate intracranial from cervical spinal lesions. Decerebrate rigidity (extension of all four limbs and opisthotonus) is often associated with brain stem compression secondary to marked intracranial hypertension or herniation. Decerebellate rigidity (extension of the front legs with hind limb flexion) indicates a cerebellar lesion, as may be seen with cerebellar herniation. Patients with decerebrate posturing have markedly altered levels of consciousness, whereas those with decerebellate posturing can be alert and aware of their surroundings. Documentation of these three categories on initial neurologic evaluation and serial re-evaluations provides the clinician with information regarding the progression of disease or a positive response to medical therapy.

Because ICP is rarely measured in veterinary medicine, one must rely on physical examination parameters that may indicate intracranial hypertension. One marker of significant intracranial hypertension is the Cushing (or CNS ischemic) response. With marked elevations in ICP, cerebral blood flow becomes limited. Carbon dioxide accumulates locally as result of decreased blood flow, which is sensed at the vasomotor center of the brain. The vasomotor center subsequently emits a massive sympathetic discharge. This causes profound peripheral vasoconstriction, an effort to elevate MAP to maintain CPP. The increased blood pressure is sensed at baroreceptors, resulting in a reflex bradycardia [14]. The combination of hypertension and bradycardia in a patient with a decreased level of consciousness should alert the clinician to the possibility of increased ICP and prompt aggressive treatment. Other less specific indicators of intracranial hypertension may include mydriasis, loss of pupillary light responses, decerebrate posturing, loss of physiologic nystagmus, and altered levels of consciousness.

Extracranial stabilization of the patient with central nervous system emergencies

The initial approach to treatment of the animal with CNS emergencies should focus on extracranial stabilization, closely followed by therapies directed toward intracranial stabilization. Extracranial stabilization involves optimizing systemic oxygenation and ventilation as well as restoring tissue perfusion to maintain CPP.

Hypoxia should be avoided at all costs in patients with intracranial disease. Studies in human patients with TBI have shown that mortality for patients with documented episodes of hypoxia after injury is double that of patients without documented hypoxia [15]. It is prudent to provide oxygen supplementation to all animals with intracranial disease when oxygenation cannot be readily determined so as to avoid the risk of progressive neurologic injury. A variety of routes by which oxygen can be supplemented exist, including oxygen cages, flow-by masks, and hoods. Intranasal and intratracheal routes should be avoided if possible when intracranial disease exists because they can elicit sneezing or coughing fits, which can transiently increase ICP. Once it has been documented that the animal can maintain the oxygen saturation of hemoglobin (SaO_2) at or greater than 97% (corresponding to a PaO_2 of 90 mm Hg) while breathing room air, this practice can be discontinued. If the SaO_2 cannot be maintained despite supplementation of oxygen in concentrations upward of 60%, intubation and positive-pressure ventilation should be considered.

Hypoventilation results in an elevated $PaCO_2$. Hypoventilation can occur because of an impaired ventilatory drive as a result of damage to the respiratory center or from sedation, thoracic pain, mechanical airway obstruction from neck or neck trauma, or respiratory muscle fatigue/paralysis. Acute elevations in $PaCO_2$ concentrations can contribute to intracranial hypertension by causing a respiratory acidosis that is sensed at central chemoreceptors. In response to this acidosis, the cerebral vasculature vasodilates, thus increasing cerebral blood volume (known as chemical autoregulation), one component of ICP [16]. $PaCO_2$ concentrations should be maintained within a normal range and not allowed to exceed 40 mm Hg in patients with intracranial disease. If this value cannot be maintained within an acceptable range, intubation alone or in combination with mechanical ventilation should be performed (Fig. 1).

The correction of tissue perfusion deficits, mainly as a result of hypovolemia, is another important stabilizing therapy in the patient with intracranial disease. Altered mental status impairing the ability to eat or drink, increased insensible losses with seizure activity, and the possibility of

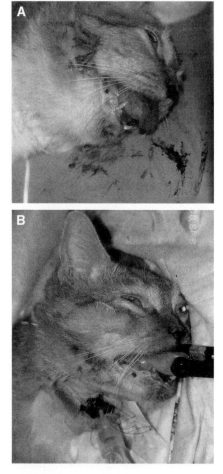

Fig. 1. (*A*) This cat was hit by a car and was presented with head injuries. Significant oral swelling and fractures to the maxilla and mandible impaired ventilation. Impaired ventilation causing respiratory acidosis can increase intracranial pressure via vasodilation of cerebral vessels. (*B*) Initial patient stabilization consisted of intubation and positive-pressure ventilation, followed by an emergency tracheostomy. The tracheostomy allowed bypass of the airway obstruction so that ventilation could be improved. Pulse oximetry during initial stabilization allowed for monitoring of oxygen saturation.

blood loss after trauma all predispose animals with intracranial disease to hypovolemia. The primary goal of fluid therapy is rapid restoration of blood pressure, such that CPP is maintained greater than 70 mm Hg. Intravenous fluid restriction should be strictly avoided, because only minimal decreases in ICP can be achieved. Fluid therapy should be directed toward restoration of euvolemia, provision of maintenance requirements, and replacement of ongoing losses while avoiding overhydration.

There is controversy regarding the best type of fluid to use when resuscitating a patient with intracranial hypertension. Acceptable options include isotonic crystalloids (Normosol-R, 0.9% sodium chloride, Abbott Laboratories, North Chicago, IL), hypertonic crystalloids (7.0%–7.5% sodium chloride), artificial colloids (dextran-70, hydroxyethyl starch), or blood products. The intact blood-brain barrier (BBB) is impermeable to ions and colloids [17]. As such, in the noninjured brain, there is minimal concern that aggressive isotonic crystalloid resuscitation may promote cerebral edema formation by redistribution into the interstitial space. With an intact BBB, the advantage of using an artificial colloid to minimize extravascular redistribution is negated with respect to the brain. In the diseased or injured brain, the BBB may be disrupted regionally or globally, making it possible for isotonic crystalloids and artificial colloids to leak or redistribute into the cerebral interstitium. Regardless, the overall benefit obtained by restoring CPP with either of these fluid types far outweighs the aforementioned risks. Aliquots of the shock dose of isotonic crystalloids (60–90 mL/kg in the dog; 45–60 mL/kg in the cat) or artificial colloids (10–20 mL/kg) should be given intravenously as rapidly as possible until the desired effect of improved tissue perfusion (based on normalization of heart rate, pulse quality, mucous membrane color, and capillary refill time) is achieved. Hypotonic crystalloid solutions (0.45% sodium chloride or 5% dextrose in water) should be strictly avoided during resuscitation because they primarily expand the intracellular fluid compartment and promote edema formation.

Hypertonic saline (7.5%) has many properties that, considered in combination, may make it a superior resuscitation fluid for patients with intracranial disease. When administered intravenously, a rapid rise in osmolarity promotes transcapillary flux of interstitial and intracellular fluid into the vasculature. The result is a rapid and pronounced volume expansion that exceeds the volume infused. The recommended dose of 7.5% sodium chloride for volume expansion is 3 to 5 mL/kg administered over 10 to 15 minutes. The peak volume-expanding effect occurs within minutes of administration [18]. Hypertonic saline is a crystalloid solution; although its volume-expanding effects are immediate, subsequent redistribution to other fluid compartments limits the duration of this effect. To prolong the duration of volume expansion, hypertonic saline can be combined with an artificial colloid [19].

After initial fluid resuscitation continued fluid therapy to address dehydration, provide maintenance requirements, and account for ongoing losses is mandatory. Many of these animals are not interested in food or water, and the use of osmotic agents to minimize cerebral edema can promote excessive free water loss from the body.

Intracranial stabilization of central nervous system emergencies

Once initial patient assessment and extracranial stabilization have occurred, medical intervention to address intracranial issues can ensue. The goals with intracranial stabilization focus on decreasing ICP and minimizing elevations in the cerebral metabolic rate (CMR). ICP can be manipulated with agents that decrease cerebral edema, optimizing cerebral blood volume and eliminating space-occupying masses. Cerebral edema is most effectively addressed with osmotically active agents, such as mannitol and hypertonic saline.

Reducing cerebral edema

Mannitol is a hyperosmolar agent that has traditionally been the osmotic agent of choice for treating cerebral edema. The recommended dose ranges from 0.5 to 1.0 g/kg as a slow bolus over 10 to 20 minutes. The osmotic effects of this drug are delayed by 15 to 30 minutes after administration. This drug promotes movement of water from the intracellular and interstitial spaces of the brain into the vasculature, inducing an osmotic diuresis, and thus reducing cerebral edema. This effect peaks 1 hour after administration and can persist for up to 6 to 8 hours after a single intravenous bolus. Mannitol has other mechanisms of action that may be beneficial in the patient with intracranial hypertension. Immediately after administration, mannitol causes a transient volume expansion and decreases blood viscosity. This rheologic effect, which persists for approximately 75 minutes, results in cerebral vascular vasoconstriction to maintain cerebral blood flow. Thus, ICP decreases secondary to a decreased cerebral blood volume despite maintained cerebral blood flow [20]. Additionally, mannitol is reported to have free radical scavenging properties that may help to limit secondary oxidative injury in the brain [21].

Risks associated with mannitol therapy include the development of a reverse osmotic shift when the BBB is disrupted, precipitation of acute tubular necrosis, and perpetuation of hypovolemia or volume depletion [22]. With the exception of its volume-depleting effect, the other two risks are largely unsubstantiated in the literature, and it is thought that the overall beneficial effects from mannitol outweigh these potential risks in the face of intracranial hypertension. Mannitol should be avoided in hypovolemic patients until intravenous fluid therapy has afforded adequate volume expansion to maintain systemic blood pressure, and thus CPP.

Hypertonic saline is an osmotically active agent that may reduce cerebral edema by the same mechanism by which volume expansion is afforded. This agent should be considered when intracranial hypertension coexists with a hypovolemic state. In this scenario, the use of mannitol perpetuates the hypovolemic state, whereas the hypertonic saline promotes volume expansion and reduces cerebral edema. Hypertonic saline encourages regional cerebral blood flow, and therefore oxygen delivery, by minimizing endothelial cell swelling and promoting arteriolar dilation [23]. It has been shown to modulate the inflammatory response in the brain by limiting cellular adhesion [24] and to decrease excitotoxicity by promoting reuptake of excitatory amino acids into the intracellular space [25]. Recently, less concentrated forms of hypertonic saline (3.0%–3.5%) have been investigated for use as a constant rate infusion in human patients with intracranial hypertension refractory to conventional therapy, with some promising results [26].

Corticosteroids have been used to reduce cerebral edema, but they are more likely to be effective when used to minimize vasogenic cerebral edema (as a result of BBB disruption) rather than cytotoxic cerebral edema. Corticosteroids have been well documented to reduce peritumor edema [27]. The use of corticosteroids in animals with TBI has fallen out of favor, however, because multiple prospective clinical trials in human head trauma patients have shown no benefit [28]. This, in combination with the many adverse effects of corticosteroids (hyperglycemia, immunosuppression, gastric ulceration, delayed wound healing, and exacerbation of a catabolic state), precludes their recommendation for use in veterinary patients with TBI.

Optimizing cerebral blood volume

Cerebral blood volume is another intracranial component that contributes to ICP. It can be manipulated with minimal invasiveness to achieve changes in ICP. Encouraging venous drainage from the brain assists in controlling ICP. This can be accomplished by avoiding jugular venous compression and by elevating the head and neck in a uniform plane. Elevation to an angle between 15° and 30° above horizontal facilitates venous outflow from the brain while maintaining arterial inflow [29]. Elevating the head and neck to a steeper angle should be avoided because this can limit arterial inflow, and thus limit oxygen delivery to the brain. When elevating the head and neck, one should take care to avoid kinking the neck because this occludes venous drainage.

Cerebral blood volume can also be manipulated by taking advantage of chemical autoregulation. Hyperventilation can be used as a short-term method to decrease intracranial blood volume, and therefore ICP, as a result of cerebral vasoconstriction in response to the respiratory alkalosis induced by acute decreases in $Paco_2$. This practice is used primarily in emergent situations in which intracranial hypertension is causing profound patient instability requiring immediate intervention or herniation appears imminent. When used, effects are immediate (within 30 seconds) and profound (affording up to a 25% reduction in ICP) but transient, because intracranial buffering returns the pH toward normal, neutralizing the cerebral vascular response [30]. Care should be taken to avoid excessive hyperventilation ($Paco_2$ no lower than 30 mm Hg) because this can worsen cerebral ischemia and secondary neurologic injury [30].

Eliminating space-occupying masses

The third mechanism by which ICP reductions can be obtained is by eliminating space-occupying masses within the cranial vault. This refers to surgical resection and/or debulking of tumors or evacuation of expansile hematomas secondary to trauma. Although this is beyond the scope of emergency clinicians, it is important to understand in concept that this may provide improvement in some animals. The decision to pursue surgical decompression should be based on CT or MRI of the brain and consultation with a neurosurgeon.

Minimizing elevation in cerebral metabolic rate

CMR determines the oxygen and nutrient requirements of the brain. Minimizing elevations in CMR is another important concern for patients with intracranial disease because this reduces demands for energy production and helps to limit secondary injury. Any seizures that develop as a result of head trauma or underlying neuropathologic changes should be tightly controlled with anticonvulsants. Hyperthermia, which can be a result of direct trauma to the thermoregulatory center; excitement; paddling; iatrogenic causes (heating pads); or pain should be avoided. Provision of analgesics to minimize excitement and paddling is recommended. Drugs that minimize cardiovascular and respiratory depression, such as butorphanol or hydromorphone, should be used. Barbiturates, propofol, and etomidate are acceptable anesthetic agents because they do not adversely affect cerebral blood flow or CMR. For these reasons, ketamine, acepromazine, and xylazine should be avoided (the reader is referred to the article on pain management of the emergency patient in this issue).

Treatment and stabilization of the seizuring animal

Animals in status epilepticus or with cluster seizures are among the most critical cases presented to emergency clinicians. Status epilepticus has been defined as an isolated seizure lasting for more than 30 minutes or multiple seizures lasting for more than 5 minutes each, without normalcy between ictal episodes [31]. Cluster seizures refer to multiple seizures in a 24-hour period. Seizures can occur as a result of intracranial diseases (eg, neoplasia, idiopathic epilepsy, meningitis, trauma) or extracranial diseases (eg, hypoglycemia, hyperammonemia, toxicity, sodium imbalance) [32]. When presented with a seizuring animal, the initial goal of the emergency clinician is to stop the current seizure activity, prevent recurrence of seizures in the immediate future, and treat any adverse effects resulting from the seizure activity.

An intravenous catheter should be placed immediately into a peripheral vein. This facilitates administration of intravenous anticonvulsant medications and allows one to obtain a small blood sample from the catheter's hub. At minimum, a blood glucose concentration should be determined from this sample to rule out hypoglycemia as a cause of seizures. Documented hypoglycemia (<60 mg/dL) should be treated with dextrose at a dose of 0.25 to 0.50 g/kg administered intravenously to alleviate seizure activity. When possible, determination of packed cell volume, total solids, sodium, calcium, and acid-base status should be obtained on an immediate basis. In the event that a catheter cannot be placed because of patient motion, an acceptable alternative is direct venipuncture with a hypodermic needle or butterfly catheter for drug administration. Once the seizure has been stopped, vascular access can be secured.

Diazepam is the anticonvulsant of choice for stopping an ongoing seizure because of its rapid onset of action and reliable efficacy. An intravenous dose of 0.5 mg/kg often results in immediate cessation of seizure activity. This dose can be repeated if seizure activity returns; however, because the effects of diazepam are short-lived, one must consider additional therapy to prevent additional seizures from occurring in the immediate future. When diazepam cannot effectively eliminate seizure activity, propofol, pentobarbital, or general anesthesia with inhalant anesthetics should be considered.

In the absence of vascular access or diazepam for injection, bilateral ocular compression can be attempted to arrest seizure activity. It has been reported that this technique may be useful for alleviating seizure activity in dogs, presumptively via a vagally mediated reflex [33]. Owners of animals with known seizure activity may also be sent home with diazepam (along with their long-term anticonvulsant medication) to be given intranasally or per rectum if seizure activity occurs at home. A recent study reported that intranasal diazepam (0.5 mg/kg) can reach therapeutic concentrations to inhibit seizure activity [34], although applying diazepam via this route during active seizures carries a danger of the owner being bitten. Alternatively, diazepam can be given per rectum in the seizuring animal (using the injectable formulation or a suppository). The recommended dose for per rectal diazepam is 1 to 2 mg/kg up to three times in a 24-hour period, not to be given within 15 minutes of the previous dose [35]. It should be stressed to owners that although this affords short-term control of seizures, further medical care is ultimately likely to be necessary to obtain better long-term seizure control.

The approach used for prevention of further seizures in the immediate future is dependent on whether or not the animal is already on anticonvulsant medications. If the animal has not been on long-term anticonvulsant medications before presentation, this author prefers loading with intravenous phenobarbital. Therapeutic serum concentrations (approximately 20 µg/mL) can be obtained by administering a cumulative phenobarbital dose of 16 to 20 mg/kg intravenously. The rate at which the loading dose is administered depends on the severity of seizures; however, in the author's practice, four doses of phenobarbital at a rate of 4 to 5 mg/kg have been given as often as every 30 minutes to effectively load the animal over 2 hours. This loading regimen can cause profound sedation; the patient should be evaluated before administration of subsequent doses and if the animal is deemed to be too sedated, the dosing interval can be lengthened. With less severe seizures, this loading can take place over the course of a day or longer.

If the animal is already receiving phenobarbital as a long-term anticonvulsant, serum drug concentrations should be drawn on presentation or as a trough value. One can use the level obtained to calculate an additional loading dose of phenobarbital to raise serum concentrations to a desired range (Fig. 2). Alternatively, particularly when serum concentrations are known to be adequate, the patient can be placed on a diazepam constant rate infusion (0.1–0.5 mg/kg/h). This infusion can be tapered in 25% increments until discontinued once the animal's seizure activity has been adequately controlled for 12 to 24 hours. The goal in treating status epilepticus or cluster seizures is to achieve a seizure-free period of at least 24 hours in that animal. Owners should be advised to hospitalize the animal for treatment and monitoring until the animal has gone without a seizure for a period of 1 day.

Three important side effects to recognize that can result from seizure activity are hyperthermia, hypoxemia, and cerebral edema. Hyperthermia occurs with seizures secondary to vigorous muscular activity for a prolonged period. In assessing the seizuring animal, a rectal temperature should be

$$\left(\frac{\text{Desired concentration}}{\text{Current concentration}} \right) \times \begin{array}{c} \text{Current} \\ \text{Dose} \end{array} = \begin{array}{c} \text{New} \\ \text{Dose} \end{array}$$

$$\begin{array}{c} \text{New} \\ \text{Dose} \end{array} - \begin{array}{c} \text{Current} \\ \text{Dose} \end{array} = \begin{array}{c} \text{Intravenous loading} \\ \text{dose to rapidly achieve} \\ \text{serum concentration} \end{array}$$

Fig. 2. This formula can be used to adjust phenobarbital dose (mg) for patients currently on phenobarbital that are presented with status epilepticus or cluster seizures. Once the animal's current serum phenobarbital concentration (µg/mL) has been determined, intravenous loading with the calculated dose (mg) can be performed to reach desired serum concentrations rapidly. Therapeutic phenobarbital concentrations range from 20 to 40 µg/mL.

obtained as soon as possible. Body temperatures in excess of 104°F should be externally cooled while seizure control is achieved. Convective cooling, for example, using a fan to create a cool breeze flowing past the animal, is one of the most effective means for rapid external cooling. When instituting external cooling, the body temperature should be reassessed approximately every 10 minutes and cooling discontinued once a temperature of 103.0°F to 103.5°F has been achieved so as to prevent hypothermia.

Hypoxemia can develop as a result of seizure activity secondary to aspiration or the development of neurogenic pulmonary edema, a form of noncardiogenic pulmonary edema. Supplementation of flow-by oxygen should be provided until it has been established that the patient is adequately oxygenating. Neurogenic pulmonary edema is characterized radiographically by a bilaterally symmetric dorsocaudal distribution of an interstitial to alveolar pulmonary pattern. It is hypothesized that neurogenic pulmonary edema occurs secondary to massive sympathetic stimulation, causing a rapid transient increase in pulmonary hydrostatic pressure, which results in transvascular fluid flux into the interstitium and alveoli [36]. Treatment of neurogenic pulmonary edema is primarily supportive with oxygen supplementation (fraction of inspired oxygen [F_{IO_2}]: 0.3–0.6). When the oxygen saturation (Sp_{O_2}) cannot be maintained at greater than 92% or the Pa_{O_2} at greater than 60 mm Hg via noninvasive means, positive-pressure ventilation with positive end-expiratory pressure may be necessary to maintain oxygenation while the edema resolves. Furosemide therapy is controversial and should only be used with caution. Bronchodilators, corticosteroids, and antibiotics are not useful for treating this condition [37]. In general, most patients with neurogenic pulmonary edema demonstrate marked improvement or continue to deteriorate and die within the first 48 hours of treatment.

Cerebral edema may result from prolonged seizure activity. Patients with status epilepticus, prolonged postictal periods, and persistently altered mentation may benefit from mannitol (0.5–1 g/kg administered intravenously over 15–20 minutes). If a positive response to therapy is noted, as evidenced by improved mentation, pupil size, or pupillary light response, additional doses can be given at 6- to 8-hour intervals as dictated by clinical signs.

Monitoring of animals with central nervous system emergencies

Monitoring of animals with CNS emergencies should emphasize evaluation of cardiovascular and respiratory function as well as serial neurologic evaluation. Early detection of hypotension, hypoxia, hypercarbia, or changes in neurologic status facilitates timely intervention and may help to improve outcome.

Cardiovascular function can be monitored noninvasively by assessing mucous membrane color, capillary refill time, heart rate and pulse quality. Indirect blood pressure can be monitored every few minutes initially, and tapered as dictated by patient stability, as a means to ensure maintenance of systemic blood pressure to maintain CPP. Continuous electrocardiographic monitoring can aid in the detection of bradycardia, which may serve as a marker for intracranial hypertension requiring immediate intervention.

Respiratory function can be monitored noninvasively with pulse oximetry. Many patients with severe intracranial disease tolerate continuous monitoring by placement of the probe on the tongue, lip, or skin. Alarms can be programmed to alert the clinician when desaturation occurs, allowing for early intervention and minimizing hypoxic causes of secondary injury. Arterial blood gas monitoring allows for assessment of adequacy of ventilation.

Re-evaluation of neurologic status should be recorded after resuscitation, hourly initially and then every 4 to 8 hours depending on patient stability. Early detection of alterations in mentation and brain stem reflexes facilitates changes in medical therapy. The Small Animal Coma Scale (also referred to as the Modified Glasgow Coma Scale) is a quantitative means to grade the severity of neurologic injury after trauma [38]. This scoring system provides an objective method to prognosticate outcome and can also be used to assess improvement or deterioration of neurologic signs when performed serially. This scoring system has been retrospectively validated and shown to correlate with 48-hour outcome in dogs with TBI [39].

If mannitol or hypertonic saline is being used, frequent assessment of electrolytes (at least twice daily) is critical to avoid hypernatremia or a host of other electrolyte abnormalities. Electrolytes, acid-base status, and blood glucose should always be assessed at least once daily in the critically ill patient, and fluid therapy should be adjusted to maintain electrolytes within normal limits. Measurement of urine output facilitates calculation of fluid ins-and-outs, such that fluid therapy can be tailored to help maintain euvolemia and hydration.

Quality nursing care is essential for management of the animal with intracranial disease. Frequent turning, provision of clean dry bedding, and physical therapy help to prevent pressure sores, urine scalding, and limb contraction. Urinary bladders may need to be expressed or an indwelling urinary catheter placed if the animal is not voiding voluntarily. Early nutritional support should be considered in these patients if they are not eating voluntarily so as to prevent a catabolic state.

By following a logical approach to CNS emergencies that is based on attentive physical evaluation, institution of timely and optimal stabilizing treatment and continued monitoring outcomes can be optimized for animals with signs and symptoms of neurologic disease or injury.

References

[1] Busija DW, Heistad DD, Marcus ML. Effects of sympathetic nerves on cerebral vessels during acute, moderate increases in arterial pressure in dogs and cats. Circ Res 1980;46: 696–702.

[2] Lang EW, Czosnka M, Mehdorn HM. Tissue oxygen reactivity and cerebral autoregulation after severe traumatic brain injury. Crit Care Med 2003;31:267–71.

[3] Bagley RS. Intracranial pressure in dogs and cats. Compend Contin Educ Pract Vet 1996;18: 605–21.

[4] The Brain Trauma Foundation. The American Association of Neurological Surgeons. The Joint Section on Neurotrauma and Critical Care. Guidelines for cerebral perfusion pressure. J Neurotrauma 2000;17:507–11.

[5] Chestnut RM. The management of severe traumatic brain injury. Emerg Med Clin N Am 1997;15:581–604.

[6] Deardon NM. Mechanisms and prevention of secondary brain damage during intensive care. Clin Neuropathol 1998;17:221–8.

[7] Hochachka PW, Mommsen TP. Protons and anaerobiosis. Science 1983;219:1391–7.

[8] Syring RS, Otto CM, Drobatz KJ. Hyperglycemia in dogs and cats with head trauma: 122 cases (1997–1999). J Am Vet Med Assoc 2001;218:1124–9.

[9] Siegel JH. The effect of associated injuries, blood loss, and oxygen debt on death and disability in blunt traumatic brain injury. The need for early physiologic predictors of severity. J Neurotrauma 1993;12:579–90.

[10] Drobatz KJ, Saunders H, Pugh CR, Hendricks JC. Noncardiogenic pulmonary edema in dogs and cats: 26 cases (1987–1993). J Am Vet Med Assoc 1995;206:1732–6.

[11] Provencio JJ, Bleck TP. Cardiovascular disorders related to neuroemergencies. In: Cruz J, editor. Neurologic and neurosurgical emergencies. Philadelphia: WB Saunders; 1998. p. 39–50.

[12] Oliver JE, Lorenz MD, Kornegay JN. Blindness, anisocoria, and abnormal eye movements. In: Handbook of veterinary neurology. 3rd edition. Philadelphia: WB Saunders; 1997. p. 274–86.

[13] Fenner WR. Diseases of the brain. In: Ettinger SJ, Feldman EC, editors. Textbook of veterinary internal medicine. 5th edition. Philadelphia: WB Saunders; 2000. p. 552–602.

[14] Ganong WF. Cardiovascular regulatory mechanisms. In: Review of medical physiology. Stamford, CT: Appleton and Lange; 1997. p. 553–66.

[15] Chestnut RM, Marshall LE, Klauber MR, et al. The role of secondary brain injury in determining outcome from severe head injury. J Trauma 1993;34:216–22.

[16] Brian JE. Carbon dioxide and the cerebral circulation. Anesthesiology 1998;88:1365–86.

[17] Zhuang J, Shackford SR, Schmoker JD, et al. Colloid infusion after brain injury: effect on intracranial pressure, cerebral blood flow, and oxygen delivery. Crit Care Med 1995;23: 140–8.

[18] Kramer GC, Perron PR, Lindsey DC, et al. Small-volume resuscitation with hypertonic saline dextran solution. Surgery 1986;100:239–46.

[19] Qureshi AI, Suarez JI. Use of hypertonic saline solutions in treatment of cerebral edema and intracranial hypertension. Crit Care Med 2000;28:3301–13.

[20] Muizelaar JP, Wei EP, Kontos HA, et al. Mannitol causes compensatory vasoconstriction and vasodilation in response to blood viscosity changes. J Neurosurg 1983;59:822–8.

[21] Mizoi K, Suzuki J, Imaizumi S, et al. Development of new cerebral protective agents: the free radical scavengers. Neurol Res 1986;8:75–80.

[22] The Brain Trauma Foundation. American Association of Neurological Surgeons, Joint Section on Neurotrauma and Critical Care. Use of mannitol. J Neurotrauma 2000;17: 521–5.

[23] Shackford SR, Schmoker JD, Zhuang J. The effect of hypertonic resuscitation on pial arteriolar tone after brain injury and shock. J Trauma 1994;37:899–908.

[24] Angle N, Hoyt DB, Cabello-Passini R, et al. Hypertonic saline resuscitation reduces neutrophil margination by suppressing neutrophil L selectin expression. J Trauma 1998;45: 7–13.

[25] Doyle JA, Davis DP, Hoyt DB. The use of hypertonic saline in the treatment of traumatic brain injury. J Trauma 2001;50:367–83.

[26] Khanna S, Davis D, Peterson B, et al. Use of hypertonic saline in the treatment of severe refractory posttraumatic intracranial hypertension in pediatric traumatic brain injury. Crit Care Med 2000;28:1144–51.

[27] Gutin PH. Corticosteroid therapy in patients with brain tumors. Natl Cancer Inst Monogr 1977;46:151–6.

[28] Bazarian JJ. Evidence based emergency medicine. Corticosteroids for traumatic brain injury. Ann Emerg Med 2002;40:515–7.

[29] Meixensberger J, Baunach S, Amschler J, et al. Influence of body position on tissue-pO2, cerebral perfusion pressure and intracranial pressure in patients with acute brain injury. Neurol Res 1997;19:249–53.

[30] The Brain Trauma Foundation. American Association of Neurological Surgeons, Joint Section on Neurotrauma and Critical Care. Hyperventilation. J Neurotrauma 2000;17: 513–20.

[31] Podell M. Seizures in dogs. Vet Clin N Am Small Anim Pract 1996;26:779–809.

[32] Platt SR, Haag M. Canine status epilepticus: a retrospective study of 50 cases. J Small Anim Pract 2002;43:151–3.

[33] Speciale J, Stahlbrodt JE. Use of ocular compression to induce vagal stimulation and aid in controlling seizures in seven dogs. J Am Vet Med Assoc 1999;214:663–5.

[34] Platt SR, Randell SC, Scott KC, et al. Comparison of plasma benzodiazepine concentrations following intranasal and intravenous administration of diazepam to dogs. Am J Vet Res 2000;61:651–4.

[35] Podell M. The use of diazepam per rectum at home for the acute management of cluster seizures in dogs. J Vet Intern Med 1995;8:68–74.

[36] Johnston SC, Darragh TM, Simon RP. Postictal pulmonary edema requires pulmonary vascular pressure increases. Epilepsia 1996;37:428–32.

[37] Drobatz KJ, Saunders HM. Noncardiogenic pulmonary edema. In: Bonagura JD, editor. Kirk's current veterinary therapy XIII: small animal practice. Philadelphia: WB Saunders; 2000. p. 810–2.

[38] Shores A. Craniocerebral trauma. In: Kirk RW, editor. Current veterinary therapy X: small animal practice. Philadelphia: WB Saunders; 1983. p. 847–54.

[39] Platt SR, Radaelli ST, McDonnell JJ. The prognostic value of the modified Glasgow Coma Scale in head trauma dogs. J Vet Intern Med 2001;17:581–4.

ELSEVIER
SAUNDERS

Vet Clin Small Anim
35 (2005) 359–373

VETERINARY
CLINICS
Small Animal Practice

Urinary Tract Emergencies

Teresa M. Rieser, VMD

VCA Newark Animal Hospital, 1360 Marrows Road, Newark, DE 19711, USA

Emergencies of the upper and lower urinary tract are commonly seen in small animal practice. The goal of this article is to discuss the most common of these emergencies, with a focus on diagnosis and treatment. This article discusses urethral obstruction in the dog and cat, acute renal failure, and uroperitoneum.

Urethral obstruction

Urethral obstruction is one of the most common emergencies seen involving the urinary system. Untreated, it can rapidly progress to a life-threatening crisis that is characterized by severe electrolyte and acid-base disturbances.

Urethral obstruction is more common in male cats and dogs than in female animals, but both sexes can be affected. The most frequent cause of obstruction is mucous plugs (in cats) or uroliths (in cats and dogs); however, obstruction can occur secondary to neoplasia as well as from strictures associated with trauma.

Most mucous plugs in cats are associated with magnesium ammonium phosphate (struvite) crystals [1]. Uroliths in cats are most commonly struvite or calcium oxalate [1,2]. In dogs, struvite and calcium oxalate uroliths are also the most prevalent [3]. Neoplasms that can result in urethral obstruction include squamous cell carcinoma, transitional cell carcinoma, and other less frequently seen tumors [4].

Regardless of the underlying cause, prolonged urethral obstruction results in fluid deficits that lead to hypovolemia and decreased tissue perfusion. The adverse effects on cardiac output, and thus tissue perfusion, are exacerbated by the profound electrolyte and acid-base disturbances seen with obstruction. In addition to azotemia, urethral obstruction is

---

E-mail address: Teresa.Rieser@vcamail.com

associated with metabolic acidosis, hyperkalemia, hyperphosphatemia, and hypocalcemia [5].

Metabolic acidosis occurs in urethral obstruction as a result of an inability to excrete hydrogen ions via the urinary system. Lactic acidosis secondary to low cardiac output may contribute to a worsening acid-base status. Profound metabolic acidosis (pH <7.2) has far-reaching effects in the body, affecting the respiratory, cardiovascular, and central nervous systems. Initially, the response of the body to acidosis is to increase the minute ventilation by increasing the respiratory rate and/or the tidal volume. Severe acidosis can predispose the patient to cardiac arrhythmias as well as to decreases in cardiac contractility and an inotropic response to catecholamines [6]. In the central nervous system (CNS), acidosis can result in neurologic signs that can range from depression to coma [6]. This may be further compounded by poor tissue perfusion and uremia.

Hyperkalemia is the electrolyte disturbance most commonly associated with urethral obstruction. Hyperkalemia occurs because of a decrease in renal excretion of potassium as well as from the shifting of potassium from the intracellular space in response to acidosis. Potassium plays a major role in the determination of resting cell membrane potential. Initially, extracellular hyperkalemia can make the cell more excitable, but as potassium elevations become severe, the resting membrane potential may become less than the threshold potential, thus making the cell unable to repolarize after depolarization [7]. Clinically, this effect is seen in muscle tissue and the conduction system of the heart [7].

The changes that are seen on the electrocardiogram (ECG) in response to hyperkalemia include bradycardia, decreased amplitude or absent P waves, a widened QRS complex, tall T waves, a shortened QT interval, and ST segment depression. Elevation in extracellular potassium also results in generalized muscle weakness. It is extremely important to remember that the severity of clinical signs does not necessarily correlate with the magnitude of change in the serum potassium concentration. Thus, a cat with a serum potassium level of 8.0 may be severely compromised, whereas another cat with a serum potassium level of 9.0 may be hemodynamically stable. Decisions about the treatment of hyperkalemia should be based on the overall clinical assessment of the patient and not just on clinical laboratory parameters.

In addition to hyperkalemia, urethral obstruction can result in ionized hypocalcemia [5,8]. This exacerbates the effects of any concomitant hyperkalemia [9]. The metabolic acidosis may ameliorate the severity of the ionized hypocalcemia because it favors a shift of calcium from the protein-bound fraction of total calcium to the ionized calcium fraction. Clinically, hypocalcemia may result in neuromuscular hyperexcitability, decreased cardiac contractility, and peripheral vasodilation [10].

The final electrolyte disturbance commonly seen with urethral obstruction is hyperphosphatemia. This occurs because of a decrease in renal clearance of phosphorus. The presence of hyperphosphatemia may contribute to the development of hypocalcemia as well as contributing to the metabolic acidosis.

Clinical signs and the initial database

The clinical signs associated with urethral obstruction include stranguria or dysuria, vocalizing, lethargy, anorexia, vomiting, excessive licking of the perineum, and diarrhea [5]. On physical examination, the most striking finding is an extremely firm bladder on abdominal palpation. In addition, the body temperature of these animals may range from hypothermic to hyperthermic. They may be bradycardic or tachycardic. They may have an elevated respiratory rate and poor peripheral pulse quality. Lethargy and depression may also be appreciated [5].

An initial database for the urethral obstruction patient should include, if possible, measurement of packed cell volume (PCV); total solids; blood urea nitrogen (BUN); blood glucose; venous blood gas; and electrolytes, including ionized calcium, potassium, sodium, and chloride. Blood pressure measurement and an ECG provide information on the cardiovascular effects of the metabolic changes, whereas a complete blood cell count (CBC) and serum chemistry profile give more extensive information regarding the patient's overall status. Survey radiographs, contrast cystography, and ultrasonography more clearly characterize the cause of the obstruction but should be withheld until the animal has been stabilized. On relief of the obstruction, a urine sample should be taken for urinalysis as well as urine culture. Urine samples should be analyzed within 60 minutes of collection to minimize the effects of time and temperature on crystal formation [11].

Treatment

The ultimate goal of treatment is to relieve the obstruction and re-establish urethral patency. The hemodynamic stability of the patient must first be addressed, however.

In addition to relieving the obstruction, therapy should be instituted for correction of acid-base abnormalities, azotemia, and electrolyte disturbances (Table 1). The mainstay in achieving these goals is fluid therapy. In the past, 0.9% sodium chloride (NaCl) has been the fluid of choice because it contains no potassium, but it may contribute to the metabolic acidosis seen in these patients. Recent data show that a balanced electrolyte solution, even with potassium, results in no clinically significant difference in acid-base or electrolyte parameters [12]. Animals that have had a urethral obstruction frequently exhibit a postobstructional diuresis as the uremia is corrected; this is especially true of animals that have been obstructed long enough to exhibit electrolyte or acid-base alterations. This is of vital importance in determining fluid rates, because the required rate is often far greater than what would be chosen for a normal animal. It is not remarkable for an

Table 1
Useful drugs for electrolyte and acid-base disturbances

Drug	Dose range	Frequency	Route	Indications
Calcium gluconate	50–100 mg/kg	PRN	IV	Hyperkalemia, hypocalcemia
Regular insulin	0.1–0.25 U/kg	Every 2–4 hours	IV	Hyperkalemia
Dextrose	0.5 g/kg	PRN	IV	Hyperkalemia
Sodium bicarbonate	0.3 × base deficit × BW (kg), give 1/3–1/2 of this amount	PRN[a]	Slow IV (15–30 minutes)	Metabolic acidosis, hyperkalemia

Abbreviations: BW, body weight; IV, intravenous; PRN, as needed.

[a] Sodium bicarbonate can result in cerebrospinal fluid acidosis and cerebral edema if given overzealously. It also lowers ionized calcium.

average-sized cat with a urethral obstruction to require a fluid rate of 40 to 50 mL/h (in a 5-kg cat, that is administration of fluids at roughly 8–10 mL/kg/h). Monitoring of urine output is invaluable in guiding changes in fluid administration rate. If the animal also has evidence of cardiac disease, fluid therapy should be administered with caution and a central venous pressure (CVP) line can also be used to guide therapy.

In animals that show hemodynamic compromise because of their acid-base and electrolyte disturbances, specific remedies are indicated in addition to fluid therapy. A number of treatment options can be used. For the hyperkalemic patient, calcium gluconate, regular insulin, and bicarbonate may all be considered.

Intravenous administration of 10% calcium gluconate at a dose of 50 to 100 mg/kg treats the cardiovascular effects of hyperkalemia and corrects the ionized hypocalcemia that is often present. Calcium does not have a direct effect on the serum potassium concentration; instead, it re-establishes a more normal difference between the resting membrane potential and the depolarization threshold in the cell, thus ameliorating the effects of the high potassium. The benefit of calcium gluconate administration is immediate [13].

Intravenous administration of regular insulin (0.1–0.25 U/kg) has a direct effect on potassium. The insulin promotes the movement of glucose intracellularly, carrying potassium with it. As the serum potassium level decreases, the resting membrane potential of the cell tends to normalize. When this drug is used, it is important to provide dextrose to the patient. In addition to administering a bolus of dextrose at the time that the insulin is given, it is advisable to supplement the intravenous fluids with dextrose, because the effects of intravenously administered regular insulin can last from 2 to 4 hours. Another approach that uses the same underlying physiology is to give just a dextrose bolus (0.5 g/kg administered intravenously, dilute 1:3); this method depends on the endogenous secretion of insulin from the patient's pancreas [13].

A final remedy for hyperkalemia is the administration of sodium bicarbonate ($0.3 \times$ base deficit $\times$ body weight (kg) $=$ total amount of bicarbonate (mEq) needed to correct pH to 7.4; administer one third to one half of this amount as an intravenous bolus over 10–15 minutes). Sodium bicarbonate lowers the extracellular potassium concentration by promoting the cellular uptake of potassium in exchange for the movement of hydrogen ions out of the cell. Sodium bicarbonate also treats the metabolic acidosis but may further lower the ionized calcium. The effects of sodium bicarbonate are seen within 30 to 60 minutes and may persist for hours after administration [13].

Once the hemodynamic stability of the patient has been addressed, specific therapy to relieve the obstruction should be undertaken. This is most commonly accomplished by placing a urinary catheter. The techniques for relief of obstruction differ in the dog and cat; thus, both are discussed. The passing of a urinary catheter in an obstructed animal is often an uncomfortable procedure. If the animal is hemodynamically stable, sedation should be used (see article in this issue on anesthetic protocols for common emergencies).

Before attempting to pass the catheter, it is worthwhile to extrude the penis and visually inspect it for any mucous plugs or grit; it is sometimes possible to relieve an obstruction by gently teasing a plug out of the tip of the penis. If a plug is not seen, the catheter should be passed. In the cat, the obstruction is initially relieved using an open-end tom-cat catheter (Kendall Co., Mansfield, MA) or a Minnesota olive-tipped catheter (EJAY International, Glendora, CA). At this point, the urethra is flushed copiously with sterile saline in an attempt to break up the plug or push it back into the urinary bladder. Under no circumstances should the catheter be forced up the urethra; this can result in trauma to the urethra and may lead to iatrogenic rupture of the urethra [14]. In addition to flushing the urethra, the penis should be retracted caudad to straighten the normal flexure of the feline urethra.

Once patency has been re-established, the bladder should be copiously flushed with sterile saline. The tom-cat catheter should not be left in the bladder. Instead, it should be replaced with a soft 3.5- or 5-French red rubber catheter (Kendall Co.) that is then connected to a closed urine collection system. To minimize injury to the wall of the bladder, avoid inserting an excessive length of catheter into the bladder. An excessively long catheter placed in the bladder can also become tied into a knot and then requires surgical removal.

In the dog, retropulsion of stones is accomplished using a different technique. A red rubber or Foley catheter is introduced into the penis up to the level of the obstruction, and the tip of the penis is occluded. The pelvic urethra is digitally compressed via the rectum, and saline flush is infused into the urethra. This flush distends the urethra and "floats" the stones. When the pressure at the pelvic urethra is removed, the stones move retrograde into the bladder. Some stones may be adhered to the bladder wall and do not float, but distention of the urethra may allow passage of the urinary catheter around the stone. At that time, a red rubber catheter can be advanced into the bladder and connected to a closed collection system.

In animals in which the obstruction cannot be relieved by catheterization, a number of alternatives may be considered. One of the first techniques that may be used is cystocentesis. Decompression of the bladder may facilitate catheterization by decreasing the pressure exerted against the urethral obstruction from the bladder side of the urethra. It is important to remember that the integrity of the bladder wall may not be normal and that urinary bladder rupture may occur, however [15]. Other options for relief of a urethral obstruction include urethrostomy, cystostomy, and voiding urohydropropulsion [16–18]. The reader is referred elsewhere for a detailed discussion of these techniques [18–20].

Once a urethral obstruction has been relieved and immediate acid-base and electrolyte issues have been addressed, the animal should be continued on intravenous fluids and the urine output should be monitored. Additional monitoring, including serial electrolytes (this may vary from every 4 hours to once daily depending on patient stability), a continuous ECG, and serial blood pressure measurements may also be appropriate. Even though an animal may have initially presented with hyperkalemia, it is not uncommon for that same animal to be hypokalemic in the days after initial stabilization. In addition, medications like phenoxybenzamine or prazosin may be started to relax the urethra and thus ameliorate urethral spasm. In the absence of bacteriuria on urinalysis, antibiotic therapy is relatively contraindicated while a urinary catheter is in place. Finally, it may be of benefit to consider pain management (see article in this issue on pain management in the emergency patient). In light of the recent insult to the renal system, it may be prudent to avoid nonsteroidal anti-inflammatory drugs (NSAIDs) and to consider other analgesic options.

Uroperitoneum

Uroperitoneum occurs when the integrity of the lower urinary tract has been broached, allowing leakage of urine into the abdomen. It is important to remember that although this may be caused by rupture of the urinary bladder, damage to other areas of the urinary tract may also result in uroperitoneum. Alternatively, damage to the upper urinary tract (kidneys and ureters) may result in uroretroperitoneum but no peritoneal cavity fluid accumulation. The most common cause of uroperitoneum is trauma; however, it can also be seen with neoplasia, prolonged urinary tract obstruction, and overzealous urinary catheter placement [21].

Clinically, animals with uroperitoneum may be presented in hemodynamic collapse. They can have metabolic acidosis, chemical peritonitis, profound azotemia, hyperkalemia, hypernatremia, and hyperphosphatemia.

When urine moves into the peritoneal cavity (or the retroperitoneal cavity), a number of important effects are seen. First, the presence of a large osmotically active particle, such as creatinine, results in the movement of water into the peritoneal cavity at the expense of the intracellular and intravascular fluid. This third spacing can result in significant volume depletion and hemodynamic compromise. Although creatinine diffuses across membranes, its movement is slower than that of smaller solutes, such as potassium and urea. The rapid movement of the smaller solutes down their concentration gradient from the peritoneum to the intravascular space results in elevated concentrations of these solutes in the blood. Sodium and chloride, which normally are found in higher concentrations in the blood than in the urine, diffuse into the peritoneum, thus furthering the contraction to the intravascular fluid compartment. The dehydration that occurs in these patients further exacerbates abnormalities by decreasing the glomerular filtration rate, and thus the excretion of urea and creatinine.

The presence of sterile urine within the peritoneal space is irritating, resulting in peritonitis, whereas the presence of infected urine can cause septic peritonitis. Metabolic acidosis results not only from hypovolemia but from failure to excrete hydrogen ions from the body. Instead, hydrogen ions accumulate in the abdominal cavity, are reabsorbed into the circulation, and result in depletion of the buffering capability of the body.

Physical examination and laboratory parameters

On physical examination, these animals may show signs of hemodynamic compromise. In addition, they may have abdominal distention, abdominal pain, and a palpable fluid wave. They may also shows signs of external trauma. The presence of a palpable urinary bladder does not rule out the possibility of uroperitoneum. If urine has extravasated into subcutaneous tissues, this may result in inflammation with pain and swelling in the affected area; this can be seen with a ruptured urethra, where urine leaks into the perineum and can then dissect down the hind limbs. Clinically, this area appears bruised, edematous, and painful.

The diagnosis of uroperitoneum is made by comparison of abdominal fluid creatinine and potassium with that of serum creatinine and potassium. In dogs, a ratio of abdominal fluid creatinine to serum creatinine of 2:1 and a ratio of abdominal fluid potassium to serum potassium of 1.4:1 are considered diagnostic for uroperitoneum [22]. In cats, the diagnostic ratios are 2:1 for creatinine and 1.9:1 for potassium [14,22]. The measurement of urea is of less use in making this diagnosis because it rapidly diffuses across membranes to reach equilibrium; this means that disparity between urea measurements in abdominal fluid and serum may not show clear-cut differences.

A number of other findings may provide supporting evidence. The initial database may include a PCV, total solids, venous blood gas, electrolytes, serum chemistry, CBC, and abdominal radiographs. These data may show metabolic acidosis, azotemia, hyperkalemia, and evidence of volume contraction. On survey radiographs, there is a loss of abdominal detail. Positive-contrast radiography is the study of choice for determining the site of urine leakage. Excretory urography is helpful in identifying leaks in the kidneys and ureters, whereas a retrourethrocystogram is helpful in identifying leaks in the urethra and urinary bladder.

Treatment

Treatment of uroperitoneum involves the correction of acid-base and electrolyte disturbances as well as definitive treatment of the rupture. As with urethral obstruction, the mainstay of therapy is fluids, with definitive therapy of hyperkalemia warranted based on clinical signs. In addition to these interventions, drainage of the abdominal cavity is important. This can be achieved by placement of a peritoneal dialysis catheter into the abdomen. Peritoneal dialysis is an excellent technique not only for the drainage of urine but for the resolution of acid-base abnormalities, azotemia, and electrolyte disturbances [23]. Placement of a urinary catheter into the bladder is of benefit in keeping the bladder decompressed.

After the metabolic disturbances have been stabilized, definitive repair of the rupture must be considered. This commonly is achieved by surgical repair, although in certain instances, such as iatrogenic bladder rupture, medical management involving decompression of the urinary bladder with an indwelling urinary catheter has been advocated [24]. The reader is referred elsewhere for a detailed discussion of surgical techniques [19,20,25].

Acute renal failure

Receiving 20% to 25% of the total blood flow in the body, the kidney is a major route for the excretion of waste products as well as the maintenance of water and electrolyte balance. Although this abundant blood flow is needed to maintain adequate renal function, it also makes the kidney especially sensitive to changes in blood flow as well as blood-borne toxins. The distribution of blood flow within the kidney is not uniform; instead, most blood flow goes to the renal cortex, whereas less than 10% of all the blood flow that the kidney receives goes to the renal medulla. This is approximately the same amount of blood as is received by resting skeletal muscle [26]. The abundance of blood flow that the kidney receives makes it especially vulnerable to the effects of toxins, and the disparity of blood flow within the kidney makes the renal medulla susceptible to ischemic insult and the cortex susceptible to toxins.

Autoregulation allows the kidney to maintain a relatively constant renal blood flow and glomerular filtration rate (GFR) over mean arterial blood pressures ranging from 70 to 170 mm Hg. Without autoregulation, relatively small increases in blood pressure would result in a marked increase in GFR and urine production. Conversely, at less than a mean arterial pressure of 70 mm Hg, renal blood flow and GFR decline in direct relation to decreases in mean arterial pressure. Thus, decreases in urine production in the hypotensive patient may reflect the effect of decreased renal blood flow and are not always evidence of oliguric or anuric renal failure.

Pathophysiology of acute renal failure

Acute renal failure is most commonly caused by an ischemic event or a bloodborne toxicant. Other conditions that can result in acute renal failure include immune-mediated disease, pyelonephritis, leptospirosis, hypercalcemia, and urinary tract obstruction.

The kidney is especially vulnerable to toxicant injury because of its abundant blood supply, whereas the processes of tubular secretion, countercurrent multiplication, and reabsorption can concentrate toxicants even further. Because the cortex of the kidney receives most renal blood flow, it is the prime target of intoxicant-induced injury. A variety of possible compounds can result in acute renal failure, including aminoglycosides, metals, snakebite and bee venoms, myoglobin, hemoglobin, certain chemotherapeutic agents, radiographic contrast agents, and ethylene glycol [27–31]. Recently, acute renal failure has been associated with lily ingestion in cats and with ingestion of raisins and grapes in dogs [32,33]. A number of different types of lilies have been implicated, including the Tiger lily, day lily, Easter lily, Stargazer lily, and Asiatic hybrid lily, but the underlying toxic insult remains unknown [32,34]. The toxic insult is also unclear in raisin and grape ingestion; however, the amount needed to cause acute renal failure is alarmingly small (0.32–0.65 oz/kg in one report [35] and 0.41–1.1 oz/kg in another report [33]).

When the systemic blood pressure drops to less than 70 mm Hg, renal blood flow decreases in a linear fashion with blood pressure. As the oxygen and energy supply to the kidney are compromised, cellular ATP and energy become depleted and cell membrane pumps fail, resulting in cell swelling because of the intracellular accumulation of sodium and water. As calcium accumulates within the cell, a number of cellular processes, including oxidative phosphorylation within the mitochondria, are deranged [36,37]. A loss of renal autoregulation occurs, which is thought to be caused by increased responsiveness to renal nerve stimulation, which, in turn, has been related to increases in intracellular calcium in the afferent arteriole cells of the glomerulus [38,39]. Cell swelling and vasoconstriction contribute to vascular stasis and predispose to the formation of microthrombi, which occlude renal vessels and further contribute to renal ischemia. The decrease of energy substrates also predisposes to the formation of oxygen-free radical species, which results in further cellular damage [36,37].

A number of events and conditions can result in renal ischemia, including shock, anesthetic-induced vasodilation and hypotension, hyperthermia, hypothermia, extensive cutaneous burns, NSAID administration, hyperviscosity/polycythemia, and disseminated intravascular coagulation (DIC) [36].

Clinical signs

The clinical signs of acute renal failure are nonspecific and include lethargy, depression, anorexia, vomiting, and diarrhea. Because the disease course of acute renal failure is brief, these animals frequently do not have weight loss. Animals with acute renal failure may be polyuric and polydipsic, but they can also be anuric or oliguric. Physical examination may reveal large painful kidneys. Laboratory data show elevations in BUN and creatinine and may show elevations in potassium and phosphorus. Calcium can be increased or decreased. Animals in acute renal failure frequently have a marked metabolic acidosis, and the CBC may show a stress leukogram. Urinalysis reveals isosthenuric urine and may show proteinuria, hematuria, glucosuria, and the presence of granular casts, which may indicate acute tubular injury [37]. The fractional excretion of sodium

$$Fe_{Na} = \frac{Urine_{Na}}{Plasma_{Na}} \times \frac{Plasma_{Creatinine}}{Urine_{Creatinine}} \times 100\%$$

in the urine may also be increased in acute renal failure; this is indicative of a significant tubular insult, because a normal animal with prerenal azotemia should be able to reabsorb more than 99% of the filtered load of urine sodium [37]. In animals with other underlying conditions that favor sodium reabsorption (eg, congestive heart failure, hepatic failure, nephritic syndrome), the fractional excretion of sodium may be normal despite tubular dysfunction [37]. Another test that may be helpful in the diagnosis of acute renal failure is carbamylated hemoglobin measurement. Carbamylated hemoglobin is the product of a reaction between hemoglobin within the red blood cells and cyanate, which equilibrates with urea in the blood. As the red blood ages, carbamylated hemoglobin accumulates and can be measured to help differentiate acute from chronic renal failure, because chronic renal failure can be expected to result in a higher carbamylated hemoglobin concentration [40,41].

Therapy

One of the main components in the treatment of acute renal failure is fluid therapy. The goal of initial fluid therapy is to correct hemodynamic abnormalities, expand the vascular volume, and correct electrolyte abnormalities. A balanced electrolyte solution is appropriate for achieving this goal. After volume expansion, fluid therapy should be continued at a rate that facilitates diuresis; usually, a rate around 5 to 6 mL/kg/h is a good starting point. Once volume replete, a crystalloid that provides free water, such as 0.45% NaCl, may be indicated. Many of the crystalloid solutions do not provide free water and therefore can contribute to an iatrogenic hypernatremia if the animal has no other source of water intake. It is extremely helpful to monitor urine output when trying to decide on the correct fluid rate. Once an animal is volume replete and normotensive, urine output should be at least 1 to 2 mL/kg/h. Daily monitoring of the patient can provide valuable information for guiding fluid therapy as well; this includes urine output, body weight, hemodynamic parameters, and serial electrolytes. If fluid therapy is not adequate, the patient may show weight loss as well as an increase in serum sodium. By contrast, an increase in body weight may be a result of the correction of volume deficits. Urine output in the polyuric renal failure patient can be voluminous, and aggressive fluid administration may be needed to stay abreast of fluid loss. By contrast, if a patient is anuric or oliguric, overzealous fluid administration can result in volume overload, pulmonary edema, and death. CVP monitoring is invaluable for the monitoring of volume status. A consistent increase in CVP is indicative of impending fluid overload. CVP can be easily done in practice but does require the placement of a central line. Central lines are also of value in the acquisition of serial blood samples as well as allowing for the administration of hypertonic solutions, including total parenteral nutrition.

Other therapies in acute renal failure are targeted at alleviating the clinical signs and underlying causes of the acute renal failure. The most common bacterial isolates from the urinary tract in dogs include *Escherichia coli* (44.1%), *Staphylococcus* spp (11.6%), *Proteus* spp (9.3%), *Klebsiella* spp (9.1%), *Enterococcus* spp (8.0%), and *Streptococcus* spp (5.4%) [42,43]; thus, reasonable antibiotic choices in pyelonephritis could include ampicillin (22 mg/kg administered intravenously three times daily) and enrofloxacin (5 mg/kg administered intravenously once daily). Because renal failure is frequently associated with increased gastric acid secretion and vomiting, drugs like ranitidine (2 mg/kg administered intravenously three times daily), famotidine (0.5 mg/kg administered intravenously twice daily), and sucralfate (0.5–1 g administered orally two to four times daily) can all be helpful. Antiemetics like metoclopramide (continuous rate infusion [CRI] at 1 mg/kg per 24 hours administered intravenously) and chlorpromazine (0.2–05 mg/kg administered intramuscularly) can also be used. Chlorpromazine can induce hypotension and therefore should not be used in a volume-depleted or already hypotensive patient. It is also important to address nutrition in these critical patients. If possible, enteral nutrition is desirable, but parenteral nutrition can be used if needed.

When faced with an oliguric or anuric acute renal failure patient, a number of therapeutic interventions can be used (Table 2), but extrarenal causes, such as hypovolemia and hypotension, must first be ruled out. Until

Table 2
Interventions in the oliguric/anuric patient

Drug	Dose range	Frequency	Route
Isotonic crystalloid	10–20 mL/kg over 15–20 minutes	PRN	IV
Furosemide	2–6 mg/kg	Q6–8h	IV
Mannitol	0.5–1.0 g/kg over 20 minutes	Q6h	IV
Dextrose	25–50 mL/kg of 10%–25% solution over 1–2 h	Q8–12h	IV

Abbreviations: h, hours; IV, intravenous; PRN, as needed; Q, every.

the animal has a blood pressure higher than 70 mm Hg and is volume expanded, aggressive therapy for anuric acute renal failure should not be pursued; instead, all efforts should be focused on normalizing blood pressure and volume status. The first therapy in the euvolemic, normotensive, anuric patient is usually fluid boluses. If an animal is volume overloaded already, a fluid bolus is contraindicated. A reasonable bolus would be isotonic crystalloid at a dose of 10 to 20 mL/kg over 15 to 20 minutes. There should be an increase in urine output within 30 to 60 minutes. Intravenous boluses of furosemide can also be given. Furosemide has been shown to exacerbate gentamicin toxicity; thus, it should not be used in cases of aminoglycoside-induced acute renal failure [37].

If urine output is still inadequate after fluid boluses and furosemide administration and the blood pressure is adequate for the production of urine, an osmotic diuretic can be tried. Osmotic diuretics should be used with extreme caution in animals with possible fluid overload. The main osmotic diuretic used is mannitol. Mannitol is an excellent osmotic diuretic and has some free radical scavenging capabilities. Mannitol is also a weak vasodilator. Mannitol is not metabolized; it is filtered at the glomerulus and excreted from the body. Therefore, if there is no GFR, mannitol remains in the vascular space and may contribute to volume overload [43]. Because of this concern, hypertonic glucose is sometimes used in place of mannitol. The advantage of hypertonic glucose is that it can be metabolized by the body; however, it does not possess the free radical scavenging abilities of mannitol and is less effective as an osmotic agent [43].

The final drug that is sometimes used in oliguric or anuric renal failure is dopamine. The use of dopamine in acute renal failure is a controversial topic. Classically, low-dose dopamine is thought to act on renal dopamine receptors to increase renal blood flow. Evidence has shown that the cat does not possess renal dopamine receptors of the same type as other species [44,45]; however, a recent study has identified a unique dopamine receptor in the feline kidney [46]. How much of a contribution this receptor makes in hemodynamic regulation of the feline kidney requires further research. In human medicine, dopamine has begun to fall out of favor as more studies have shown that dopamine does not prevent or reverse acute renal failure and does not improve patient outcome [47,48]. The author does not use dopamine at a "kidney" dose in acute renal failure.

Peritoneal dialysis and hemodialysis should also be considered in the acute renal failure patient [23,49,50]. This is especially true of the anuric acute renal failure patient, but the decision to pursue dialysis should not be made in the eleventh hour. Peritoneal dialysis is a viable technique for the private practice setting, but it is labor-intensive and can result in complications, including septic peritonitis and electrolyte imbalances [23]. Hemodialysis, although still fairly limited in veterinary medicine because of its lack of availability as well as expense, is being more widely used than ever before and is an excellent option for acute renal failure patients.

New directions

Research is constantly being conducted to find better treatment options for acute renal failure. On the horizon are calcium channel blockers. In the human literature, the use of calcium channel blockers, such as diltiazem, for the prevention and treatment of acute renal failure is a topic of debate, but some evidence does support their use in acute renal failure [51,52]. In veterinary medicine, the use of diltiazem in the treatment of acute renal failure is also under investigation, but not enough evidence is present at this time to warrant its routine use in acute renal failure (Karol Mathews, DVM, DVSc, personal communication, 2004).

References

[1] Houston DM, Moore AEP, Favrin MG, et al. Feline urethral plugs and bladder uroliths: a review of 5484 submissions 1998–2003. Can Vet J 2003;44(12):974–7.

[2] Thumchai R, Lulich J, Osborne CA, et al. Epizootiologic evaluation of urolithiasis in cats: 3498 cases (1982–1992). J Am Vet Med Assoc 1996;208:547–51.

[3] Ling GV, Franti CE, Ruby AL, et al. Urolithiasis in dogs. I: mineral prevalence and interrelations of mineral composition, age, and sex. Am J Vet Res 1998;59:624–9.

[4] Krawiec DR. Urethral diseases of dogs and cats. In: Osborne CA, Finco DR, editors. Canine and feline nephrology and urology. Baltimore: Williams & Wilkins; 1995. p. 718–25.

[5] Lee JL, Drobatz KJ. Characterization of the clinical characteristics, electrolytes, acid-base, and renal parameters in male cats with urethral obstruction. J Vet Emerg Crit Care 2003; 134(4):227–33.

[6] Rose BD, Post TW. Metabolic acidosis. In: Clinical physiology of acid-base and electrolyte disorders. 5th edition. New York: McGraw-Hill; 2001. p. 578–646.

[7] Rose BD, Post TW. Introduction to disorders of potassium balance. In: Clinical physiology of acid-base and electrolyte Disorders. 5th edition. New York: McGraw-Hill; 2001. p. 822–35.

[8] Drobatz KJ, Hughes D. Concentration of ionized calcium in plasma from cats with urethral obstruction. J Am Vet Med Assoc 1997;211(11):1392–5.

[9] Rose BD, Post TW. Hyperkalemia. In: Clinical physiology of acid-base and electrolyte disorders. 5th edition. New York: McGraw-Hill; 2001. p. 888–930.

[10] Zaloga GP, Robert PR. Calcium, magnesium, and phosphorus disorders. In: Shoemaker WC, Ayres SM, Grenvik A, et al, editors. Textbook of critical care. Philadelphia: WB Saunders; 2000. p. 862–75.

[11] Albasan H, Lulich JP, Osborne CA, et al. Effects of storage time and temperature on pH, specific gravity, and crystal formation in urine samples from dogs and cats. J Am Vet Med Assoc 2003;222:176–9.

[12] Cole SG, Drobatz KJ. Influence of crystalloid type on acid-base and electrolyte status in cats with urethral obstruction [abstract]. In: Proceedings of the Ninth International Veterinary Emergency and Critical Care Symposium, New Orleans, 2004. p. 766.

[13] Phillips SL, Polzin DJ. Clinical disorders of potassium homeostasis: hyperkalemia and hypokalemia. Vet Clin North Am Small Anim Pract 1998;28(3):545–64.

[14] Aumann M, Worth LT, Drobatz KJ. Uroperitoneum in cats: 26 cases (1986–1995). J Am Anim Hosp Assoc 1998;34(4):315–24.

[15] Osborne CA, Kruger JM, Lulich JP, et al. Disorders of the feline lower urinary tract. In: Osborne CA, Finco DR, editors. Canine and feline nephrology and urology. Baltimore: Williams & Wilkins; 1995. p. 625–80.

[16] Lekcharoensuk C, Osborne CA, Lulich JP. Evaluation of trends in frequency of urethrostomy for treatment of urethral obstruction in cats. J Am Vet Med Assoc 2002; 221:502–5.

[17] Stiffler KS, McCrackin Stevenson MA, Cornell KK, et al. Clinical use of low-profile cystostomy tubes in four dogs and a cat. J Am Vet Med Assoc 2003;223:325–9.

[18] Lulich JP, Osborne CA, Carlson M, et al. Nonsurgical removal of urocystoliths in dogs and cats by voiding urohydropropulsion. J Am Vet Med Assoc 1993;203:660–3.

[19] Waldron DR. Urinary bladder. In: Slatter D, editor. Textbook of small animal surgery. Philadelphia: WB Saunders; 2003. p. 1629–37.

[20] Bjorling DE. The urethra. In: Slatter D, editor. Textbook of small animal surgery. Philadelphia: WB Saunders; 2003. p. 1638–51.

[21] Gannon KM, Moses L. Uroabdomen in dogs and cats. Compend Contin Educ Pract Vet 2002;24(8):604–12.

[22] Schmeidt C, Tobias KM, Otto CM. Evaluation of abdominal fluid: peripheral blood creatinine and potassium ratios for diagnosis of uroperitoneum in dogs. J Vet Emerg Crit Care 2001;11(4):275–80.

[23] Dzyban LA, Labato MA, Ross LA, et al. Peritoneal dialysis: a tool in veterinary critical care. J Vet Emerg Crit Care 2000;10(2):91–102.

[24] Osborne CA, Sanderson SL, Lulich JP, et al. Medical management of iatrogenic rents in the wall of the feline urinary bladder. Vet Clin N Am Small Anim Pract 1996;26(3):551–62.

[25] McLoughlin MA, Bjorling DE. Ureters. In: Slatter D, editor. Textbook of small animal surgery. Philadelphia: WB Saunders; 2003. p. 1619–28.

[26] Rieser TM, Otto CM. Regulation of renal hemodynamics and the nitric oxide-arginine pathway. J Vet Emerg Crit Care 1997;8(1):7–18.

[27] Frazier DL, Aucoin DP, Riviere JE. Gentamicin pharmacokinetics and nephrotoxicity in naturally acquired and experimentally induced disease in dogs. J Am Vet Med Assoc 1988; 192(1):57–63.

[28] Geor RJ. Drug-induced nephrotoxicity: recognition and prevention. Compend Contin Educ Pract Vet 2000;22(9):876–8.

[29] Gookin JL, Riviere JE, Gilger BC, et al. Acute renal failure in four cats treated with paromomycin. J Am Vet Med Assoc 1999;215(12):1821–3.

[30] Lane IF, Grauer GF, Fettman MJ. Acute renal failure. Part I. Risk factors, prevention and strategies for protection. Compend Contin Educ Pract Vet 1994;16(1):15–29.

[31] Puig J, Vilafranca M, Font A, et al. Acute intrinsic renal failure and blood coagulation disorders after a snakebite in a dog. J Small Anim Pract 1995;36(7):333–6.

[32] Langston CE. Acute renal failure caused by lily ingestion in six cats. J Am Vet Med Assoc 2002;220(1):49–52.

[33] Gwaltney-Brant S, Holding JK, Donaldson CW, et al. Renal failure associated with ingestion of grapes or raisins [letter]. J Am Vet Med Assoc 2001;218(10):1555–6.

[34] Stokes JE, Forrester SD. New and unusual causes of acute renal failure in dogs and cats. Vet Clin N Am Small Anim Pract 2004;34(4):909–22.

[35] Mazzaferro EM, Eubig PA, Hackett TB, et al. Acute renal failure associated with raisin or grape ingestion in 4 dogs. J Vet Emerg Crit Care 2004;14(3):203–12.

[36] Binns SH. Pathogenesis and pathophysiology of ischemic injury in cases of acute renal failure. Compend Contin Educ Pract Vet 1994;16(1):31–43.

[37] Grauer GF, Lane IF. Acute renal failure: ischemic and chemical nephrosis. In: Osborne CA, Finco DR, editors. Canine and feline nephrology and urology. Baltimore: Williams & Wilkins; 1995. p. 441–59.

[38] Schrier RW, Wang W, Poole B, et al. Acute renal failure: definitions, diagnosis, pathogenesis, and therapy. J Clin Invest 2004;114(1):5–14.

[39] Conger JD, Robinette JB, Schrier RW. Smooth muscle calcium and endothelium-derived relaxing factor in the abnormal vascular responses of acute renal failure. J Clin Invest 1988; 82:532–7.

[40] Vaden SL, Gookin J, Trogdon M, et al. Use of carbamylated hemoglobin concentration to differentiate acute from chronic renal failure in dogs. Am J Vet Res 1997;58(11):1193–6.

[41] Heiene R, Vuilliet PR, Williams RL, et al. Use of capillary electrophoresis to quantitate carbamylated hemoglobin concentrations in dogs with renal failure. Am J Vet Res 2001; 62(8):1302–6.

[42] Ling GV, Norris CR, Franti CE, et al. Interrelations of organism prevalence, specimen collection method, and host age, sex, and breed among 8,354 canine urinary tract infections (1969–1995). J Vet Intern Med 2001;15:341–7.

[43] Lane IF, Graur GF, Fettman MJ. Acute renal failure. Part II. Diagnosis, management and prognosis. Compend Contin Educ Pract Vet 1994;16(5):625–45.

[44] Clark KL, Robertson MJ, Drew GM. Do renal tubular dopamine receptors mediate dopamine-induced diuresis in the anesthetized cat? J Cardiovasc Pharm 1991;17:267–76.

[45] Wohl JS, Schwartz DD, Flournoy S, et al. Renal hemodynamic and diuretic effects of low-dose dopamine in the cat. In: Proceedings of the Seventh International Veterinary Emergency and Critical Care Symposium, Orlando, 2000. p. 14–24.

[46] Flourney S, Wohl JS, Albrecht-Schmitt TJ, et al. Pharmacologic identification of a putative D1 dopamine receptor in feline kidneys. J Vet Pharmacol Ther 2003;26(4):283–90.

[47] Kellum JA, Decker J. Use of dopamine in acute renal failure: a meta-analysis. Crit Care Med 2002;30(8):1934–6.

[48] Debaveye YA, Berghe GH. Is there still a place for dopamine in the modern intensive care unit? Anesth Analg 2004;98(2):461–8.

[49] Langston CE, Cowgill LD, Spano JA. Applications and outcome of hemodialysis in cats: a review of 29 cases. J Vet Intern Med 1997;11:348–55.

[50] Cowgill LD, Langston CE. Role of hemodialysis in the management of dogs and cats with renal failure. Vet Clin N Am Small Anim Pract 1996;26(6):1347–78.

[51] Schramm L, Heidbreder E, Lukes M, et al. Endotoxin-induced acute renal failure in the rat: effects of urodilatin and diltiazem on renal function. Clin Nephrol 1996;46(2):117–24.

[52] Schramm L, Heidbreder E, Schaar J, et al. Toxic acute renal failure in the rat: effects of diltiazem and urodilatin on renal function. Nephron 1994;68(4):454–61.

VETERINARY
CLINICS
Small Animal Practice

ELSEVIER
SAUNDERS

Vet Clin Small Anim
35 (2005) 375–396

Approach to the Acute Abdomen

Matthew W. Beal, DVM

College of Veterinary Medicine, Michigan State University, D208 Veterinary Medical Center,
Michigan State University, East Lansing, MI 48824–1314, USA

Acute abdomen refers to the acute onset of abdominal pain. The underlying etiology of acute abdomen in the small animal patient may be minor and transient or an immediately life-threatening process. An understanding of the mechanisms of abdominal pain and an efficient approach to stabilization and diagnosis can facilitate rapid identification of the underlying etiology, and thus the institution of problem-specific treatment.

Neuroanatomy and the perception of abdominal pain

Stimulation of nociceptors (a highly specialized subset of sensory neurons that respond to intense stimuli) in and around the abdomen and abdominal wall is responsible for the initiation of abdominal pain [1]. Aδ and C-polymodal (CPM) fiber nociceptors are critical to the perception of the acute abdominal pain common to dogs and cats with acute intra-abdominal pathologic findings. Aδ fiber nociceptors specialize in detection of dangerous mechanical and thermal stimuli and in triggering rapid nociceptive responses. CPM fiber nociceptors respond to strong mechanical and chemical stimuli; in contrast to Aδ fiber nociceptors, CPM fiber nociceptors mediate dull or slow pain [2,3]. Somatic pain arising from abdominal wall injury or surgery is mediated by Aδ and CPM fiber nociceptors, whereas visceral pain arising directly from the hollow or parenchymal organs of the abdomen is primarily mediated by CPM fiber nociceptors [4,5].

Various stimuli common to abdominal pathologic findings seen clinically in the dog and the cat can activate nociceptors. These include the mechanical forces, such as tension, stretch, and shear, that may be seen in a dog with gastric dilatation-volvulus syndrome as well as the chemical stimuli from inflammatory mediators, ischemia, and chemical irritants seen in patients with various types of peritonitis. Inflammatory mediators not only stimulate CPM fiber nociceptors but may recruit silent nociceptors [6].

E-mail address: bealmatt@cvm.msu.edu

These various stimuli result in opening of nonspecific sodium and calcium channels, with subsequent depolarization of the membrane and, ultimately, opening of voltage-gated sodium channels (if depolarization is sufficient). The opening of these channels leads to the generation of an action potential that travels afferently through CPM fibers and Aδ fibers to the dorsal root ganglion and, subsequently, to the dorsal root of the spinal cord [1]. These signals are then transmitted through spinothalamic and spinoreticulothalamic tracts to the thalamus and, ultimately, to the cerebral cortex, where conscious perception of pain occurs [1].

Clinical signs, history, and physical examination of the patient with acute abdomen

Initial client contact in emergency practice is usually limited to triage, which includes the presenting complaint and a major body systems assessment to identify immediately life-threatening problems. Briefly, triage should include assessment of the cardiovascular (mucous membrane color, capillary refill time, and pulse rate and quality), respiratory (rate and effort), and central nervous (level of consciousness) systems. Triage should take no longer than 30 seconds. If the patient is judged to be unstable or requires further assessment, it should be moved to the treatment area for further evaluation of vital physiologic parameters (blood pressure, oxygen saturation [SpO_2] of hemoglobin, and ECG) and institution of treatment. If the patient is judged to be stable, further historical questioning and a complete physical examination may proceed as described elsewhere in this article.

Clinical signs that may be noticed by the owners of a patient presented with acute abdomen are listed in Box 1.

The patient's history should be obtained from the client presenting the patient with a complaint of abdominal pain or abdomen-related illness and should proceed in complete detail as it would for any other disease process. Questioning regarding patient history should proceed in the following format, with specific questioning directed to an exploration of the symptoms of acute abdomen or abdomen-related illness:

Presenting complaint
   What is the major problem(s)?
Last normal
   When was the patient last normal? This line of questioning, along with a past 6-month history, helps to determine the chronicity of a problem that may be manifesting acutely.
Progression of illness
   Chronologic documentation of the progression of the current problem(s) from the date that the patient was last normal should be recorded. This line of questioning may overlap with inquiries about systemic manifestations of the disease.

Box 1. Clinical signs commonly reported historically in small animals with acute abdomen

Gastrointestinal manifestations
  Vomiting
  Retching
  Regurgitation
  Diarrhea
  Painful defecation
Miscellaneous manifestations
  Anorexia
  "Praying" position
  Restlessness
  Icterus
Cardiorespiratory manifestations
  Panting
  Lethargy
  Collapse
Abdominal manifestations
  Abdominal distention
  Abdominal tenderness
  Abdominal wall bruising
Urogenital manifestations
  Vaginal discharge
  Stranguria
  Pollakiuria
  Painful defecation
  Anuria

Systemic manifestations of the disease
  A specific exploration into the systemic manifestations of the disease, including but not limited to vomiting, diarrhea, polyuria/polydipsia, anorexia, polyphagia, restlessness, panting, coughing, sneezing, defecation habits, and urination habits, should be undertaken.
Current and previous medications
  A list of dose, route, and frequency of all current medications as well as types of medications that have been administered in the past month but that the patient is not currently receiving should be provided. Heartworm and flea/tick preventatives should be documented if the patient is receiving these medications.
Past 6 months
  A concise line of questioning should be directed toward the 6 months before the last normal date. This line of questioning is designed to

determine the chronicity of the current illness or the presence or absence of comorbid conditions. Topics may include changes in body weight, an increase or decrease in water consumption, and changes in appetite or activity level as well as others. Determining chronicity helps to narrow the list of possible etiologies for the underlying problem and to determine whether the current problem is truly acute or an acute manifestation of a chronic disease.

Previous medical conditions

A list of all documented bouts of illness or injury known to have occurred during the life of the patient, including past medical and/or surgical history, should be provided. Additional topics should include the presence of any allergies or adverse reactions to foods or medications; history of receipt of whole blood or blood product transfusion; and reproductive status of the patient, including last estrus cycle and breeding history if applicable.

Diet

Specifics of the current diet, including type, quantity, and frequency of feeding, should be recorded.

The physical examination of the patient with acute abdomen or a complaint potentially related to intra-abdominal disease should focus first on the major body systems (cardiovascular, respiratory, and central nervous systems) and on abdominal palpation to facilitate the identification and early initiation of treatment for immediately life-threatening problems as stated previously.

Specific abdominal palpation techniques that may help in assessment of the patient with acute abdomen include identification of whether the pain is focal, regional, or diffuse. Focal abdominal pain is commonly seen in conditions like small bowel obstruction caused by a foreign body, mild pancreatitis, and intussusception. Regional abdominal pain is more common in conditions like pyometra and moderate to severe pancreatitis or cholecystitis. Diffuse abdominal pain is common in conditions involving the entire peritoneum, such as peritonitis (chemical, septic, and inflammatory) and diffuse enteritis (parvoviral enteritis). Thorough abdominal palpation should also include assessment of the size of the liver, spleen, and kidneys; presence of a mass effect anywhere in the abdomen; bladder size; assessment of small bowel loops and the colon for pain, gas or fluid distention, thickening, or a foreign body; gentle ballottement for assessment of a fluid wave; and finally, assessment of the spine for the presence of pain that could be interpreted as originating in the abdomen. In addition to palpation, the abdomen should be visually inspected for the presence of distention, periumbilical bruising, or inguinal bruising suggesting peritoneal or retroperitoneal injury or disease. Intermittently, animals with abdominal pain may assume the "praying position," with the forelimbs flat on the ground and the rear limbs extended and standing. In the author's experience, the praying position is a specific sign of significant abdominal pathologic change and should be taken seriously.

Careful attention must also be paid to the other body systems to take full diagnostic advantage of the physical examination. For example, rectal examination of a patient with acute abdomen may reveal melena, indicating upper gastrointestinal hemorrhage; acholic feces could indicate biliary obstruction; and a painful and unilaterally enlarged prostate could indicate the presence of a prostatic abscess. Similarly, peripheral lymphadenopathy in a patient with acute abdomen and splenomegaly may be suggestive of lymphoma or various infectious diseases. Oral examination, including assessment of the sublingual region for a linear foreign body, should also be undertaken. Overall, there is no diagnostic substitute for a complete physical examination.

Specific etiology of acute abdomen and acute abdomen in trauma

Acute abdomen may result from specific injury or disease of the peritoneal or retroperitoneal structures, diaphragm, or body wall constituents. Pain referred from other sites (especially the spine) is also frequently mistaken for abdominal pain. The numerous etiologies of acute abdomen are best illustrated through an anatomic/body systems approach (Box 2); however, the list is narrowed through structured and thorough historical questioning, complete physical examination, and appropriate diagnostic testing. In today's technologic world, we must not trivialize the value of the medical history and physical examination.

Historical examination and physical examination should allow the clinician to recognize the likelihood that a given patient has sustained trauma. Trauma associated with acute abdomen is a unique situation and should prompt an already narrowed list of differential diagnoses (Box 3). It is critical to recognize that trauma is most often a whole body problem (polytrauma) involving multiple body systems. Similarly, it is not uncommon for trauma-associated acute abdomen to result from multiple injuries, for example, concurrent uroperitoneum and hemoperitoneum.

Initial stabilization and management

Stabilization of the patient with acute abdomen should initially be focused on restoring abnormalities identified on the assessment of major body systems to normal, thus maximizing the delivery of oxygen to the tissues. Perfusion abnormalities, including hypovolemic or septic/distributive shock, as well as oxygenation abnormalities caused by concurrent pulmonary and/or pleural space disease are commonly identified in animals with acute abdomen. This scenario is especially common in the trauma patient. Oxygen therapy initially administered by means of a mask, flow-by

Box 2. Etiology of acute abdomen in the dog and cat

Urologic system
  Bladder
    Disruption*
    Neoplasia
    Urolithiasis
    Obstruction*
    Infection
  Urethra
    Disruption
    Neoplasia
    Urolithiasis
    Obstruction
  Ureter(s)
    Disruption
    Neoplasia
    Urolithiasis
    Obstruction
  Renal pelvis
    Disruption
    Urolithiasis
    Infection (pyelonephritis)
  Kidney
    Infection
    Neoplasia
    Acute nephritis
    Renal ischemia
Hemolymphatic
  Spleen
    Neoplasia*
    Torsion
    Infarction
    Splenitis
    Abscess
    Hematoma
    Laceration
  Lymph nodes
    Reactive lymphadenopathy
    Lymphadenitis
    Neoplastic infiltrate
Genital
  Male

Prostate
  Prostatitis
  Abscess
  Cyst
  Neoplasia
  Testicular torsion (abdominal)
Female
  Uterus
    Pyometra*
    Torsion
    Acute metritis
    Neoplasia
    Dystocia
    Rupture
  Ovary(ies)
    Ovarian neoplasia
    Ovarian cyst
Peritoneum/retroperitoneum/vascular
  Peritonitis
    Septic*
    Chemical
      Uroperitoneum*
      Bile
    Pancreatitis*
  Hemoperitoneum*
  Hemoretroperitoneum
  Disseminated neoplasia
  Vascular
    Mesenteric avulsion
    Mesenteric volvulus
    Mesenteric artery thrombosis
    Portal vein thrombosis
Gastrointestinal system
  Stomach
    Gastric dilatation-volvulus (GDV)*
    Gastric dilatation (GD)*
    Ulceration/perforation
    Gastroesophageal reflux
    Neoplasia
    Obstruction*
    Foreign body*
    Ischemia
    Acute gastritis

Small bowel
   Obstruction*
   Foreign body*
   Ulceration/perforation
   Gastroduodenal intussusception
   Intussusception
   Ischemia
   Neoplasia
   Enteritis*
   Ileocecocolic intussusception
Large bowel
   Neoplasia
   Torsion
   Ulceration/perforation
   Ischemia
   Colitis
   Obstruction
   Ileus
   Cecal inversion
   Typhlitis
Hepatobiliary
  Hepatic
    Hepatic lobar torsion
    Hepatic hematoma
    Hepatic abscess
    Hepatitis
    Laceration
    Cholangiohepatitis
  Biliary
    Biliary obstruction
    Cholecystitis
    Gallbladder mucocele
    Cholelithiasis
    Biliary disruption
      Common bile duct
      Gallbladder
      Hepatic duct
Pancreatic
  Pancreatitis*
  Abscess
  Neoplasia
  Pseudocyst
  Necrosis caused by ischemia

Mesenteric
  Mesentery
    Rent with herniation
    Neoplasia
Body wall/skin and subcutaneous tissue
  Body wall
    Prepubic tendon avulsion
    Penetrating injury
    Hematoma
    Hernia
    Abscess
    Neoplasia
  Skin and subcutaneous tissue
    Penetrating injury
    Abscess
Referred pain and acute abdomen
    Intervertebral disc disease*
    Discospondylitis
    Spinal neoplasia
    Fracture/luxation
    Pelvic trauma

Common conditions are indicated by an asterisk.

techniques, hood, or cage is indicated in all animals with perfusion abnormalities, and certainly in patients with a measured Spo_2 less than 92%.

Vascular access is critical to the delivery of life-saving fluid and drug therapy. Emergency vascular access is best achieved using a large-diameter over-the-needle catheter placed in a peripheral vein. If possible, blood should be collected directly from the catheter hub to facilitate later diagnostic testing. The author prefers to collect, at minimum, packed cell volume (PCV) and/or total solids (TS), venous blood gas, electrolytes, blood glucose, and blood urea nitrogen (BUN) or Azostix (Bayer Corp., Elkhart, IN) measurements. When possible, the author also prefers to collect samples (before fluid therapy) for a complete blood cell count (CBC), blood typing, serum biochemical profile, and coagulation profile (or activated clotting time [ACT]) as well as an additional sample in a serum separator tube for miscellaneous diagnostic testing. By no means are all these samples run on all patients; however, early sample collection prevents unnecessary phlebotomy at a later time. Through the use of Microtainer (Becton Dickinson, Franklin Lakes, NJ) 0.5-mL blood collection tubes for small patients, the volume of blood collected can be as little as 3 to 4 mL for all these diagnostic tests. Urine should be collected as early as possible in the

---

Box 3. Etiology of trauma-associated acute abdomen

Hemoperitoneum
  Splenic injury
  Hepatic injury
  Vascular avulsion
  Miscellaneous injuries
Hemoretroperitoneum
  Renal avulsion
  Other vascular disruption
Uroperitoneum
  Bladder disruption
  Urethral disruption
  Ureteral disruption
  Renal pelvis or kidney disruption
Uroretroperitoneum
  Ureteral disruption
  Renal pelvis or kidney disruption
Bile peritonitis
  Bile duct disruption
  Gallbladder disruption
  Hepatic duct disruption
Septic peritonitis
  Penetrating injury
  Gastrointestinal disruption
  Gastrointestinal ischemia
  Urinary tract disruption with urinary tract infection
Hernias
  Prepubic tendon avulsion
  Diaphragmatic hernia
  Other body wall hernia
Mesenteric injury
  Mesenteric avulsion
  Mesenteric rent with herniation of bowel
Traumatic pancreatitis

---

course of diagnostics and therapy. Urine specific gravity is of greatest value when the sample is collected before the institution of fluid therapy; however, therapy should never be withheld while waiting to collect a urine specimen.

It is critical that intravascular volume be restored before the initiation of inotropic support or the use of pressor agents in patients with underlying perfusion abnormalities. Isotonic balanced crystalloid fluids, such as Normosol-R (Abbott Laboratories, North Chicago, IL) and lactated Ringer's solution (LRS; Abbott Laboratories) as well as 0.9% sodium chloride (Abbott Laboratories) are appropriate resuscitation fluids for restoring intravascular volume in the hypovolemic patient. Fluid therapy should be given to effect. Some animals may not need the "shock dose" of fluids (90 mL/kg/h), whereas others need a larger volume delivered more rapidly. The author prefers to start with an initial bolus of 25 to 30 mL/kg delivered over 15 minutes, followed by reassessment and adjustment of the dose and rate as needed to restore vital physiologic parameters (heart rate, capillary refill time, mucous membrane color, blood pressure, urine output, bicarbonate or base excess, and lactate) to normal.

Based on the clinical situation, judicious use of synthetic colloids, such as 6% hetastarch (5–20 mL/kg; Baxter Health Care Corp, Deerfield, IL) may provide more rapid and sustained volume expansion. Fresh whole blood or packed red blood cells may be used as resuscitation fluids for the patient with evidence of acute hemorrhage based on physical examination and initial diagnostic testing. Because of its volume of distribution, cost, and availability, fresh-frozen plasma is best used for the management of coagulopathy rather than for the replacement of albumin. For a more complete discussion of this topic, the reader is referred to the article on assessment and treatment of perfusion abnormalities in this issue.

Some patients with acute abdomen display signs of sepsis, severe sepsis, or septic shock. There is currently evidence in the human literature to suggest that early antibiotic therapy within 1 hour of recognition of severe sepsis can improve survival [7]. Cultures should ideally be taken before antibiotic therapy is initiated. In cases of septic peritonitis, antibiotics should be initiated after collection of an abdominal fluid sample for cytologic examination and culture. Empiric antibiotic therapy should be directed on the basis of cytologic examination and Gram staining of specimens.

Diagnostic workup for the patient with acute abdomen

The diagnostic workup for the patient with acute abdomen includes a combination of historical findings, physical examination findings, diagnostic imaging techniques, abdominal fluid analysis, laboratory findings, and, if necessary, exploratory abdominal surgery.

Detection and retrieval of abdominal fluid accumulations

Abdominal effusion is a clinical finding in many animals with acute abdomen because of alterations in capillary hydrostatic pressure, oncotic pressure, vascular permeability, lymphatic drainage, or any combination thereof. Retrieval of a fluid sample from the abdomen with subsequent analysis and culture is critical for the accurate diagnosis of the underlying condition. Fluid retrieval is generally accomplished through abdominocentesis, four-quadrant abdominocentesis, ultrasound-guided abdominocentesis, abdominal paracentesis using a peritoneal dialysis catheter, or diagnostic peritoneal lavage (DPL).

If there is a strong suspicion of abdominal effusion based on physical examination and abdominal palpation findings, the patient should be placed in left lateral recumbency and the area surrounding the umbilicus subjected to clipping and full surgical preparation. Strict asepsis should be practiced at all times. A site should be chosen that is 2 to 3 cm caudal to the umbilicus and 2 to 3 cm left of the midline for sampling. The site should ideally be draped, and abdominocentesis should be performed using a needle and syringe advancing perpendicular to the skin, the subcutaneous tissues, and, finally, the abdominal wall. The syringe should be aspirated intermittently as it is advanced. If a sample is retrieved, it should be placed in an EDTA tube for cytologic analysis, a serum tube for chemical analysis, and another sterile tube for culture. If the sample appears to be blood, it should be placed in an ACT tube or serum tube to evaluate for clotting. If the specimen was retrieved from the abdominal cavity (versus the spleen or another vascular structure), it generally does not clot unless the hemorrhage is peracute. Some clinicians prefer to use an over-the-needle catheter for abdominocentesis, whereas others prefer to use an open system (just needles). The author prefers a closed system because it does not introduce air into the peritoneal cavity, a condition that may make additional diagnostic testing more difficult to interpret. Standing abdominocentesis puts the patient at risk for splenic injury when compared with abdominocentesis performed in lateral recumbency.

If single-quadrant abdominocentesis is unsuccessful, four-quadrant abdominocentesis is performed. Using this technique, abdominocentesis is repeated in areas 2 to 3 cm cranial and lateral to the umbilicus and caudal and lateral to the umbilicus as illustrated in Fig. 1.

If abdominal fluid is still suspected but not easily retrieved, ultrasonography may be used to image areas of the peritoneum likely to contain fluid and to guide abdominocentesis for the retrieval of a diagnostic specimen. A technique called the FAST (focused abdominal sonogram for trauma) scan was recently adapted from the human medical field and applied to dogs that had sustained trauma in an effort to identify abdominal fluid accumulations. This technique calls for transverse and longitudinal views taken from four sites around the abdomen, including the subxiphoid, ventral midline over the bladder, and areas over the most gravity-dependent areas of the right and left flanks [8]. The technique was shown to be sensitive for the diagnosis of abdominal fluid accumulations after trauma when performed by clinicians with minimal ultrasonographic training [8].

Abdominal paracentesis using a peritoneal dialysis catheter is a more sensitive method for the detection and retrieval of intra-abdominal fluid and detection of intra-abdominal illness or disease than abdominocentesis and four-quadrant abdominocentesis [9]. This procedure is generally performed with the patient heavily sedated and placed in left lateral or dorsal recumbency. The urinary bladder should be expressed or catheterized before this procedure. The abdomen is subjected to surgical preparation, and a local anesthetic (lidocaine) is infused just caudal to the umbilicus to

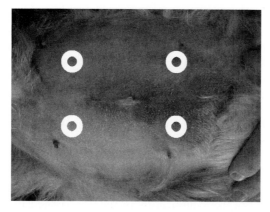

Fig. 1. Landmarks (circles) for four-quadrant abdominocentesis in the dog and cat. The patient is positioned in left lateral recumbency with the head to the right of the image.

include all planes of the body wall. A 1- to 2-cm skin incision is made, and blunt dissection is performed to reveal the linea alba. The linea is grasped with forceps or hemostats and incised to create a 0.5- to 1-cm opening in the abdomen. Through this incision, a peritoneal dialysis catheter is placed and directed in a dorsocaudal direction (toward the pelvic inlet). Various catheters are available; however, the author prefers one with numerous side holes present on the catheter to provide an increased surface area for the retrieval of a fluid sample. Once the catheter is in place, gentle negative pressure is applied to the catheter with a syringe and a fluid sample is retrieved. If a sample is not collected, repositioning and gentle ballottement of the abdomen may aid in retrieval of a sample. DPL with warm 0.9% sodium chloride (20–22 mL/kg) may be performed if a fluid sample is not retrieved. DPL presents an advantage over abdominal paracentesis methods using a dialysis catheter in that lavage fluid encounters all surfaces of the peritoneum. When a fluid sample is retrieved, it is representative of what is happening throughout the peritoneum. For example, a focal peritonitis caused by a penetrating foreign body that is walled off by omentum may be detected by DPL and missed by abdominocentesis, four-quadrant abdominocentesis, or paracentesis with a dialysis catheter. The author prefers peritoneal lavage to rule out septic peritonitis in animals with acute abdomen. Fluid retrieved by peritoneal lavage must be evaluated in light of the effect that dilution has on the sample, thus precluding significant biochemical testing of that fluid.

Cytologic abdominal fluid analysis for the patient with acute abdomen

Fluid analysis of samples collected from dogs with acute abdomen should include cytologic examination, cell count, biochemical evaluation, and culture. Cytologic examination may aid in the differentiation of conditions, including but not limited to septic peritonitis and various causes of nonseptic peritonitis (eg, pancreatitis, various types of neoplasia, bile peritonitis). Direct smears of the fluid sample may be diagnostic; however, centrifugation with subsequent examination of the pellet is frequently more rewarding and allows more nucleated cells to be evaluated. Samples retrieved from peritoneal lavage procedures should be centrifuged before cytologic analysis. The author prefers to prepare slides for Romanowsky type staining (Diff-Quick Stain Kit; Imeb, San Marcos, CA) as well as Gram staining procedures if bacteria are seen on initial cytologic examination. Performing a cell count and total protein concentration analysis of the abdominal fluid sample allows the clinician to characterize the sample as a transudate, modified transudate, or exudate. This, in concert with specific cytologic findings, may aid in the identification of the underlying cause of illness.

Cytologic evaluation of abdominal fluid samples has been the diagnostic test of choice for the acute diagnosis of septic peritonitis in dogs and cats. Cytologic evaluation alone is considered to be 57% to 87% accurate in making the diagnosis [10–13]. Although extracellular infectious agents are suggestive of peritonitis, aspiration of a bowel loop may also yield these findings. The presence of phagocytosed infectious agents is critical to making this diagnosis. Septic peritonitis is always a surgical emergency.

The presence of phagocytosed golden-green-blue granular pigment along with a vigorous inflammatory response is the traditional cytologic finding confirming bile peritonitis; however, a recent report detailed cases of bile peritonitis in dogs in which there was no evidence of bile pigment seen cytologically; instead, a fibrillar mucinous material was seen in concert with total bilirubin in the abdominal fluid twice that of the serum. Biliary tract disruption was subsequently confirmed in these patients [14].

The abdominal fluid characteristics of common causes of acute abdomen are listed in Table 1.

Biochemical abdominal fluid analysis and culture

Biochemical analysis of abdominal effusions is helpful in determining the underlying etiology of acute abdomen and has received research attention in the past 5 years.

A recent study evaluated the utility of blood glucose gradients between the abdominal fluid and the blood in an effort to find a highly sensitive and specific mechanism for the rapid diagnosis of septic peritonitis [13]. Biochemical tests like glucose determination must be performed on samples acquired directly from the peritoneum rather than from DPL samples. The authors concluded that a gradient of greater than 20 mg/dL between the blood and the abdominal fluid (the abdominal fluid is less than the blood) was 100% sensitive and specific in dogs for the diagnosis of septic peritonitis. In cats, the same gradient was 86% sensitive and 100% specific

Table 1
Characteristics of common causes of abdominal effusion in acute abdomen

Diagnosis	Cytologic characteristics	Fluid characteristics	Biochemical analysis	Course of treatment
Septic peritonitis	Septic suppurative inflammation with intracellular infectious agents	Exudate most commonly	Abdominal fluid BG/serum BG gradient >20 mg/dL	Emergency surgery
Pancreatitis	Nonseptic suppurative inflammation	Modified transudate to exudate		Supportive measures, possible surgery
Bile peritonitis	Nonseptic suppurative inflammation plus phagocytosed bile pigment or mucinous substance	Exudate most commonly	[Total bilirubin] abdominal fluid/[total bilirubin] serum >2.0 is sensitive indicator	Emergency surgery
Hemoperitoneum	Evidence of hemorrhage, may contain platelets if acute; erythrophagocytosis may be observed	Exudate		Possible surgery depending on cause, most traumatic hemoabdomen cases do not require surgical intervention
Uroperitoneum	Suppurative inflammation with or without evidence of sepsis if animal has concurrent urinary tract infection	Modified transudate	[Creatinine] abdominal fluid/[creatinine] serum >2.0 [K+] abdominal fluid/[K+] serum >1.4 (dogs)/1.9 (cats)	Emergency surgery or urinary diversion

Abbreviation: BG, blood glucose.

for the diagnosis of septic peritonitis. This study should be interpreted with some caution because of the small sample size, however [13].

Evaluation of the ratio of abdominal fluid creatinine to peripheral blood creatinine and abdominal fluid potassium to peripheral blood potassium is useful for the diagnosis of uroperitoneum. Abdominal fluid creatinine–to–peripheral blood creatinine ratios of greater than 2.0 in the dog and cat are highly sensitive and specific indicators of uroperitoneum. An abdominal fluid potassium–to–peripheral blood potassium ratio of 1.4 in dogs and 1.9 in cats is also supportive. To maximize the diagnostic value of these tests, both ratios should be performed on fluid samples [15,16]. A positive diagnosis of uroperitoneum should trigger the initiation of retrograde urethrocystography and/or excretory urography to determine the site of urinary tract disruption.

There have been many anecdotal reports and some experimental evidence supporting assessment of the ratio of abdominal fluid amylase/lipase concentrations to that in the serum to provide supportive evidence for a diagnosis of pancreatitis [17–21]. At this time, additional investigation in clinical small animal patients is necessary to validate this information.

The ratio of abdominal fluid total bilirubin to that in the serum (>2.0) has been used to support a diagnosis of biliary tract disruption in dogs and seems to be a sensitive indicator of this condition [14,22]. To the author's knowledge, however, the effect of conditions like hemolysis in an abdominal fluid sample on the total bilirubin of that sample or the assessment of total bilirubin in samples from clinical patients without bile peritonitis has not yet been evaluated. As a result, use of the ratio of total bilirubin concentration in abdominal fluid to that in the serum as a predictor of biliary tract disruption requires further objective investigation before it can be considered a specific predictor of this condition.

In the future, additional testing of abdominal fluid samples to identify markers of neoplasia and other causes of acute abdomen may aid the attending clinician in identifying the underlying condition.

Samples of abdominal fluid from patients with acute abdomen should be saved for aerobic and anaerobic culture. Decisions to pursue culture should be based on cytologic analysis. It is the author's practice to culture abdominal fluid samples that contain evidence of an inflammatory process without an obvious underlying cause. Bacterial culture should always be performed on samples with cytologic evidence of infectious agents.

Imaging of the patient with acute abdomen

Diagnostic imaging is an invaluable resource for identification of the underlying cause of acute abdomen in dogs and cats. Abdominal radiographs, thoracic radiographs, abdominal ultrasound, CT, and MRI may aid in the identification of the underlying condition. It is imperative to achieve patient stability and to use analgesic and sedative techniques before initiation of potentially stressful imaging procedures. Oxygen supplementation should be administered during imaging procedures for any animal with signs of respiratory compromise or shock.

Radiography is an accessible diagnostic tool for most veterinary practitioners, and abdominal radiography is a valuable tool in the examination of the acute abdomen patient. It is extremely important that image quality is adequate to assess all intra-abdominal structures and the surrounding tissues. Table 2 includes a list of common radiographic findings in animals with acute abdomen and their possible causes. Special radiographic studies, including positive-contrast studies of the gastrointestinal system and urinary tract, are valuable in the diagnosis of various causes of acute abdomen. Upper gastrointestinal studies are "functional" studies, and thus are the most appropriate diagnostic test for ruling out small bowel obstruction in dogs and cats. For dogs and cats in which there is no evidence of gastrointestinal disruption, 30% barium sulfate suspension (Liquid E-Z-Paque; E-Z-EM Canada Inc., subsidiary of EZEM, Westbury, NY) may be administered via a nasogastric or orogastric tube at a dose of 10 to 12 mL/kg. Lateral and ventrodorsal radiographic views may then be taken at 0, 15, 30, 60, 90, 120, or 180 minutes after administration or when the contrast agent has left the small bowel [23]. For animals with the possibility of gastrointestinal tract disruption, an iodinated contrast agent, such as diatrizoate sodium (Hypaque Sodium Oral Powder, Nycomed, Princeton, NJ), may be administered as a 30% solution at a dose of 2 to 20 mL/kg. Small intestinal transit time is 3 to 4 hours in dogs and 1 to 2 hours (up to 3–4 hours) in cats. Iodinated contrast agents decrease small intestinal transit time.

Thoracic radiographs are indicated for all dogs and cats with acute abdomen in concert with a history or physical examination evidence of cardiorespiratory disease or decreased oxygenation indices. Aspiration pneumonia is not uncommon in the critically ill patient with vomiting or regurgitation, and acute lung injury or the acute respiratory distress syndrome (ARDS) may occur secondary to numerous conditions that also result in acute abdomen. Finally, the author performs thoracic radiographs on all adult or geriatric patients with acute abdomen to help evaluate for evidence of neoplastic disease.

Abdominal ultrasound has gained popularity in recent years as a tool for assessment of the patient with acute abdomen. Unlike abdominal radiography, abdominal ultrasonography allows the operator to evaluate the entire organ rather than only its silhouette. Abdominal ultrasound is complementary to abdominal radiography and frequently allows the list of differential diagnoses to be narrowed and, occasionally, a diagnosis to be made. In addition, ultrasound guidance may be used to retrieve peritoneal and retroperitoneal fluid accumulations and to aspirate or biopsy various abdominal structures and pathologic findings. Features like Doppler ultrasonography can be used to assess for the presence or absence of blood

Table 2
Common radiographic findings and their diagnostic significance in the dog and cat with acute abdomen

Radiographic finding	Possible cause	Miscellaneous information
Free peritoneal gas	Disrupted hollow viscus, abdominal wall disruption, open abdominocentesis	Consider horizontal beam radiography, indication for emergency laparotomy
Gas compartmentalization of stomach	GDV	Indication for emergency laparotomy
Gas distention of stomach	Gastric dilatation, aerophagia	
Diffuse small bowel gas or fluid distention >2.5 rib widths	Mesenteric volvulus	Indication for emergency laparotomy
Segmental gas or fluid-distended small bowel >2.5 rib widths	Small bowel obstruction or ileus	Indication for additional imaging or emergency laparotomy
Gas in duodenum with displacement to right and widening of duodenal-pyloric angle plus poor serosal detail in cranial abdomen	Pancreatitis	Consider abdominal ultrasound
Gas-distended colon	Ileus, diarrhea, colonic torsion (rare)	
Small bowel plication (accordion) with "C"-shaped small intestinal gas pockets	Linear foreign body (LFB)	Indication for emergency laparotomy, evaluate for sublingual LFB
Cranial gastric axis displacement	Microhepatica, caudal abdominal mass	Consider abdominal ultrasound
Caudal gastric displacement	Hepatomegaly caused by infiltrative, inflammatory/infectious, or neoplastic disease	Consider abdominal ultrasound

Splenomegaly	Infiltrative/infectious/inflammatory disease/splenic torsion/splenic venous thrombosis/neoplasia/passive congestion associated with sedation	Consider abdominal ultrasound to assess blood flow and appearance of splenic architecture and vasculature, consider exploratory laparotomy
Prostatomegaly	Benign prostatic hyperplasia (BPH)/prostatic neoplasia/prostatitis/prostatic abscess/prostatic cyst	Consider rectal examination and abdominal ultrasound for further assessment
Uterine distention	Pyometra/mucometra/hydrometra/pregnancy	Consider ovariohysterectomy
Renomegaly	Infiltrative/neoplastic/infectious/obstructive disease/inflammatory disease leading to acute renal failure	Consider abdominal ultrasound, excretory urogram
Bladder distention	Obstructive disease/neurologic dysfunction	Consider abdominal ultrasound and cystourethrogram
Loss of peritoneal serosal margin detail	Abdominal effusion, emaciation, peritonitis, carcinomatosis, immature fat	Consider abdominal ultrasound and abdominocentesis or DPL
Loss of retroperitoneal detail	Retroperitoneal effusion	Consider ultrasound-guided fluid retrieval and excretory urogram
Mass effect in peritoneum or retroperitoneum	Neoplasia, abscess, cyst, granuloma, hematoma	Consider abdominal ultrasound and thoracic radiography

Abbreviations: **BPH**, benign prostatic hyperplasia; **DPL**, diagnostic peritoneal lavage; **GDV**, gastric dilatation-volvulus; **LFB**, linear foreign body.

flow. Ultrasound can be a valuable diagnostic tool in the hands of a formally trained operator. Diagnostic utility is severely limited and misdiagnosis is extremely common, however, when ultrasonography is performed by individuals without extensive training and experience. Overall, the diagnostic utility of abdominal ultrasonography is quite operator dependent.

CT is a widely used tool for evaluation of people with acute abdomen, especially in patients with a history of abdominal trauma. At this point, the use of CT for assessment of acute abdomen and its value in comparison to other diagnostic tests in the dog have not been prospectively evaluated.

Surgical evaluation of the acute abdomen patient

Abdominal exploration is the ultimate diagnostic and therapeutic intervention for the patient with acute abdomen. A decision to perform exploratory surgery on the dog or cat with acute abdomen is frequently based on a culmination of historical and physical examination findings, appropriate laboratory data, and results of imaging studies and ancillary diagnostic tests, such as DPL. Frequently, a presumptive diagnosis has been made, and a clear indication for surgical intervention has been identified before abdominal exploration. Surgical exploration may also be indicated for patients with acute abdomen when symptoms are persistent or severe and a diagnosis has not been established. Clients should be warned of the possibility of a "negative" exploration, one in which a definitive cause for acute abdomen cannot be identified. Even a negative exploration may have diagnostic value after biopsies are taken, however. Abdominal exploration should be performed through an incision from the xiphoid to the pubis so as to gain adequate exposure for a complete and systematic evaluation of the abdomen. Definitive therapy should be initiated for inciting causes of acute abdomen. In addition, biopsies should be taken of all grossly abnormal tissues and all small bowel segments in animals with a history of vomiting or diarrhea without an obvious cause. Large bowel biopsies are indicated only in patients with gross pathologic findings or specific signs localizing the condition to the large bowel.

Wounds or crushing injuries over the abdomen warrant special consideration. Wounds over body cavities frequently follow the iceberg analogy. What is seen on the surface is a small component of what lies beneath. Evaluation of the patient with any wounds over the abdominal cavity should always include surgical exploration of those wounds. It is generally accepted that simple probing of wounds over a body cavity is ineffective in identifying penetrating injury because of the motion of the skin, subcutaneous tissues, and muscular layers over one another. All bite wounds should be explored surgically, opened to allow adequate exposure for exploration, debrided, lavaged, closed using appropriate drainage techniques, or left open to heal by second intention. Wounds found to penetrate into the abdominal cavity warrant local wound care as previously mentioned, followed by exploration through a ventral midline laparotomy. It should be noted that even nonpenetrating wounds can result in severe intra-abdominal injury. The most common clinical cause of this situation is crushing injury as a result of bite wounds. Abdominal exploration is never an improper diagnostic test in this scenario.

Postoperative patients may develop or redevelop acute abdomen with pain that is perhaps more severe than expected after surgery or not responsive to appropriate analgesic techniques. In these scenarios, diagnostic testing should be initiated just as described previously to move proactively to identify the underlying cause, such as dehiscence of an enterotomy site, mesenteric volvulus, or pancreatitis.

Early enteral nutritional support maximizes the likelihood of a positive outcome in patients with acute abdomen. Anesthesia and abdominal surgery in particular offer the unique opportunity to initiate early enteral nutritional support through placement of esophagostomy, gastrostomy, or jejunostomy feeding tubes. An esophagostomy or gastrostomy tube is an excellent choice for feeding patients that are not vomiting. Esophagostomy tubes have an advantage over gastrostomy tubes in that if the tube becomes dislodged, it (unlike a gastrostomy tube) does not result in life-threatening pathologic conditions (eg, septic peritonitis). Gastrostomy tubes have the advantage of offering a portal not only for feeding but for gastric decompression, however. The author prefers surgical placement of a gastrostomy tube in dogs undergoing abdominal exploration that have evidence of gastric atony and vomiting or regurgitation. Jejunostomy tubes bypass the stomach and are indicated in patients that have persistent vomiting (eg, dogs with pancreatitis) or decreased gastric motility. When placed appropriately and evaluated daily, the jejunostomy tube is well tolerated. Premature dislodgment of a jejunostomy tube or leakage around the ostomy site can result in cellulitis, body wall abscessation, or septic peritonitis. Care of any enteral feeding device should include daily visual inspection, ostomy care, and replacement of a sterile dressing. If enteral nutrition is not tolerated, parenteral nutritional support can be used to supplement or provide complete caloric requirements.

Summary

Acute abdomen is a common clinical complaint identified in small animal patients. Success results from a proactive approach to management, including rapid stabilization of major body systems, early identification of the inciting problem(s), attention to comorbid conditions, and timely definitive therapy.

References

[1] Woolf CJ. Pain: moving from symptom control toward mechanism specific pharmacologic management. Ann Intern Med 2004;140:441–51.

[2] LaMotte RH, Campbell JN. Comparison of responses of warm and nociceptive C-fiber afferents in monkey with human judgments of thermal pain. J Neurophysiol 1978;41:509–28.

[3] Perl ER. Sensitization of nociceptors and its relation to sensation. In: Bonica JJ, Albe-Fessard D, editors. Advances in pain research and therapy, vol. 1. New York: Raven Press; 1976. p. 17–28.

[4] Cervero F. Mechanisms of visceral pain. In: Lipton S, Miles J, editors. Persistant pain; modern methods of treatment. vol. 4. New York: Grune and Stratton; 1983. p. 1–19.

[5] Janig W, Morrison JFB. Functional properties of spinal visceral afferents supplying abdominal and pelvic organs with special emphasis on visceral nociception. In: Cervero F, Morrison JF, editors. Visceral sensation. Amsterdam: Elsevier; 1986. p. 87–114.

[6] Buena L, Fioramonti J. Visceral perception: inflammatory and non-inflammatory mediators. Gut 2002;51(Suppl 1):i19–23.

[7] Dellinger RP, Carlet JM, Masur H, et al. Surviving sepsis campaign guidelines for management of severe sepsis and septic shock. Crit Care Med 2004;32(3):858–73.

[8] Boysen SR, Rozanski EA, Tidwell AS, et al. Focused abdominal sonogram for trauma (FAST) in 100 dogs. In: Proceedings of the Ninth International Veterinary Emergency and Critical Care Symposium, New Orleans, LA, 2003. San Antonio (TX): Veterinary Emergency and Critical Care Society. p. 765.

[9] Crowe DT. Diagnostic abdominal paracentesis techniques: clinical evaluation in 129 dogs and cats. J Am Anim Hosp Assoc 1984;20:223–30.

[10] Mueller MG, Ludwig LL, Barton LJ. Use of closed-suction drains to treat generalized peritonitis in dogs and cats: 40 cases (1997–1999). J Am Vet Med Assoc 2001;219:789–94.

[11] Lanz OI, Ellison GW, Bellah JR, et al. Surgical treatment of septic peritonitis without abdominal drainage in 28 dogs. J Am Anim Hosp Assoc 2001;37:87–92.

[12] Hardie EM, Rawlings CA, Calvert CA. Severe sepsis in selected small animal surgical patients. J Am Anim Hosp Assoc 1986;22:33–41.

[13] Bonczynski JJ, Ludwig LL, Barton LJ, et al. Comparison of peritoneal fluid and peripheral blood pH, bicarbonate, glucose, and lactate concentration as a diagnostic tool for septic peritonitis in dogs and cats. Vet Surg 2003;32:161–6.

[14] Owens SD, Gossett R, McElhaney MR, et al. Three cases of canine bile peritonitis with mucinous material in abdominal fluid as the prominent cytologic finding. Vet Clin Pathol 2003;32(3):114–20.

[15] Aumann M, Worth LT, Drobatz KJ. Uroperitoneum in cats. J Am Anim Hosp Assoc 1998;34:315–24.

[16] Schmiedt C, Tobias KM, Otto CM. Evaluation of abdominal fluid: peripheral blood creatinine and potassium ratios for diagnosis of uroperitoneum in dogs. J Vet Emerg Crit Care 2001;11(4):275–80.

[17] Connally HE. Cytology and fluid analysis of the acute abdomen. Clin Tech Small Anim Pract 2003;18(1):39–44.

[18] Crowe DT. The first steps in handling the acute abdomen patient. Vet Med 1988;83:652.

[19] Kolata RJ. Diagnostic abdominal paracentesis and lavage: experimental and clinical evaluations in the dog. J Am Vet Med Assoc 1976;168:697–9.

[20] Machiedo GW, Brown CS, Lavigne JE, et al. The use of peritoneal lavage in the diagnosis of experimental acute pancreatitis. Surg Gynecol Obstet 1975;140:889–92.

[21] Kerry RL, Glas WW. Traumatic injury of the pancreas and duodenum: a clinical and experimental study. Arch Surg 1962;85:813–6.

[22] Ludwig LL, McLoughlin MA, Graves TK, et al. Surgical treatment of bile peritonitis in 24 dogs and 2 cats: a retrospective study. 1987–1994. Vet Surg 1997;26:90–8.

[23] Moon M, Myer W. Gastrointestinal contrast radiology in small animals. Semin Vet Med Surg (Small Anim) 1986;1:121–43.

ELSEVIER
SAUNDERS

Vet Clin Small Anim
35 (2005) 397–420

VETERINARY
CLINICS
Small Animal Practice

Reproductive Emergencies

L. Ari Jutkowitz, VMD

*Department of Small Animal Clinical Sciences, College of Veterinary Medicine,
Michigan State University, East Lansing, MI 48824–1314, USA*

Reproductive problems often arise after normal business hours, so it is not uncommon for them to fall into the domain of the emergency veterinarian. Because most owners lack medical knowledge, they frequently look to the veterinarian to answer questions and to identify potential problems. The emergency clinician must therefore be familiar with normal reproductive behavior in addition to the common emergencies that may arise. With this goal, the events surrounding normal parturition as well as the common complications that may develop during this period are reviewed in this article.

Normal parturition

Normal gestation length in the dog may range from 57 to 72 days from the time of first breeding, with an average length of 65 days [1]. The reason for this apparent variability is that female dogs may stand to be bred as early as 11 days before and as late as 3 days after ovulation [2]. Additionally, canine sperm may survive for 6 to 11 days [1,3] in the female reproductive tract. Thus, there may be considerable variation between the breeding dates and the actual time of fertilization. If the date of the preovulatory luteinizing hormone (LH) peak is known, gestation length becomes less variable, ranging from 64 to 66 days [1]. Because cats are induced ovulators, there is generally less variability in gestation length, which ranges from 63 to 65 days. Ovulation may not take place after the first breeding, however, so in the event of multiple breedings, uncertainties with regard to gestation length may still be present.

As the whelping date approaches, a number of clues may point toward impending parturition. Mammary development, vulvar enlargement, mucous vaginal discharge, and relaxation of the pelvic ligaments are early signs of approaching parturition. Onset of lactation may be noted in primiparous

---

E-mail address: jutkowit@cvm.msu.edu

vetsmall.theclinics.com

bitches within 24 hours of parturition but may occur several days before parturition in multiparous bitches. A sudden drop in body temperature ($>2°F$) is generally noted within 24 hours of parturition [4] in dogs and cats as a result of decreases in progesterone levels, but this finding is not always reliable. In one recent study, nadir temperature occurred longer than 48 hours before parturition in 24% of dogs and an appreciable drop in temperature ($>1°F$) was not seen in 35% of dogs [5]. Because the drop in temperature may be transient, twice-daily monitoring is required. Serum progesterone levels typically decrease to less than 2 ng/mL within 24 to 48 hours of parturition [3,6] and thus may be used to predict parturition. Progesterone assays are also useful in confirming the presence of primary uterine inertia in bitches at risk and in deciding that a planned cesarian section may proceed safely.

Maturation of the fetal pituitary-adrenal axis and release of corticotropin are believed to be the initiating events for parturition [3,7]. Release of cortisol from the fetal adrenal glands leads to synthesis and release of prostaglandin $F_{2\alpha}$ ($PGF_{2\alpha}$) in the placenta and uterus. $PGF_{2\alpha}$ causes regression of the corpus luteum and a sudden drop in progesterone levels. With a decrease in progesterone levels, inhibition of myometrial contractions is removed, leading to uterine contractions, placental separation, and progressive dilation of the cervix.

Normal parturition proceeds in three stages. The first stage is characterized by subclinical uterine contractions and progressive dilation of the cervix. During this stage, which typically lasts for 6 to 12 hours, bitches may show signs of restlessness, apprehension, panting, nesting behaviors, hiding, and anorexia. Queens may be tachypneic, restless, and vocal or may lie purring in their nesting boxes. Active expulsion of the fetuses occurs during the second stage of labor. As the fetuses are forced into the birth canal, mechanoreceptors in the female reproductive tract generate afferent signals (Ferguson's reflex) that result in increased release of oxytocin from the posterior pituitary, thereby increasing the intensity of uterine contractions. The presence of a fetus in the cervix also induces reflex abdominal contractions that aid in parturition. The first fetus is usually delivered within 1 hour of the onset of stage 2 labor in cats and within 4 hours in dogs, with subsequent deliveries every 15 minutes to 3 hours [7,8]. Active straining generally results in expulsion of a fetus within 15 minutes. The entire process generally occurs over 2 to 12 hours but may take as long as 24 hours with large litter sizes in the dog. Normal parturition lengths of up to 42 hours have been reported in the cat [9], but clinical experience urges caution in dismissing these cases without careful evaluation for fetal distress (Fig. 1). The third stage of labor results in expulsion of the placenta. One placenta should be identified for each fetus delivered. Placentas are usually still attached to the fetus by the umbilical cord and emerge with the fetus but may emerge within 15 minutes to several hours if they become detached. Because fetuses are delivered from uterine horns alternately, it is not uncommon to have two

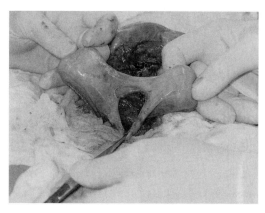

Fig. 1. Uterine rupture in a cat diagnosed 36 hours after the delivery of a healthy kitten. Two fetuses were present within the abdominal cavity. No signs of straining were noted after delivery of the first kitten.

fetuses emerge before their placentas are passed. Lochia, a greenish vaginal discharge, indicates placental separation and is typically seen shortly before the onset of stage 2 labor. After parturition, the discharge gradually becomes reddish brown, decreasing in volume over 4 to 6 weeks as uterine involution takes place.

Each puppy or kitten emerges covered by the amniotic membranes. The chorioallantois typically ruptures during the birthing process or is chewed by the dam as it begins to protrude through the birth canal. The bitch or queen removes the amnion from the neonate by chewing or licking thoroughly, and this also serves to clean the newborn and stimulate respiration. The umbilical cord is severed by biting, and the placenta is typically swallowed. Diarrhea may result if too many placentas are consumed. If the dam fails to care for her newborns, the owner must intervene, removing the amnion and carefully cleaning and drying the neonate with a soft dry towel. Fluid may be removed from the oral and nasal passages with a bulb syringe if needed. The umbilicus should be clamped, transected, and ligated approximately 1 to 2 cm from the newborn's body and then disinfected with iodine.

Dystocia

Dystocia (Greek *dys* [difficult], *tokos* [birth]) is defined as the inability to expel fetuses through the birth canal during parturition and may result from maternal or fetal factors that prevent delivery from taking place (Box 1). Dystocia related to maternal factors may be further classified based on whether it results from myometrial failure (physiologic) or obstruction of the birth canal (morphologic). Uterine inertia is the most common cause of dystocia [4,10–12], seen when the myometrium produces only weak and infrequent contractions that fail to expel a normal fetus through a normal

Box 1. Causes of dystocia

Maternal
  Physiologic
    Primary uterine inertia
    Hereditary
    Stress/environmental disturbances
    Old age
    Obesity
    Systemic disease
    Uterine overdistention (eg, large litter size, fetuses too big)
    Uterine underdistention (eg, small litter size, inadequate
      fetal fluids)
    Estrogen/progesterone balance
    Calcium/magnesium balance
    Inadequate oxytocin secretion
    Prematurity
  Secondary uterine inertia
  Morphologic
    Primary (eg, birth canal too small)
    Secondary (eg, abnormal influence on or within birth canal)
      Pelvic fractures
      Uterine torsion
      Uterine rupture
      Uterine herniation
      Uterine prolapse
      Mass-like lesions of pelvic canal, uterus, vagina, or vulva
        (eg, hyperplasia, neoplasia, hematoma, abscess)
      Fibrosis of uterus, cervix, or vagina
      Vaginal septum
  Fetal
    Malpresentation
    Oversize (eg, single fetus pregnancy)
    Fetal death
    Fetal malformations

birth canal. Primary uterine inertia is considered complete when gestation has exceeded its expected length with no evidence of progression into active labor. Occasionally, a dog initiates parturition and expels one or more healthy fetuses but then subsequently fails to deliver the remaining fetuses as a result of myometrial fatigue, and this may be referred to as primary partial uterine inertia. Uterine inertia may also be considered secondary if myometrial failure results from prolonged attempts to expel an obstructed fetus and persists after relief of obstruction. Morphologic causes of dystocia are those in which an anatomic abnormality of the bitch or queen results in obstruction of the birth canal. Primary morphologic abnormalities are commonly seen in narrow-hipped dogs like Bulldogs, Boston Terriers, and Scottish Terriers, where the birth canal is too small to allow passage of a fetus that is considered to be of normal size for the breed [13]. Secondary morphologic causes of dystocia result from an abnormal influence on or within the birth canal (eg, pelvic fractures) that leads to obstruction.

Fetal factors that may result in dystocia include malpresentations, oversize, fetal malformations, and fetal death. Malpresentations are reported to be the second most common cause of dystocia in dogs and cats [4,10–12]. Some of the commonly described malpresentations include transverse presentation, lateral or ventral flexion of the neck, anterior presentation with flexion of one or both forelimbs, posterior presentation with retention of both hind limbs, and simultaneous presentation of two fetuses. It should be noted that posterior presentations are considered to be a normal variation in dogs and cats, occurring in approximately 40% of deliveries [4]. Fetal oversize is another potential cause of dystocia, most commonly seen with single pup pregnancies. Because maternal size largely dictates the size of the offspring, mating between dogs of dissimilar sizes is not a common cause of fetal oversize. Fetal death is an infrequent cause of dystocia, increasing the likelihood of malpresentation because of failure to rotate and extend the head and legs, which commonly occurs immediately before parturition. Fetal malformations are another potential cause of dystocia, with anasarca (generalized subcutaneous edema), hydrocephalus, cerebral and cerebrospinal hernias, abdominal hernias, duplications, and rib cage malformations among the more commonly noted [10,11,14].

A number of breeds have been reported to have a higher prevalence of dystocia. Congenitally narrowed birth canals are seen in many brachycephalic and terrier breeds, such as Bulldogs, Boston Terriers, and Scottish Terriers, and their fetuses may have comparatively large heads, predisposing them to maternal-fetal disproportion [13]. Bulldogs also tend to have slack abdominal musculature that may limit their ability to lift the fetus up toward the birth canal. Many of the small and toy breeds have also been overrepresented in retrospective studies, including Chihuahuas, Pekinese, Yorkshire Terriers, Dachshunds, and Poodles [4]. Golden Retrievers, Labrador Retrievers, and German Shepherds are also heavily featured in retrospective studies, but this is more likely related to the popularity of these breeds than to a true breed predisposition. In feline dystocia, breed and cranial conformation have also been significantly associated with dystocia, with Siamese and Persians heavily overrepresented. In one study looking at the association between cranial conformation and dystocia, the prevalence of dystocia was 10% in dolichocephalic breeds (eg, Siamese, Cornish Rex), 7.3% in brachycephalic breeds (eg, Persian, British Shorthair), and only 2.3% in mesocephalic cats [12]. Uterine inertia and malpresentations were still the most commonly reported causes of dystocia in these breeds.

When an animal is brought in for suspected dystocia (Box 2), it is important to obtain an accurate breeding history. Questions to be asked should include any previous whelping history, the earliest and latest possible breeding dates, the male animal used, the time of temperature drop (if noted), the time of onset of whelping, the frequency and intensity of expulsive efforts, the number and viability of puppies or kittens already delivered, and any interventions used.

A complete physical examination should be performed to rule out the possibility of systemic illness. Abdominal palpation may be helpful to assess the size and tone of the uterus, to estimate the number of remaining fetuses, and to evaluate for the presence of a fetus in the birth canal. If there is no fetus in the pelvic inlet, the animal is not ready to whelp/queen or the uterine horn is unable to expel the fetus. The vulva should be examined for the presence of discharge. Greenish vaginal discharge (lochia) indicates placental separation, and dystocia should be suspected if parturition does not proceed within 2 to 3 hours. Digital examination with a sterile well-lubricated glove should be performed to assess for the degree of cervical dilation (if reachable), fetal position, and the presence of any vaginal or cervical anomalies. If a fetus can be palpated, presentation and viability may be assessed. Gentle feathering of the dorsal vaginal wall should stimulate reflex contractions and can be helpful in assessing their strength.

If a fetus is lodged within the birth canal, digital manipulation should be attempted. The fetus may be grasped around the head and neck, around the pelvis, or around the proximal portions of the hind limbs, depending on fetal presentation. Excessive traction should never be applied to a single

---

Box 2. Criteria for the suspicion of dystocia

1. A definite cause is visible (ie, fetus lodged in birth canal, pelvic fractures).
2. Gestation is prolonged (>70 days) with no evidence of labor.
3. Temperature has dropped to lower than 100°F and returned to normal with no evidence of labor.
4. Green vaginal discharge (indicates placental separation) or fetal fluids are seen, and 2 hours have elapsed without expulsion of fetuses.
5. Strong and persistent contractions fail to result in the delivery of a puppy within 30 minutes.
6. Weak and infrequent contractions fail to produce a fetus within 4 hours.
7. More than 4 hours have elapsed since the birth of a puppy, with no evidence of ongoing labor.
8. Signs of systemic illness or severe pain are present.

extremity because of the ease with which these may be avulsed. With the dam restrained in a standing position, traction is applied in a posterior-ventral direction. The fetus may be gently rocked back and forth and twisted diagonally to free shoulders and hips "locked" in the pelvic canal. If flexion of the head or extremities is preventing delivery, a finger may be used to extend them. One cannot overemphasize the importance of using copious amounts of sterile lubricant (KY Jelly; Johnson & Johnson, New Brunswick, NJ) during obstetric maneuvers, applied digitally or infused around the fetus using a red rubber catheter.

Radiographs should next be obtained in any animal experiencing dystocia. Radiographs are accurate for assessing the number, size, location, and position of fetuses as well as maternal pelvic morphology and the general status of the abdomen. Fetal viability is more difficult to assess from radiographs unless evidence of fetal decomposition is present. The first signs of decomposition to develop include intrafetal gas patterns and awkward fetal postures, such as hyperextension of the extremities, visible by 6 hours postmortem. Collapse of the spinal column because of loss of muscular support and overlapping of the bones of the skull are generally visible by 48 hours postmortem. As more time elapses, accumulation of large amounts of intrauterine gas may occur [15,16]. Ultrasound may be a more useful tool for assessment of fetal viability, fetal malformations, and fetal distress. Normal fetal heart rates have been reported at 180 to 245 beats per minute (bpm) in dogs and up to approximately 265 bpm in cats [17]. Deceleration of fetal heart rates to less than 180 bpm and the presence of fetal bowel movements on ultrasound have been shown to correlate with severe fetal distress and may indicate a need for rapid intervention [18].

Medical management should be considered if there is no evidence of obstruction and fetal and pelvic size appear normal. Calcium gluconate and oxytocin are the agents of choice in medical management of dystocia. Oxytocin is a peptide hormone that increases the frequency and strength of uterine contractions by promoting influx of calcium into myometrial cells. Oxytocin also promotes postpartum uterine involution, aids in control of uterine hemorrhage, and assists in expulsion of retained placentas. The dose of oxytocin has traditionally been reported at 5 to 20 U administered intra-muscularly in the dog and 2 to 4 U administered intramuscularly in the cat. With an increase in the use of uterine contraction monitoring in veterinary patients, however, there is a growing body of evidence to suggest that traditional doses may be too high, potentially causing uterine tetany, inef-fective contractions, and decreased fetal blood flow. Recent data [5,6] suggest that doses of 0.5 to 2 U are effective in increasing the frequency and quality of contraction. The oxytocin dose may be repeated in 30 minutes if expulsion of a fetus has not resulted. If labor proceeds and a fetus is delivered, oxytocin may be repeated every 30 minutes as needed to assist in expulsion of the remaining fetuses. Oxytocin is contraindicated in obstructive dystocia and uterine inertia secondary to overstretching. Postpartum injections of oxytocin should be reserved for cases in which a retained placenta is suspected.

Because myometrial contractility is dependent on the influx of extracellular calcium into myometrial cells [19,20], calcium gluconate has been used for many years as an uterotonic agent. Its use should be considered if weak infrequent contractions are noted [5,6], if the initial oxytocin dose was nonproductive [3], or when laboratory work reveals hypocalcemia. Retrospective studies have indicated that many patients failing to respond to oxytocin alone may respond to a combination of calcium and oxytocin [4,11]. The dose for calcium gluconate (10% solution) is 22 mg/kg (50–150 mg/kg if hypocalcemic) diluted in saline and given subcutaneously or added to intravenous fluids and given slowly while monitoring an ECG for arrhythmias. Subcutaneous administration has been reported to result in irritation and potential granuloma formation, although this is an infrequent complication. Dextrose infusion should also be initiated if hypoglycemia is evident on laboratory work.

The prognosis for medical management of dystocia is guarded, with success rates of 20% to 40% in the veterinary literature [4,10–12]. Additionally, stillbirth rates have been shown to rise when dystocia is allowed to continue for longer than 4.5 to 6 hours [4,10] from the time of onset of second-stage labor in the dog. For these reasons, the decision to proceed to cesarian section should not be delayed if the response to medical management is poor or unlikely to result in successful delivery (Box 3).

An anesthetic protocol for cesarian section should be selected with the goal of maximizing the survival of the neonates and dam. Attempts should be made to minimize exposure of the fetus to anesthetics by keeping the time from induction to delivery as short as possible. Ideally, the dam should be clipped and prepared before induction, equipment should be laid out, and the surgeon should be scrubbed and ready. Induction agents should be given to effect. Regional techniques, such as line blocks and epidurals, may help to minimize the need for other drugs. A line block can be performed using lidocaine, 2 mg/kg, infused along the ventral midline [21,22]. Alternately, epidural lidocaine may be administered in dogs at a dose of 2 to 3 mg/kg, not to exceed a total volume of 6 mL [21]. Neonates are poorly able to metabolize anesthetics, so drugs with a short duration of action that are rapidly metabolized by the dam (eg, propofol) or drugs that are reversible (narcotics) should be used. Propofol (4–6 mg/kg administered intravenously) or mask induction is most commonly used for cesarian section at this time and has been associated with reduced neonatal mortality in dogs. Anesthetic agents that have been associated with increased neonatal mortality include thiopental, ketamine, xylazine, medetomidine, and methoxyflurane [23–25]. After induction, the lowest possible concentration of inhalant should be administered until delivery of the puppies. Excessive use of inhalant anesthetics is associated with maternal vasodilation, decreased uterine blood flow, and neonatal depression. Once the puppies are removed, the inhalant

---

Box 3. Indications for cesarian section

1. Complete primary uterine inertia (consider at 70th day of gestation)
2. Partial primary uterine inertia or secondary uterine inertia; consider cesarian section if large numbers of fetuses remain and response to drugs is unsatisfactory
3. Fetal oversize
4. Gross abnormalities of maternal pelvis (eg, fractures, masses)
5. Fetal malformations
6. Malpresentation that is not amenable to manipulation (eg, transverse presentation)
7. Past history of dystocia or cesarian section; consider planned cesarian section just before full term
8. Fetal putrefaction
9. Maternal evidence of systemic illness
10. Suspicion of uterine torsion, rupture, prolapse, or herniation
11. Evidence of fetal distress with poor response to medical intervention

---

concentration may be increased if needed and additional analgesics given to the dam. Intravenous fluids should always be administered before and during the procedure to avoid hypotension and decreased fetal blood flow. Pregnant animals may be more susceptible to aspiration pneumonia as a result of delayed gastric emptying. In one prospective multicenter study, 56% of maternal mortalities were related to aspiration pneumonia [23]. Extra care should therefore be taken with airway protection during induction and recovery, particularly if a full stomach is seen on radiographs, and tilting the surgical table in a head down position during surgery should be avoided.

Two techniques have been described for surgical management of dystocia. In the traditional cesarian section or hysterotomy, fetuses are removed one at time from a single incision in the uterine body. Alternately, en bloc ovariohysterectomy may be performed, removing the entire uterus and handing it to a team of assistants for neonatal resuscitation. En bloc ovariohysterectomy may be considered any time disease of the uterus is present (eg, torsion, metritis, fetal putrefaction); surgical speed is required because of the critical condition of the dam; morphologic abnormalities, such as pelvic fractures, prevent future delivery; or an owner does not plan to breed the animal again. Lactation is not adversely affected by ovariohysterectomy, and neonatal survival rates are comparable to those obtained with conventional cesarian section [26]. When performing the en bloc technique, it is critical that the time from the clamping of the uterine artery to the time of newborn extraction is kept to a minimum (30–60 seconds) to minimize the degree of fetal hypoxia and maximize survival. In recent studies, neonatal survival rates after surgical treatment of dystocia have been reported at 92% at birth, with 80% still alive 7 days after the cesarian section [23,24].

Neonatal resuscitation

A warm (90°F) incubator, hemostats, suture material, suction bulb syringes, emergency drugs, and an adequate supply of soft dry towels should be prepared beforehand. As each puppy is handed off, the umbilical cord should be clamped and ligated 1 to 2 cm from the umbilicus. Fetal fluids and amnion should be removed by rubbing briskly with a soft clean towel. The oral cavity and nares may be suctioned with a bulb syringe. The old practice of "swinging" puppies to clear their airways is best avoided because of the potential for cerebral hemorrhage as a result of concussive injury. If vigorous rubbing is not successful at stimulating respiration, positive-pressure ventilation may be initiated with a snug-fitting mask, keeping the neonate's head and neck extended to ensure adequate inflation of the lungs. Alternately, intubation may be accomplished using a catheter or small uncuffed endotracheal tube. Because isoflurane is minimally metabolized, ventilation is the primary route of elimination. Thus, the depressant effects of isoflurane cannot be reversed until the neonate breathes. Cardiac massage may be instituted if a heart beat cannot be detected once warming and ventilation measures have been instituted. Epinephrine (0.1 mg/kg) may be given intratracheally, intraosseously, or intravenously if cardiac massage is unsuccessful. Naloxone (0.1 mg/kg) should be considered if the dam received opioid analgesics as part of the anesthetic regimen [27]. Although doxapram (Dopram) is routinely administered in many practices as a respiratory stimulant, it is not used for this purpose in the resuscitation of human neonates [28] and there is no evidence to support its use in veterinary patients. Because its effect is diminished when the brain is hypoxic, it is unlikely to be helpful in the apneic newborn [27]. Additionally, there is evidence that doxapram may result in significant decreases in cerebral blood flow that could be detrimental in vulnerable hypoxic newborns [29,30].

Fetal and uterine monitoring

Perinatal monitoring systems are now commercially available (Whelpwise; Veterinary Perinatal Specialties, Wheat Ridge, CO) and are being increasingly used for monitoring and periparturient management of high-risk pregnancies (ie, older dogs, prior history of dystocia, large or small litter size, expensive breedings). Monitoring systems consist of the following equipment: (1) a tocodynamometer attached to a clipped area of the caudal abdomen, which senses changes in intrauterine and intra-amniotic pressure; (2) a recorder worn in a small backpack, which records the uterine contraction patterns; and (3) a modem for transferring these data to the perinatal service. Owners are also provided handheld Doppler units and are taught to monitor fetal heart rates for evidence of fetal distress.

Uterine monitoring is generally initiated approximately 1 week before the due date, and recordings are taken at home twice daily. The frequency of recording is increased once first-stage labor is entered. Obstetric personnel, available 24 hours a day, interpret the recordings and communicate the results to the client's veterinarian. In this way, much of the guesswork is taken out of management of parturition by providing objective data on the frequency and strength of uterine contractions and allowing definitive diagnosis of uterine inertia and uterine obstructive patterns. Medical treatments using oxytocin and calcium gluconate can be used more accurately, because the effects of these drugs may be directly measured. The decision to proceed to surgery may also be made in a more timely fashion if medical management fails to induce effective uterine contractions, a uterine obstructive pattern develops, or evidence of fetal distress is noted. Correspondingly, studies in bitches after uterine and fetal monitoring have shown significantly lower stillbirth rates (2.5%–3.7%) than previously reported [5,6].

Hemorrhage

Severe uterine hemorrhage (hematometra) and uterine bleeding between heat cycles (metrorrhagia) are uncommon problems in dogs and cats. Differential diagnoses include uterine vessel tear secondary to obstetric trauma, inherited or acquired coagulopathies [31,32], uterine or vaginal masses, subinvolution of placental sites [33], cystic endometrial hyperplasia or pyometra [34], endometritis, uterine serosal inclusion cysts [35], uterine torsion [36], and prepubertal metrorrhagia [37]. If postpartum hemorrhage is mild but persistent and the animal is otherwise clinically normal, oxytocin may be given to hasten resolution by promoting uterine involution. For severe hemorrhage or hemorrhage unrelated to whelping, further investigation is needed. Measurement of baseline packed cell volume (PCV) and total solids (TS), a minimum database (complete blood cell count [CBC], serum biochemistry, and urinalysis), and coagulation testing should be performed. Remember that the hematocrit in the periparturient dog normally decreases to approximately 30%. Evidence of severe anemia in conjunction with clinical signs, such as tachycardia, tachypnea, anorexia, weakness, or altered mentation, may indicate a need for packed red blood cell transfusion, however. Fresh-frozen plasma transfusion should be considered if clotting times are prolonged. Vaginal cytologic examination may help to raise the index of suspicion for endometritis or pyometra, and ultrasound may be helpful to identify mass lesions or other uterine abnormalities. Depending on the cause of the bleeding, or if a definitive cause is not identified, ovariohysterectomy may be indicated.

Uterine prolapse

Uterine prolapse is a rare postpartum complication reported more commonly in cats than in dogs [38,39]. It is generally only seen during or immediately after parturition, because the cervix must be open for prolapse to occur. Reported causes include severe tenesmus during or after parturition, incomplete placental separation, relaxation or atony of the uterus, and excessive relaxation of the pelvic and perineal regions [38]. If the uterus prolapses into the cranial vagina, nonspecific signs of abdominal pain and straining may be noted. In the case of complete uterine prolapse, a large mass of tissue protrudes visibly through the vaginal orifice, with varying degrees of tissue edema, ulceration, and necrosis, depending on the duration and severity of the prolapse. Symptoms of hemorrhagic shock frequently develop after uterine prolapse as a result of ovarian or uterine vessel rupture and may necessitate emergency laparotomy (Fig. 2).

Treatment consists of initially lubricating and protecting the exposed tissues while the animal is treated with intravenous fluids to correct shock. Blood transfusion may be required if severe hemorrhage has occurred. Systemic antibiotics should be administered in any patient in which tissue necrosis is seen. Once the animal is stable, general anesthesia is administered to allow reduction of the prolapse. If uterine tissues are relatively healthy and no further fetuses are present, the tissues should be gently cleaned, lubricated, and then replaced manually. A test tube may be used to invert and reduce the uterus, and hydropulsion with a red rubber catheter and sterile saline may enable proper positioning of the uterine horns. If the prolapse cannot be reduced because of severe tissue edema, a dorsal episiotomy may be performed to facilitate reduction. Oxytocin should be administered after reduction to promote uterine involution. Planned laparotomy should be considered after reduction to ensure proper positioning of the uterine horns and assess the integrity of the uterine vessels. If there is any evidence of

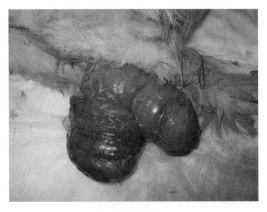

Fig. 2. Uterine prolapse in a cat.

compromised tissue viability or if further breeding is not desired, an ovariohysterectomy should be performed.

In cases in which manual reduction is unsuccessful, surgical reduction may be necessary, allowing the surgeon to apply traction from the abdomen while an assistant applies external pressure. Once reduced, the uterus may then be pexied to the ventrolateral body wall to prevent recurrence. If reduction is not possible because of severe tissue swelling or necrosis, amputation of the traumatized external tissue may be needed before the remainder can be reduced. The urethra should be catheterized during this process to prevent accidental trauma. After resection of the necrotic segment, the remaining tissue is reduced and a laparotomy is performed to complete the ovariohysterectomy.

Uterine torsion

Uterine torsion is a complication of pregnancy that has been reported infrequently in dogs and cats. Although it typically occurs in multiparous animals late in pregnancy or at the time of parturition, uterine torsion has also been reported in nonpregnant nulliparous animals and as a complication of pyometra [36,40]. The cause of uterine torsion is unknown, but contributing factors may include excessive fetal movement, lack of uterine tone, lack of fetal fluids, and previous stretching of the broad ligament in multiparous animals. Uterine torsions most commonly involve a single uterine horn twisted at its base, but torsions of both horns or the uterine body have also been described [36]. Clinical signs are variable and include abdominal pain, shock, hypothermia, hemorrhagic vaginal discharge, dystocia (with continuous straining), vomiting, and restlessness. Torsions of 180° may persist for weeks without clinical signs until labor ensues [41].

Radiography or ultrasonography may show evidence of a fluid-filled uterus, fetal death, or peritoneal effusion, but results may be nonspecific. Exploratory surgery is usually required for definitive diagnosis and treatment. As with other forms of torsion, uterine torsion should not be corrected before ovariohysterectomy to prevent release of endotoxins and inflammatory mediators contained within the compromised tissue [42]. The prognosis is generally good if shock is corrected and surgery is performed in a timely fashion.

Mastitis

Mastitis is a postpartum complication seen in dogs and cats that results from bacterial infection of the mammary glands. Bacteria most commonly enter through the nipple as a result of nursing, trauma, or poor hygiene but may also be spread hematogenously. In mild cases, discomfort, swelling, and inflammation may be seen, whereas in severe cases, signs of systemic illness, such as fever, anorexia, and lethargy, frequently develop. Dogs often refuse to allow their young to nurse and may be reluctant to lie down. Severe mastitis often progresses to abscessation and necrosis.

A diagnosis of mastitis is generally based on history and clinical signs (fever and swollen painful glands in the postpartum animal), but a baseline CBC and chemistry testing as well as milk cytologic testing and culture are useful for assessing the severity of illness and appropriateness of antibiotic selection. Milk expressed from the gland may be purulent, stringy, hemorrhagic, or gray, and cytologic examination typically shows large numbers of white blood cells and intracellular bacteria. The most common bacteria isolated on culture include *Escherichia coli*, staphylococci, and streptococci.

Treatment is initiated immediately with broad-spectrum antibiotics. Amoxicillin-clavulanic acid (Clavamox, Augmentin) or cephalexin (Keflex) is a good first choice; both are safe for nursing neonates. Trimethoprim-sulfamethoxazole ([TMZ-SMP], Tribrissen), chloramphenicol, and clinda-mycin (Antirobe) are other useful antibiotics reported to achieve high concentrations in milk [43]. Other measures that may be useful in the management of mastitis include warm compresses, hydrotherapy, and frequent milk stripping. If a fluctuant abscess pocket is identified on palpation, early lancing and flushing may limit the degree of skin necrosis that follows. Large ruptured mammary abscesses may be successfully managed as open wounds with warm compresses, hydrotherapy, and systemic antibiotics, but in these cases, mastectomy may provide a more rapid and cosmetic resolution of the problem.

Endometritis

Endometritis is a bacterial infection of the uterus that is generally seen within the first 3 days (up to 1 week) after whelping, although it may develop during pregnancy as well. Potential causes include retained fetuses or placentas, abortions, uterine trauma secondary to dystocia or obstetric manipulation, and ascending infection from the vaginal canal. Typical signs include fever, lethargy, anorexia, vomiting, diarrhea, poor lactation, neglect of offspring, and a foul-smelling vaginal discharge. Just as in the nonpregnant dog, any purulent vaginal discharge noted during or after pregnancy is abnormal and should prompt investigation.

Laboratory work abnormalities consistent with sepsis may be seen, including leukocytosis with a left shift or leukopenia, thrombocytopenia, elevated liver values, and hypoalbuminemia. Coagulation testing should be performed to rule out disseminated intravascular coagulation. Radiography or ultrasound is indicated to evaluate for fetal death, retained placentas, or evidence of uterine enlargement. Cytologic examination of vaginal discharge typically shows degenerate neutrophils and macrophages with intracellular bacteria. The most common organisms associated with uterine infections include staphylococci, streptococci, *E coli*, *Salmonella*, *Campylobacter*, and *Chlamydia* [44].

An animal suspected of having septic metritis should be treated aggressively with intravenous fluids. Broad-spectrum antibiotic combinations, such as ampicillin-enrofloxacin, ampicillin-aminoglycoside, or cefazolin-aminoglycoside-metronidazole, should be administered. After stabilization, ovariohysterectomy is the treatment of choice for metritis. If the animal is not showing signs of sepsis and the owner wishes to use it for breeding purposes in the future, evacuation of the uterine contents using $PGF_{2\alpha}$ (Lutalyse) may also be attempted in conjunction with broad-spectrum antibiotics (see section on pyometra for protocol). Potential complications of $PGF_{2\alpha}$ include vomiting, abdominal discomfort, uterine rupture, and septic peritonitis. Because $PGF_{2\alpha}$ treatment may require several days to achieve a good effect, animals that are severely ill should always be treated with ovariohysterectomy. Ovariohysterectomy is also the best choice when the animal is not intended for future breeding or if the health of the dam is a higher priority than possible future breedings.

Eclampsia

Eclampsia or puerperal tetany is a life-threatening condition that results from the development of hypocalcemia in the periparturient period. It is one of the more common complaints noted after parturition, accounting for 23% of periparturient emergencies in one study [45]. Eclampsia is believed to result from the loss of calcium through lactation and fetal skeletal mineralization in excess of that entering the extracellular fluid through gastrointestinal absorption and bone resorption. Other factors, such as inadequate diet or parathyroid atrophy resulting from oversupplementation of calcium, may also contribute, although the diet in affected animals was not significantly different from that in nonaffected animals in retrospective studies [45,46]. An increasing ratio of litter size to maternal body weight has also been identified as a significant factor in the development of periparturient hypocalcemia [45].

Eclampsia is most commonly seen in small dogs, first-time whelpings, and dogs with large litter sizes. It typically develops 2 to 4 weeks after parturition [45,47] but is occasionally seen in late gestation [46]. Clinical signs in dogs most commonly include stiff gait, trembling, twitching, seizures, tachycardia, panting, and hyperthermia, but approximately 20% of dogs may present with atypical signs, such as whining, vomiting, diarrhea, and behavior changes [45]. If untreated, death may result from respiratory impairment or from hyperthermia and cerebral edema. Cats may demonstrate clinical signs similar to those of dogs but, unlike dogs, are more prone to hypothermia and may present with hyperexcitability, hypersensitivity, or flaccid paralysis in place of clonic-tonic muscle spasms [46].

A diagnosis of eclampsia is made on the basis of history and physical examination findings in conjunction with low total or ionized calcium levels. Ionized calcium represents the physiologically active portion of calcium within the body and is involved in muscular contraction as well as neurologic and cardiovascular function. Ionized calcium levels are thus believed to be a more sensitive indicator of extracellular calcium levels than total calcium and typically fall to less than 0.8 mmol/L in dogs with eclampsia (reference range: 1.2–1.4 mmol/L). In one study [48], however, total calcium levels were found to be decreased in all dogs with eclampsia, suggesting that total calcium levels may provide sufficient information in this disease if an ionized calcium measurement is not available.

Animals presented with eclampsia should have an intravenous catheter placed and intravenous fluids administered to address fever, dehydration, and tachycardia. Calcium gluconate (10%) should immediately be administered intravenously slowly to effect. Most animals have tremors controlled at doses ranging from 0.5 to 1.5 mL/kg. ECG should be monitored during calcium administration, and the infusion should be stopped if bradycardia or arrhythmias develop. Ionized calcium levels should be rechecked after administration to make sure that ionized calcium levels remain within the normal range. Temperature should be carefully monitored in animals presenting with tremors, and active cooling measures (eg, cool fluids, wetting the hair coat, and fan blowing over the animal) should be instituted for patients with severe hyperthermia. Body temperature generally falls quickly once tremors are controlled, so active cooling measures should be discontinued once the animal's temperature falls below 103°F. Oral calcium carbonate (Tums) supplementation should be continued at a dose of 100 mg/kg/d throughout lactation. Up to 20% of dogs [47] may have recurrence of eclampsia despite supplementation if puppies are allowed to nurse, so bottle feeding and early weaning of the puppies are recommended.

Supplementation of calcium before whelping is not recommended because this may downregulate parathyroid hormone secretion, decreasing intestinal calcium absorption and increasing the risk of eclampsia during lactation. Instead, calcium administration (100 mg/kg/d divided) should be instituted after whelping in dogs at risk and dogs with a previous history of eclampsia.

Pyometra

Pyometra, the accumulation of purulent exudate within the uterine lumen, is a hormonally mediated disease seen during diestrus in dogs and cats. It is typically but not always [49] preceded by cystic endometrial hyperplasia (CEH), an abnormal uterine response to progesterone. During diestrus, a period of approximately 70 days when the uterus is under the influence of progesterone produced by the corpus luteum, dogs with CEH develop excessive proliferation of mucus-producing glands, leading to endometrial thickening. Increased glandular activity in conjunction with decreased myometrial activity may lead to fluid accumulation in the uterus, referred to as mucometra or hydrometra at this stage, depending on the viscosity of the fluid. With continued progesterone stimulation, the uterine response may become inflammatory, with infiltration of lymphocytes and plasma cells into the endometrium. CEH typically resolves once progesterone levels decrease at the end of diestrus but may worsen with subsequent cycles.

Estrogen by itself does not cause CEH or pyometra but may contribute to its development. In one experimental study, CEH could not be produced by exogenous administration of estrogen to ovariectomized dogs but did develop when estrogen was given in conjunction with progesterone [50]. Estrogen is therefore believed to enhance the stimulatory effects of progesterone on the uterus, but the mechanism by which this occurs is poorly understood [51]. Thus, exogenous estrogen (eg, mismate shots, diethylstilbestrol) given during estrus or diestrus may greatly increase the risk of developing pyometra and has been implicated as one of the most common factors in the development of pyometra in young animals [52].

The changes associated with CEH set up a favorable environment for secondary bacterial infection. The most common source of these bacteria is from the normal vaginal vault flora, which may enter through the open cervix during proestrus and estrus. Vaginal populations of bacteria have not been shown to differ between dogs that develop pyometra and those that do not [53], suggesting opportunistic invasion of the abnormal progesterone-primed uterus. There is some evidence to suggest that high progesterone levels may decrease phagocytic activity within the uterus and that estrogen may promote the inhibitory actions of progesterone on uterine bactericidal activity [54]. *E coli* is the bacterium most commonly isolated from dogs and cats with pyometra, possibly as a result of its ability to adhere to receptors in the progesterone-primed uterus [55]. Other bacteria commonly implicated in the development of pyometra include *Staphylococcus*, *Streptococcus*, *Klebsiella*, *Pseudomonas*, and *Proteus* [56–60]. During pyometra, release of bacterial endotoxin occurs and may indirectly account for many of the adverse effects associated with pyometra, including cardiovascular collapse, altered renal function, hepatocellular injury, and disseminated intravascular coagulation. Blood endotoxin levels have been shown to be significantly different between healthy dogs and dogs with pyometra, and higher endotoxin levels were associated with a worse outcome in one study [58]. Endotoxin levels decreased significantly in all dogs after surgery.

Pyometra is considered to be a disease of middle-aged to older dogs that have been through numerous heat cycles and have therefore undergone repetitive progesterone stimulation of the uterus. Progesterone levels in dogs with pyometra were not shown to be different from those of unaffected dogs [61], possibly explaining why repetitive cycles (ie, older dogs) are necessary to cause disease. An increasing frequency of pyometra has been reported in younger dogs, however. In a study of 57 bitches with pyometra that were treated with $PGF_{2\alpha}$, the mean age was 2.5 years [52]. Pyometra is also seen in cats but less frequently than in dogs, because cats are induced ovulators that require intercourse before luteal activity and progesterone secretion occur. The use of megestrol acetate (Ovaban) and the presence of retained corpora lutea [52,56,57] are factors that have been associated with an increased likelihood of developing pyometra in cats.

Historical findings in animals presenting with pyometra classically include vulvar discharge, anorexia, depression, polyuria, polydipsia, vomiting, and diarrhea. Signs typically develop 1 to 2 months after estrus. If signs are recognized early, the animal may appear otherwise healthy. The longer it takes for signs to be recognized by the owner, the more likely it is that severe signs of dehydration, sepsis, or shock as well as death will occur. The fact that most closed-cervix pyometras present with more severe symptoms than open-cervix pyometras likely reflects the lack of an obvious sign that owners can recognize, leading to a prolonged clinical course before veterinary attention is sought.

On physical examination, purulent vulvar discharge is often the most obvious sign. The uterus may be palpably enlarged, depending on uterine turgor, the size of the animal, and the degree of abdominal relaxation. Caution should be taken during palpation to avoid rupture of the friable uterus. Rectal temperature is often normal but may be elevated as a result of uterine inflammation and septicemia. With decompensatory septic shock, hypotension, hypothermia, tachycardia, pale mucous membranes, and prolonged capillary refill time may be noted.

Anemia of chronic disease is a common finding in animals with pyometra, occurring in approximately 70% of cases [62]. The anemia is generally non-regenerative, normocytic, and normochromic but may progress to a micro-cytic and hypochromic anemia, especially when there is concurrent blood loss. Leukocytosis is another common finding, often exceeding $30,000/\mu L$, accompanied by a left shift. Normal or only mildly elevated white blood cell counts may be seen in dogs with open pyometra, however [52]. Serum chemistry frequently shows hyperproteinemia secondary to dehydration, although hypoalbuminemia may also result from sepsis. Hyperglycemia may be seen initially because of catecholamine release and peripheral insulin resistance. As sepsis progresses, decreased gluconeogenesis, depletion of glycogen stores, and increased peripheral glucose use may result in hypoglycemia. Elevations in alanine aminotransferase and alkaline phos-phatase may occur secondary to hepatocellular damage from hypovolemia or sepsis. Azotemia is another frequent finding reported in 12% to 37% of animals with pyometra [56,59] and may be prerenal or renal in origin. One study identified a 75% incidence of renal dysfunction in dogs with pyometra. Tubulointerstitial nephritis was the lesion seen most commonly on renal biopsy, but lesion severity did not correlate with degree of functional loss [59]. Endotoxemia is believed to result in reversible renal tubular damage, reducing the sensitivity of the renal tubules to the effects of antidiuretic hormone (ADH) and leading to decreased concentrating ability. Urine specific gravity may be concentrated early in the course of disease as a result of dehydration but frequently becomes isosthenuric (1.007–1.017) or hyposthenuric (1.001–1.006) because of the effects of endotoxin on the renal tubules. This can make it challenging to distinguish renal from prerenal causes of azotemia, but seeing decreases in BUN and creatinine immediately after fluid therapy would support a prerenal cause. Azotemia unresponsive to fluid therapy suggests acute tubular necrosis and may carry a more guarded prognosis, although renal values may improve after ovariohysterectomy. Concurrent urinary tract infections have been reported in 22% to 72% [55,56,59] of animals with pyometra and should be suspected if pyuria, hematuria, or proteinuria is seen on urinalysis. Cystocentesis should not be performed before surgery because of the risk of puncturing the infected uterus, but a sample for cystocentesis may be collected at the time of surgery.

Vaginal cytologic examination typically shows large numbers of degenerative neutrophils with intracellular bacteria. Vaginoscopy may be helpful in determining the origin of the discharge but is not routinely performed in the emergency setting. Anterior vaginal cultures using a shielded swab may be valuable for determining antibiotic sensitivity when managing pyometra medically. Vaginal and uterine cultures have been reported to be negative in 10% to 30% of cases [56,60,63].

Radiographs frequently show a large tubular structure in the caudoventral abdomen, and loss of abdominal detail may be present if uterine rupture has occurred. An inability to identify the uterus on radiographs does not rule out pyometra, because drainage associated with open pyometra may prevent significant distention from being appreciable. Pregnancy is one of the most important differential diagnoses for pyometra and cannot be differentiated from pyometra radiographically until approximately day 42, when fetal skeletal mineralization is sufficient to be detected. Ultrasound may therefore be a more accurate way to assess the uterus, allowing visualization of the uterine size, wall thickness, and presence of fluid and fetal structures.

Once pyometra has been diagnosed, ovariohysterectomy is strongly recommended unless the owner desires the animal solely for breeding purposes. Before inducing anesthesia, aggressive fluid therapy should be directed toward correction of shock, electrolyte and acid-base abnormalities, and hypoglycemia. Crystalloids, such as lactated Ringer's solution, are initially a good choice, with colloidal solutions, such as hetastarch, added if hypoalbuminemia and decreased oncotic pressure are a concern. Hypertonic saline has also been shown to be a beneficial adjunct therapy in patients with septic shock undergoing ovariohysterectomy for pyometra [64]. Fresh-frozen plasma (10 mL/kg) may be indicated if coagulation testing reveals prolonged clotting times. Broad-spectrum antibiotics should be administered before surgery and continued for 10 days after surgery. Once the animal is relatively stable, surgery should be performed. Severe clinical signs associated with pyometra are related to septicemia and endotoxemia; consequently, they do not resolve until the source of infection is removed.

At the time of surgery, the uterus may be large and friable, and caution should be taken to avoid uterine laceration on entry or accidental rupture or spillage during manipulation of the uterus. The uterus should be exteriorized and packed off with laparotomy sponges to avoid abdominal contamination and then removed using a triple-clamp technique. The uterine stump should not be oversewn because this may increase the risk of abscessation by "walling off" a portion of the infected stump. Rather, the stump should be gently cleaned and lavaged before closure. In the event of accidental abdominal contamination, copious lavage with sterile saline should be performed. The prognosis for surgically managed pyometra is generally good, with a reported survival of approximately 92% in dogs and cats [56,58]. The development of severe generalized peritonitis resulting from uterine rupture carries a more guarded prognosis, however, frequently necessitating closed-suction drain placement or management using open abdominal drainage techniques to maximize the chances for a positive outcome.

Medical management of pyometra is generally discouraged because of the possibility of severe complications, adverse effects, and a high recurrence rate. If an animal is valued solely for breeding purposes, however, and if signs of systemic illness are mild, medical therapy may be attempted. $PGF_{2\alpha}$ (Lutalyse) is currently the medical therapy of choice, resulting in resolution of pyometra in 75% to 100% of dogs and cats with open-cervix pyometra and successful breeding in approximately 90% [52,60,63,65,66]. Actions of $PGF_{2\alpha}$ include contraction of the myometrium and relaxation of the cervix, leading to evacuation of the uterine contents. The luteolytic effects of $PGF_{2\alpha}$ may also result in decreased progesterone levels, removing some of the stimulus for CEH. Considerations for deciding on medical versus surgical management should include age and reproductive status of the animal, severity of illness, and the type of pyometra (open or closed cervix). Medical management should be strongly discouraged in older animals or animals not intended for breeding. Additionally, because $PGF_{2\alpha}$ generally does not result in clinical improvement for at least 48 hours [60], surgical management is still the treatment of choice for severely ill animals. $PGF_{2\alpha}$ should also be used with caution in animals with closed-cervix pyometra because of the increased risk of uterine rupture and the possibility of retrograde expulsion of exudate through the oviducts into the abdomen. When used in these animals, success rates of 25% to 41% have been reported [52,60,65].

$PGF_{2\alpha}$ is typically administered subcutaneously at a dose of 0.1 to 0.25 mg/kg once daily for 5 days. Only naturally occurring $PGF_{2\alpha}$ (Lutalyse) should be used, because the synthetic analogues are more potent and could be fatal at this dose range. The lower dose is often used initially to assess an individual animal's response before increasing the dose if needed. Because positive blood cultures have been reported after treatment [60], antibiotic therapy should be started empirically using amoxicillin-clavulanate

(Clavamox, Augmentin), enrofloxacin (Baytril), or TMZ-SMP (Tribrissen) and then continued for 14 days based on the results of anterior vaginal cultures. $PGF_{2\alpha}$ is associated with a number of adverse effects that are commonly seen after injection. Initial signs may include restlessness, panting, and pacing, followed by hypersalivation, tachycardia, abdominal pain, fever, or vomiting. Cats may additionally show signs of mydriasis, vocalizing, excessive grooming, tenesmus, or lordosis [63]. Symptoms typically last for 30 to 60 minutes after injection and decrease in severity with subsequent injections. Variable evidence of uterine evacuation may be seen after injections. Because of the risk of complications and adverse effects, animals should be hospitalized during medical management of pyometra for observation and supportive care. Resolution of clinical signs, clearing and ultimate cessation of vaginal discharge, decrease in uterine size, and resolution of neutrophilia are indications of a good response to medical management. In contrast, persistent symptoms of tachycardia, tachypnea, fever, hypothermia, depressed mentation, abdominal pain, and vomiting should raise concerns about the possibility of uterine rupture or peritonitis and should prompt immediate attention. Recently, a low-dose protocol for $PGF_{2\alpha}$ (0.02 mg/kg administered subcutaneously three times daily for 8 days) has been used successfully with fewer reported side effects [66].

Animals treated with $PGF_{2\alpha}$ should be rechecked 2 weeks after completion of treatment. The presence of purulent discharge, fever, neutrophilia, or uterine enlargement is an indication for a second 5-day course of treatment. Retrospective reports indicate that approximately 64% of dogs [52] and 95% of cats [63] with open-cervix pyometra have a good outcome after a single course of therapy, with 93% of dogs having a good response after a second 5-day course. Recurrence has been reported in up to 77% of dogs within 27 months of initial therapy [67]. Therefore, breeding is recommended on the first cycle after treatment so as to maximize the reproductive potential of the bitch and to minimize the possibility of recurrence. Once the animal is no longer used for breeding, an ovariohysterectomy should be performed.

References

[1] Concannon P, Whaley S, Lein D, et al. Canine gestation length: variation related to time of mating and fertile life of sperm. Am J Vet Res 1983;44:1819–21.
[2] Johnson CA. Disorders of pregnancy. Vet Clin N Am Small Anim Pract 1986;16:477–82.
[3] Feldman EC, Nelson RW. Breeding, pregnancy, and parturition. In: Canine and feline endocrinology and reproduction. Philadelphia: WB Saunders; 1987. p. 547–71.
[4] Gaudet DA. Retrospective study of 128 cases of canine dystocia. J Am Anim Hosp Assoc 1985;21:813–8.
[5] Copley K. Comparison of traditional methods for evaluating parturition in the bitch versus using external fetal and uterine monitoring. In: Proceedings of the Society of Theriogenology Annual Conference, Colorado Springs, CO, 2002. Society of Theriogenology. p. 375–82.
[6] Davidson AP. Uterine and fetal monitoring in the bitch. Vet Clin N Am Small Anim Pract 2001;31:305–13.

rtrt

rt2

rtrt

rtrt

[7] Concannon PW, McCann JP, Temple M. Biology and endocrinology of ovulation, pregnancy, and parturition in the dog. J Reprod Fertil Suppl 1989;39:3–25.

[8] Linde-Forsberg C, Eneroth A. Parturition. In: Simpson GM, editor. Manual of small animal reproduction and neonatology. Cheltenham: British Small Animal Veterinary Association; 1998. p. 127–42.

[9] Root MV, Johnston SD, Olson PN. Estrous length, pregnancy rate, gestation and parturition lengths, litter size, and juvenile mortality in the domestic cat. J Am Anim Hosp Assoc 1995;31:429–33.

[10] Darvelid AW, Linde-Forsberg C. Dystocia in the bitch: a retrospective study of 182 cases. J Small Anim Pract 1994;35:402–7.

[11] Eckstrand C, Linde-Forsberg C. Dystocia in the cat: a retrospective study of 155 cases. J Small Anim Pract 1994;35:459–64.

[12] Gunn-Moore DA, Thrusfield MV. Feline dystocia: prevalence, and association with cranial conformation and breed. Vet Rec 1995;136:350–3.

[13] Cruz R, Alvarado MS, Sandoval JE, et al. Prenatal sonographic diagnosis of fetal death and hydranencephaly in two Chihuahua fetuses. Vet Radiol Ultrasound 2003;44:589–92.

[14] Eneroth A, Linde-Forsberg C, Uhlhorn M, et al. Radiographic pelvimetry for assessment of dystocia in bitches: a clinical study of two terrier breeds. J Small Anim Pract 1999;40:257–64.

[15] Farrow CS, Morgan JP, Story EC. Late term fetal death in the dog: early radiographic diagnosis. J Am Vet Radiol 1976;17:11–7.

[16] Farrow CS. Maternal-fetal evaluation in suspected canine dystocia: a radiographic perspective. Can Vet J 1978;19:24–6.

[17] Verstegen JP, Silva LDM, Onclin K, et al. Echocardiographic study of heart rate in dog and cat fetuses in utero. J Reprod Fertil Suppl 1993;47:175–80.

[18] Zone MA, Wanke MM. Diagnosis of canine fetal health by ultrasonography. J Reprod Fertil Suppl 2001;57:215–9.

[19] Wray S, Kupittayanant S, Shmygol A, et al. The physiological basis of uterine contractility: a short review. Exp Physiol 2001;86:239–46.

[20] Wray S, Jones K, Kupittayanant S, et al. Calcium signaling and uterine contractility. J Soc Gynecol Investig 2003;10:252–64.

[21] Pascoe PJ, Moon PF. Periparturient and neonatal anesthesia. Vet Clin N Am Small Anim Pract 2001;31:315–41.

[22] Gilroy BA, DeYoung DJ. Caesarian section: anesthetic management and surgical technique. Vet Clin N Am Small Anim Pract 1986;16:483–93.

[23] Moon PF, Erb HN, Ludders JW, et al. Perioperative management and mortality rates of dogs undergoing cesarian section in the United States and Canada. J Am Vet Med Assoc 1998;213:365–9.

[24] Moon-Massat PF, Erb HN. Perioperative factors associated with puppy vigor after delivery by cesarian section. J Am Anim Hosp Assoc 2002;38:90–6.

[25] Funkquist PME, Nyman GC, Lofgren AMJ, et al. Use of propofol-isoflurane as an anesthetic regimen for cesarian section in dogs. J Am Vet Med Assoc 1997;211:313–7.

[26] Robbins MA, Mullen HS. En bloc ovariohysterectomy as a treatment for dystocia in dogs and cats. Vet Surg 1994;23:48–52.

[27] Moon PF, Massat BJ, Pascoe PJ. Neonatal critical care. Vet Clin N Am Small Anim Pract 2001;31:343–67.

[28] Kattwinkel J, Niermeyer S, Nadkarni V, et al. Resuscitation of the newly born infant: an advisory statement from the Pediatric Working Group of the International Liaison Committee on Resuscitation. Circulation 1999;99:1927–38.

[29] Roll C, Horsch S. Effects of doxapram on cerebral blood flow velocity in preterm infants. Neuropediatrics 2004;35:126–9.

[30] Miletich DJ, Ivankovich AD, Albrecht RF, et al. The effects of doxapram on cerebral blood flow and peripheral hemodynamics in the anesthetized and unanesthetized goat. Anesth Analg 1976;55:279–85.

[31] Wheeler SL, Weingand KW, Thrall MA, et al. Persistent uterine and vaginal hemorrhage in a beagle with factor VII deficiency. J Am Vet Med Assoc 1984;185:447–8.

[32] Padgett SL, Stokes JE, Tucker RL, et al. Hematometra secondary to anticoagulant rodenticide toxicity. J Am Anim Hosp Assoc 1998;34:437–9.

[33] Dickie MB, Arbeiter K. Diagnosis and therapy of the subinvolution of placental sites in the bitch. J Reprod Fertil Suppl 1993;47:471–5.

[34] Troxel MT, Cornetta AM, Pastor KF, et al. Severe hematometra in a dog with cystic endometrial hyperplasia/pyometra complex. J Am Anim Hosp Assoc 2002;38:85–9.

[35] Arnold S, Hubler M, Hauser B, et al. Uterine serosal inclusion cysts in a bitch. J Small Anim Pract 1996;37:235–7.

[36] Shull RM, Johnston SD, Johnston GR, et al. Bilateral torsion of uterine horns in a non-gravid bitch. J Am Vet Med Assoc 1978;172:601–3.

[37] Joshi BP, Humor A. Prepubertal metrorrhagia in bitches: a case study. Indian Vet J 1991;68: 879–80.

[38] Wallace LJ, Henry JD, Clifford JH. Manual reduction of uterine prolapse in a domestic cat. Vet Med Small Anim Clin 1970;65:595–6.

[39] Maxson FB, Krausnick KE. Dystocia with uterine prolapse in a Siamese cat. Vet Med Small Anim Clin 1969;64:1065–6.

[40] Homer BL, Altman NH, Tenzer NB. Left horn uterine torsion in a non-gravid nulliparous bitch. J Am Vet Med Assoc 1980;176:633–4.

[41] Biller DS, Haibel GK. Torsion of the uterus in a cat. J Am Vet Med Assoc 1987;191: 1128–9.

[42] Ridyard AE, Welsh EA, Gunn-Moore DA. Successful treatment of uterine torsion in a cat with severe metabolic and haemostatic complications. J Feline Med Surg 2000;2:115–9.

[43] Feldman EC, Nelson RW. Periparturient diseases. In: Canine and feline endocrinology and reproduction. Philadelphia: WB Saunders; 1987. p. 572–91.

[44] Boothe DM. Treatment of bacterial infections. In: Small animal clinical pharmacology and therapeutics. Philadelphia: WB Saunders; 2001. p. 175–221.

[45] Drobatz KJ, Casey KK. Eclampsia in dogs: 31 cases (1995–1998). J Am Vet Med Assoc 2000; 217:216–9.

[46] Fascetti AJ, Hickman MA. Preparturient hypocalcemia in four cats. J Am Vet Med Assoc 1999;215:1127–9.

[47] Austad R, Bjerkas E. Eclampsia in the bitch. J Small Anim Pract 1976;17:793–8.

[48] Aroch I, Srebro H, Shpigel NY. Serum electrolyte concentrations in bitches with eclampsia. Vet Rec 1999;145:318–20.

[49] De Bosschere H, Ducatelle R, Vermeirsch H, et al. Cystic endometrial hyperplasia-pyometra complex in the bitch: should the two entities be disconnected? Theriogenology 2001;55: 1509–19.

[50] Dow C. Experimental reproduction of the cystic hyperplasia-pyometra complex in the bitch. J Pathol Bacteriol 1959;78:267–78.

[51] De Cock H, Ducatalle R, Tilmant K, et al. Possible role of insulin-like growth factor-I in the pathogenesis of cystic endometrial hyperplasia pyometra complex in the bitch. Theriogenology 2002;57:2271–87.

[52] Nelson RW, Feldman EC. Pyometra. Vet Clin N Am Small Anim Pract 1986;16:561–75.

[53] Olsen P, Mather E. Canine vaginal and uterine bacterial flora. J Am Vet Med Assoc 1978; 172:708–11.

[54] Matsuda H, Okuda K, Fukui K, et al. Inhibitory effect of estradiol-17β and progesterone on bactericidal activity in uteri of rabbits infected with Escherichia coli. Infect Immun 1985;48: 652–7.

[55] Sandholm M, Vesenius H, Kivisto AK. Pathogenesis of canine pyometra. J Am Vet Med Assoc 1975;167:1006–10.

[56] Kenney KJ, Matthiesen DT, Brown NO, et al. Pyometra in cats: 183 cases (1979–1984). J Am Vet Med Assoc 1987;191:1130–2.

[57] Potter K, Hancock DH, Gallina AM. Clinical and pathologic features of endometrial hyperplasia, pyometra, and endometritis in cats: 79 cases(1980–1985). J Am Vet Med Assoc 1991;198:1427–31.
[58] Okano S, Tagawa M, Takase K. Relationship of the blood endotoxin concentration and prognosis in dogs with pyometra. J Vet Med Sci 1998;60:1265–7.
[59] Stone EA, Littman MP, Robertson JL, et al. Renal dysfunction in dogs with pyometra. J Am Vet Med Assoc 1988;193:457–64.
[60] Nelson RW, Feldman EC, Stabenfeldt GH. Treatment of canine pyometra and endometritis with prostaglandin $F_{2\alpha}$. J Am Vet Med Assoc 1982;181:899–903.
[61] Chaffaux S, Thibier M. Peripheral plasma concentrations of progesterone in dogs with pyometra. Ann Rec Vet 1978;9:587–92.
[62] de Schepper J, Van Der Stock J, Capiau E. Anaemia and leucocytosis in one hundred and twelve dogs with pyometra. J Small Anim Pract 1987;28:137–45.
[63] Davidson AP, Feldman EC, Nelson RW. Treatment of pyometra in cats using prostaglandin $F_{2\alpha}$:21 cases (1982–1990). J Am Vet Med Assoc 1992;200:825–8.
[64] Fantoni DT, Auler JOC, Futema F, et al. Intravenous administration of hypertonic sodium chloride solution with dextran or isotonic sodium chloride solution for treatment of septic shock secondary to pyometra in dogs. J Am Vet Med Assoc 1999;215:1283–7.
[65] Memon MA, Mickelson WD. Diagnosis and treatment of closed cervix pyometra in a bitch. J Am Vet Med Assoc 1993;203:509–12.
[66] Hubler M, Arnold S, Casal M, et al. Use of a low dose prostaglandin F_2 alpha in bitches. Schweiz Arch Tierheilkd 1991;133:323–9.
[67] Meyers-Wallen VN, Goldschmidt MH, Flickinger GL. Prostaglandin $F_{2\alpha}$ treatment of canine pyometra. J Am Vet Med Assoc 1986;189:1557–61.

ELSEVIER
SAUNDERS

Vet Clin Small Anim
35 (2005) 421–434

VETERINARY
CLINICS
Small Animal Practice

Pediatric Emergencies

Maureen Mcmichael, DVM

*Department of Small Animal Medicine and Surgery, College of Veterinary Medicine,
Texas A&M University, Mail Stop 4474, College Station, TX 77843–4474, USA*

In human medicine, neonatology is a distinct specialty from pediatrics. Veterinarians, however, are expected to treat animals from birth (and before) to geriatric stages. It is imperative for veterinarians to know normal neonate and pediatric biochemical, hematologic, radiographic, and physical examination values and to realize that many of these differ from adult values. In veterinary medicine, the term *neonate* encompasses birth to 2 weeks of age and the term *pediatric* refers to animals between 2 weeks and 6 months of age. This article reviews normal findings in neonatal and pediatric patients and discusses several common syndromes in this age group.

Pediatric and neonatal patients are afflicted with some of the same disease processes as adults, but because of their unique physiologic systems, they differ significantly in several key areas of diagnosis, monitoring, and treatment. Hemodynamic parameters, drug dosages, laboratory data, and diagnostic imaging differ significantly compared with those of adults of the same species, making interpretation a challenge. Veterinarians must be familiar with normal values in this age group to be able to assess disease processes accurately.

Initial examination and catheterization

The normal neonate should have a strong suckle reflex and should nurse and sleep constantly during the first 2 to 3 weeks. Constant crying occurs if they are prevented from nursing or do not ingest enough milk. Generally, puppies and kittens sleep after nursing if a sufficient amount was ingested. Weight gain should be progressive, with kittens gaining approximately 7 to 10 g/d. Puppies should gain 1 g/lb of anticipated adult weight per day [1]. If there is any question about milk supply in the dam, the puppies should be

E-mail address: mmcmichael@cvm.tamu.edu

doi:10.1016/j.cvsm.2004.10.004
vetsmall.theclinics.com

weighed before and after feeding on a gram scale to ensure weight gain indicative of sufficient milk ingestion.

Nutrition is crucial to neonatal health, and if an insufficient amount of milk is being ingested, there are several options. A surrogate dam is ideal if the biologic dam is unavailable, but this is often difficult to arrange. Bottle feeding and tube feeding are other options. A human infant bottle is preferred for puppies because they often cannot latch onto the smaller "kitten" nipple supplied with most replacement formulas. Tube feeding is done using a 5-French red rubber catheter for neonates weighing less than 300 g and an 8- to 10-French catheter for larger neonates and should only be done by experienced personnel [2]. Nutrition must be addressed early in neonates.

Normal body temperature in puppies is 96°F to 97°F for the first 1 to 2 weeks of life and should increase to 100°F by the end of the first month. Normal body temperature in kittens is 98°F at birth and increases to 100°F by the end of the first week [2].

Physical examination of all neonates includes an oral examination to check for a cleft palate, abdominal palpation to check for an umbilical hernia, skull palpation to check for an open fontanel, and verification of the presence of patent urogenital openings. Pain sensation is present at birth, and analgesia is essential for all procedures that are anticipated to be painful [3]. Normal heart rate (200 beats per minute [bpm]) and respiratory rate (15–35 bpm) are higher in neonates than in adults. By day 12 to 14, the eyes open, and vision normalizes by the end of the first month. A menace reflex is not present until 2 to 3 months of age [3]. In male dogs, the testes do not descend until 4 to 6 weeks of age.

When venous access is required, the intravenous route is preferred, and intravenous catheterization should be attempted first. Neonates often require small-gauge catheters (ie, 24 gauge), which can burr easily when being driven through the skin. A small skin puncture with a 20-gauge needle (while the skin is kept elevated) can be made, and the catheter can then be fed through the skin hole. This can prevent burring. If attempts at intravenous catheter placement fail, an intraosseous catheter should be placed. An intraosseous catheter can be inserted in the proximal femur or humerus using an 18- to 22-gauge spinal needle or an 18- to 25-gauge hypodermic needle. An intraosseous catheter can be used for fluid and blood administration [4]. The area must be prepared in a sterile manner, and the needle is inserted into the bone parallel to the long axis of the bone. Gently aspirate to ensure patency, and secure with a sterile bandage. An intraosseous catheter is ideal for neonates, which have a large portion of "red" marrow compared with adults, which have more "yellow" marrow consisting of fat. Intravenous access must be established as soon as possible, ideally within 2 hours, and the intraosseous catheter should be removed to minimize intraosseous infection. Intraosseous catheter complications correlate with duration of use [5].

Fluid requirements

Neonates have higher fluid requirements than adults for several reasons. They have a higher percentage of total body water, a greater surface area–to–body weight ratio, a higher metabolic rate, a decreased renal concentrating ability, and decreased body fat. Although dehydration is common, overhydration is also a serious concern, because the kidneys cannot dilute urine to rid the body of excess water [6]. The best way to monitor for under- or overhydration is to have an accurate pediatric gram scale and weigh the patient three to four times per day. Baseline thoracic radiographs are also helpful. Because the heart takes up so much of the thoracic cavity and normal neonate lungs have more interstitial fluid than adults, it can be difficult to diagnose fluid overload without baseline radiographs. Other ways to monitor fluid therapy include checking hematocrit (HCT) and total solid values. Bear in mind that the HCT decreases in normal neonates from day 1 to 28 and that total solids are lower than in adults (see section on laboratory values).

I suggest a fluid bolus of 30 to 40 mL/kg in moderately dehydrated neonates, followed by a constant rate infusion (CRI) of warm crystalloids at a rate of 80 to 100 mL/kg/d. Keep in mind that a liter of fluids warmed to 104°F cools down to room temperature (70°F) within approximately 10 minutes. A fluid warmer that is placed in the line is a good option to keep the fluids warmed. Lactated Ringer's solution may be ideal, because lactate is the preferred metabolic fuel in the neonate during times of hypoglycemia [7,8].

Laboratory values

The HCT decreases from 47.5% at birth to 29.9% by day 28 in puppies. This decrease is normal and is thought to be caused by the change from a relatively hypoxic environment to an oxygen-rich environment [9]. By the end of the first month, the HCT starts to increase again. The decrease may be caused by a lack of iron, because the nadir occurs just before weaning to solid foods containing iron. Kittens also have an HCT nadir at 4 to 6 weeks of age of 27% [10]. Knowledge of this normal decrease in HCT is essential during treatment of any neonate, and during this time, a rise in the HCT is usually indicative of significant dehydration.

Concentrations of clotting factors and antithrombin are decreased at birth but increase to normal values by the end of the first week. Prothrombin time is increased to approximately 1.3 times adult values and normalizes by 7 days. Partial thromboplastin time is also increased (1.8 times adult values) but decreases to 1.6 times adult values on day 7 [11].

In the biochemical profile, there are slight increases in bilirubin (0.5 mg/dL, normal adult range: 0–0.4 mg/dL) and dramatic increases in liver enzymes at birth in puppies. Serum alkaline phosphatase (ALP; 3845 IU/L, normal adult range: 4–107 IU/L) and γ-glutamyltransferase (GGT; 1111 IU/L, normal adult range: 0–7 IU/L) are more than 20 times greater than adult values [12]. In kittens, the ALP (123 IU/L, normal adult range: 9–42 IU/L) is three times that seen in adults. It is unclear why the liver enzymes can get so high, but colostrum is a rich source of ALP and GGT and is thought to be contributory. In fact, in goats, increases in ALP and GGT are used as indicators of successful transfer of colostrum. Bile acids are normal in puppies at birth and in kittens at 2 weeks of age [12].

Serum blood urea nitrogen (BUN), creatinine, albumin, cholesterol, and total protein are lower in neonates than in adults. Lower creatinine is thought to be caused by decreased muscle mass, and lower BUN and cholesterol are thought to be a result of immature liver function [12]. Knowledge of these values is crucial to prevent a misdiagnosis of liver disease in the neonate (elevated liver enzymes and low levels of BUN, cholesterol, and albumin can all mimic liver dysfunction).

Bone growth causes elevations in calcium and phosphorous in the young. Urine is isosthenuric in neonates, because the capacity to concentrate and dilute urine is limited in this age group [6]. This becomes a key point during fluid resuscitation attempts, because overhydration is just as much a concern as underhydration. Mean arterial pressure (MAP) is lower (49 mm Hg at 1 month of age in puppies) and normalizes (94 mm Hg) by 9 months of age [13]. Central venous pressure is higher (8 cm H_2O) at 1 month of age in puppies but decreases (2 cm H_2O) by 9 months of age [14].

Imaging and pharmacology

Radiographs can be challenging to interpret in pediatric patients if the veterinarian is not familiar with the normal anatomic differences in the young. The thymus is located in the cranial thorax on the left side and can mimic a mediastinal mass or lung consolidation on thoracic radiographs. The heart takes up more space in the thorax than it does in adults and can falsely appear enlarged. The lung parenchyma has increased water content and appears more opaque in neonates [14]. There is an absence of costochondral mineralization, causing the liver to seem to protrude further from under the rib cage than expected and making a misdiagnosis of hepatomegaly more likely. There is loss of abdominal detail because of lack of fat and a small amount of abdominal effusion, and these can hamper interpretation [14].

Differences in body fat, total protein, and albumin (a protein to which many drugs bind) and immature renal and hepatic mechanisms all contribute to differences in drug metabolism in neonates. Renal clearance of drugs is decreased in neonates. Hepatic clearance is more complicated. Drugs requiring activation via hepatic metabolism have lower plasma concentrations, whereas drugs requiring metabolism for excretion have higher plasma concentrations [15–17]. There are differences in the maturity of components of the autonomic nervous system, which can make it difficult to dose cardiac and autonomic drugs. The blood-brain barrier is more permeable in neonates, allowing drugs that do not normally cross over to enter the central nervous system (CNS) [15].

Oral drug absorption is significantly higher in the first 72 hours because of increased permeability of the gastrointestinal tract. Intestinal flora is sensitive to disruption by oral antimicrobials, and this route should be avoided in neonates. Intravenous routes seem to be the most predictable and are preferred over intramuscular or subcutaneous routes [6].

Aminoglycosides have been shown to cause histologic damage to the kidneys in neonates. Because neonate urine is isosthenuric and neonates have decreased levels of BUN and creatinine, it is difficult to monitor for renal damage, and aminoglycosides should be avoided [18]. Chloramphenicol can cause significant changes in hematopoietic parameters and should also be avoided in this age group [15,19]. Tetracyclines should be avoided because of skeletal growth abnormalities and staining of the teeth. Fluoroquinolones (eg, enrofloxacin [Baytril]) can cause destructive lesions in the cartilage of long bones [6]. Sulfonamides (eg, trimethoprim/sulfadiazine [Tribrissen]) can suppress the bone marrow [6]. Metronidazole is the preferred drug for giardiasis and anaerobes. The dose should be decreased or the dosing interval increased in neonates. β-lactam antibiotics (ie, cephalosporins) seem to be safe in neonates, but the dose interval should be increased to every 12 hours rather than every 8 hours [6].

Cardiovascular drugs (eg, epinephrine, dopamine, dobutamine) can be quite difficult to dose in neonates because of individual variations in the maturity of the autonomic nervous system. Response to treatment and continuous monitoring of hemodynamic variables are essential when using these drugs. Elevations in heart rate after administration of dopamine, dobutamine, or isoproterenol cannot be predicted until 9 to 10 weeks of age, and the response to atropine or lidocaine is decreased in the neonate [20–22].

A normal neonate respiratory rate is approximately two to three times higher than that of adults because of higher airway resistance and higher oxygen demand. Drugs that depress respiration should be avoided in neonates. Neonates have a lower percentage of contractile fibers in their myocardium than adults and do not have the ability to increase cardiac output by increasing contractility (ie, stroke volume). Because cardiac output is equal to stroke volume times heart rate, neonates must increase their heart rate to increase their cardiac output [23]. Neonates are dependent on a high heart rate to increase cardiac output, and drugs that depress heart rate should be avoided. Renal excretion of many drugs (eg, diazepam, digoxin) is diminished, thus increasing the half-life of the drug in circulation [6]. Thiopental can cause an increased response in neonates because of their lower percentage of body fat and decreased hepatic clearance. These drugs (ie, decreased clearance, increased response) should be administered at a reduced dose in neonates [1]. Opioids are a good choice for analgesia because of their reversibility, but the animal must be monitored closely because of the propensity of these drugs to depress heart and respiratory rates.

Hypoglycemia

Immature glucose feedback mechanisms make hypoglycemia a concern in neonates. There is inefficient hepatic gluconeogenesis, decreased liver glycogen stores, and loss of glucose in the urine. Urinary glucose re-absorption does not normalize until approximately 3 weeks of age in puppies [24,25]. The brain requires glucose for energy in the neonate, and brain damage can occur with prolonged hypoglycemia [25]. The fetal and neonatal myocardium uses carbohydrate (glucose) for energy rather than the long-chain fatty acids used by the adult myocardium [26]. In summary, neonates have an increased demand for, an increased loss of, and a decreased ability to synthesize glucose compared with adults.

Clinical signs of hypoglycemia can be challenging to recognize because of inefficient counterregulatory hormone release during hypoglycemia in neonates [25]. In adults, the counterregulatory hormones are released (ie, cortisol, growth hormone, glucagon, epinephrine) in response to low blood glucose and facilitate euglycemia by increasing gluconeogenesis and antagonizing insulin. Clinical signs of hypoglycemia, if seen, may include lethargy and anorexia. Vomiting, diarrhea, infection, and decreased intake all contribute to hypoglycemia in neonates. Infusions of 12.5% dextrose (ie, dilute 50% dextrose 1:4) at a rate of 1 mL/kg followed by a CRI of isotonic fluids supplemented with 1.25% to 5.0% dextrose are required to treat this condition. It is important to remember that any bolus of dextrose should be followed by a CRI that is supplemented or there is a risk of rebound hypoglycemia [27]. In addition, some neonates may have refractory hypoglycemia and may only respond to hourly boluses of dextrose in addition to a CRI of crystalloid with supplemental dextrose. Consider carnitine supplementation in these cases because it improved hypoglycemia in some studies.

Hypovolemia and dehydration

Hypovolemia results in decreased perfusion and subsequent decreases in oxygen delivery to tissues. Hypovolemia most commonly occurs in neo-nates as a result of diarrhea, vomiting, or decreased intake. In adults, hypovolemia is compensated or partially compensated for by increasing the heart rate, concentrating the urine, and decreasing urine output. In neonates, compensatory mechanisms may not be adequate or even existent. Contractile elements make up a smaller portion of the fetal myocardium (30%) compared with the adult myocardium (60%), making it difficult for the fetus to increase cardiac contractility in response to hypovolemia. Neonates also have immaturity of the sympathetic nerve fibers in the myocardium and cannot maximally increase their heart rate in response to hypovolemia. Complete maturation of the autonomic nervous system does not occur until after 8 weeks of age in puppies [23,28].

MAP is lower (49 mm Hg) in normal neonates at 2 months of age and normalizes (94 mm Hg) by 9 months of age [29]. The muscular component of the arterial wall seems to be immature at birth and is thought to be the cause of the relatively low MAP. In adults, the kidneys autoregulate blood pressure over a wide range of systemic arterial pressures. Neonates cannot do this, and the glomerular filtration rate (GFR) decreases as the systemic blood pressure decreases, making restoration of fluid volume critical in neonates [29].

Immature kidneys are incapable of concentrating urine in response to hypovolemia [30]. Appropriate concentration and dilution of urine are not seen until approximately 10 weeks of age [27,31]. The capacity to concentrate urine increases almost linearly with age during the first year of life in human beings [32]. Inefficient countercurrent mechanisms, decreased sodium resorption in the thick ascending loop of Henle, relatively short loops of Henle, and decreased urea concentration are thought to be causative [32]. Simultaneously, BUN and creatinine are lower in neonates than in adults, making monitoring of azotemia challenging.

Skin has an increased fat and decreased water content in neonates compared with adults; therefore, skin turgor cannot be used to assess dehydration. Mucous membranes remain moist in the face of severe dehydration in neonates and cannot be used to assess it adequately.

Because of neonatal fluid requirements (higher than in adults) and increased losses (eg, decreased renal concentrating ability, higher respiratory rate, higher metabolic rate), dehydration can rapidly progress to hypovolemia and shock if not adequately treated. The most common causes of hypovolemia in neonates are gastrointestinal disturbances (eg, vomiting, anorexia, diarrhea) and inadequate feeding. The most common cause of diarrhea in neonatal puppies and kittens is owner overfeeding with formula.

Because of the difficulties in adequately assessing hypovolemia in neonates, there are some assumptions that should be made. One should assume that all neonates with severe diarrhea, inadequate intake, or severe vomiting are dehydrated and potentially hypovolemic and that treatment should be initiated immediately. Treatment of hypovolemia includes fluid therapy, monitoring of electrolyte and glucose status, and nutritional support. I suggest weighing the patient at least every 12 hours, preferably every 8 hours. Dehydration is likely when the urine specific gravity reaches 1.020, and this should be monitored as an indicator of rehydration [33]. I start with a bolus of warm isotonic fluids at a rate of 45 mL/kg in severely dehydrated or hypovolemic animals. This is followed by a CRI of maintenance fluids (80 mL/kg/d), together with losses. Losses can be estimated (ie, 2 tablespoons of diarrhea is equal to 30 mL of fluid). If the neonate is hypoglycemic or not able to eat, dextrose is added to the intravenous fluids at the lowest amount that maintains normoglycemia (ie, start with 1.25% dextrose).

Sepsis

Neonatal sepsis is most often secondary to wounds, such as tail docking and umbilical cord ligation, or respiratory and gastrointestinal infections. Clinical signs, as in hypovolemia, are often subtle, and sepsis can be difficult to detect in this population for this reason. Some clinical signs that may be associated with sepsis include crying and reluctance to nurse, decreased urine output, and cold extremities. In human patients, three serial C-reactive protein (CRP) levels had a negative predictive value of 99% in neonatal sepsis. Neonates with a suspicion of sepsis had CRP levels evaluated on initial presentation and then 24 and 48 hours later. The positive predictive value of elevated CRP levels is low, however [34].

Aggressive fluid resuscitation is associated with decreased mortality in children with sepsis and in several animal models of sepsis [35]. Large volumes of fluid are often needed in septic patients because of increased capillary permeability (increased losses) and vasodilation. I start with a bolus of warm isotonic fluids at a rate of 45 mL/kg and monitor serial checks of perfusion via mucous membrane color (should be less pale), pulse quality (should get stronger), extremity temperature (should go up), lactate levels (should go down), and mentation. I often give a CRI of fresh or fresh-frozen plasma from a well-vaccinated adult dog to attempt to augment "immunity," and some have advocated giving serum from a vaccinated adult subcutaneously [36]. One study in kittens showed that intraperitoneal and subcutaneous administration of adult cat serum in three 5-mL increments (at birth, 12 hours, and 24 hours) resulted in IgG concentrations equivalent to those seen in kittens that suckled normally [37]. Frequent electrolyte and blood glucose checks are essential, with supplementation as needed. Warmth and nutrition are addressed as well.

Septic neonates that have been adequately fluid resuscitated and continue to be hypoperfused (ie, cold extremities, high lactate levels, low urine output) may benefit from inotropic support. Because of variations in the maturity of the autonomic nervous system, all inotropic drugs need to be individually tailored to each animal. Acceptable end points of perfusion include increases in extremity temperature, decreases in lactate levels, increased urine production, and improvement in attitude.

Ideally, a culture and sensitivity sample from the area of concern is submitted before beginning antibiotics. Broad-spectrum antibiotics may be required if the source of infection cannot be identified. First-generation cephalosporins are a good choice in the neonate and provide coverage for gram-positive and some gram-negative organisms.

Oxygen therapy should be kept at or below a fraction of inspired oxygen (FIO_2) of 0.4 to avoid oxygen toxicity, which is even more of a concern in neonates than in adults. Excess oxygen supplementation in neonates can cause retrolental fibroplasia, which can lead to permanent blindness [38].

Sepsis can be difficult to detect in neonates. An index of suspicion should be maintained for all neonates with risk factors, and treatment should be instituted rapidly and aggressively. In human beings, the incidence of pediatric sepsis is highest in premature newborns. Respiratory infections (37%) and primary bacteremia (25%) were the most common infections [39].

Respiratory distress of the newborn

According to the most recent guidelines on neonatal resuscitation, "ventilation of the lungs is the single most effective step in cardiopulmonary resuscitation of the compromised infant" [40]. The respiratory distress encountered at birth may be caused by pulmonary hypertension, decreased surfactant levels (prematurity), aspiration of meconium, or excess fluid in the airways. Congenital defects may cause persistent pulmonary hypertension and respiratory distress that is refractory to treatment.

Emergency treatment of a newborn in respiratory distress includes reversal of any drugs that were used during anesthesia if a cesarean section was performed. Bulb suctioning of the airways can help to clear out any accumulated fluid. Aggressive suctioning of the airways (ie, with a suctioning device) should be avoided, because it can cause a vagal response or laryngospasm. Gentle rubbing of the neonate all over can also help to stimulate respirations. Shaking or hitting the newborn is contraindicated and can cause loss of surfactant among other complications. Doxapram hydrochloride can be given under the tongue to stimulate respirations in a newborn with no respiratory drive.

Before birth, pulmonary arteries in the fetus have a higher percentage of smooth muscle than do those in the adult [41]. The elevated pulmonary vascular resistance that results causes shunting of blood from the pulmonary trunk through the patent ductus arteriosus to the aorta into the systemic circulation. Blood also reaches the systemic circulation via the foramen ovale. At birth, physical expansion of the lungs causes release of prostacyclin, which increases pulmonary blood flow through pulmonary vasodilation [42]. Nitric oxide contributes to pulmonary vasodilation and is thought to be released in response to oxygenation at birth [42].

Surfactant reduces the tension of the air-fluid interface of the alveoli and prevents collapse. It is essential to improve compliance (ie, reduce stiffness), and thus the work of breathing. Surfactant is released at birth in response to lung inflation [42]. Dramatic decreases in pulmonary vascular resistance and adequate surfactant synthesis and release are essential to neonatal survival at birth. The two most important interventions for respiratory distress at birth are oxygenation and lung expansion. These maximize the release of prostacyclin and nitric oxide and surfactant release.

Oxygen should be supplied via a face mask or endotracheal tube, because adequate lung expansion is crucial for pulmonary blood flow. A tight-fitting face mask is often easier than intubation of a newborn and can be life saving [40]. Although adequate lung expansion is essential for survival, over-expansion can cause damage; thus, it is essential to use the minimal amount of pressure for ventilation. I use an Ambu bag (Galls Emergency Medical Products, Carlsbad, CA) designed for pediatric use and intubate and ventilate if there are no spontaneous respirations at birth. The neonate should be ventilated at 40 to 60 bpm, and this should be done for approximately 30 seconds before cardiac compressions are started if required. If the chest is not expanding, check the seal on the face mask or the endotracheal tube placement, resuction the airway, or consider opening the mouth slightly in animals with small or stenotic nares (ie, bulldog pups).

Cardiopulmonary cerebral resuscitation

Cardiac compressions are recommended in human beings when the heart rate remains less than 60 bpm after 30 seconds of effective ventilation [40]. They are performed with the thumb and forefinger on either side of the thorax, with approximately 100 to 120 compressions per minute. In a piglet model of cardiac arrest, it was shown that thoracic compressions actually cause cardiac compression (versus generalized thoracic compression seen in larger animals). Intravenous access is ideal for delivery of drugs for resuscitation, but intraosseous routes also work well. Neonates have a higher proportion of red marrow than adults (who have more yellow fat marrow), making the intraosseous route ideal in the young. When an intraosseous catheter is placed, it is essential to remove it as soon as possible. In human patients, complications of intraosseous catheters are kept to a minimum by removing them within 2 hours. The goal is to use the intraosseous catheter as a bridge to increase volume and make placement of an intravenous catheter possible.

Epinephrine has both α- and β-adrenergic activity and is the first-line drug during cardiopulmonary arrest. It is started after 30 seconds of chest compressions while the animal is effectively ventilated [40]. The dose is 0.01 mg/kg for the first dose and then 0.1 mg/kg for subsequent doses. Recently, vasopressin has been advocated for cardiopulmonary arrest in human beings with asystole [43]. In a pediatric porcine model, vasopressin combined with epinephrine was superior for resuscitation compared with either drug alone [44]. Vasopressin is an accepted treatment for children with vasodilatory shock after cardiac surgery and for neonatal congestive heart failure [45,46]. It was also successful in a case series as a rescue therapy for children after prolonged cardiac arrest [47]. Vasopressin can be administered intravenously, via the endotracheal tube, or through an intraosseous catheter. The suggested dose of vasopressin for cardiopulmonary cerebral resuscitation (CPCR) is 0.8 U/kg of body weight intravenously.

Acidosis caused by decreased perfusion (ie, lactic acidosis) and decreased ventilation (ie, respiratory acidosis) is common during cardiopulmonary arrest and ideally should be addressed by treating the primary problems (ie, increasing perfusion and ventilation). Severe acidosis can decrease myocardial contractility, which could be critical in neonates, which have a lower percentage of myocardial contractile fibers than adults. It can also blunt responses to catecholamines, which is critical in neonates, which have a lower percentage of sympathetic fibers in their myocardium compared with adults. The use of buffers (eg, sodium bicarbonate) is controversial because they increase sodium levels, cause hyperosmolality, can cause paradoxic CNS and intracellular acidosis, and increase carbon dioxide. The guidelines from the American Heart Association Manual on Neonatal Advanced Life Support in human beings do not recommend bicarbonate as front-line therapy because of lack of evidence for its efficacy [48].

Glucose is the main energy substrate of the neonatal brain and myocardium and should be monitored frequently during an arrest and supplemented as needed [23]. Ionized calcium has been shown to be low in human neonates [49]. Neonates also have an increased requirement for calcium for contractility compared with adults. Calcium is not recommended for cardiopulmonary arrest in human neonates, however [48].

Head trauma

Children have a higher percentage of diffuse brain injury during trauma compared with adults, and this is thought to be a result of their greater head-to-torso ratio [50]. The neonatal brain also has a higher water content, lacks complete axonal myelinization, and may be more susceptible to hypoxia and hypotension than the adult brain [51]. There may also be a greater susceptibility to apoptosis and delayed cell death during head trauma in children compared with adults [50]. With all head trauma cases, the goals are to improve oxygen delivery, decrease intracranial pressure (ICP), and maximize cerebral perfusion pressure (CPP). Children have a lower ICP as well as a lower MAP compared with adults. Puppies also have a lower MAP, although the author is unaware of ICP values in normal puppies [52].

Because the CPP is equal to the MAP minus the ICP, it can be seen that the MAP must be kept high and the ICP kept low to maximize the CPP. Appropriate fluid therapy to keep the systolic blood pressure greater than 90 mm Hg is suggested in adult head trauma and has been associated with improved survival. Because the CPP depends on adequate cardiac output and adequate ventilation, these should be optimized in head trauma patients. Hyper- and hypoventilation should be avoided in favor of normocarbia. Hyperventilation to reduce the $Paco_2$ to less than 35 mm Hg may be helpful as a temporary bridge (usually to surgery to remove a subdural hemorrhage) in an emergency patient with impending signs of brain herniation. The resulting vasoconstriction caused by the hyperventilation can decrease the CPP in the healthy brain (because of intact autoregulation), leading to decreased oxygen delivery and hypoxia. Once volume has been addressed (ie, fluid therapy), vasopressors may be administered in human patients if the MAP is still low.

Seizures after head trauma seem to be more common in children than in adults and can occur with minimal brain damage. Elevation of the head to 30° has been suggested, but this must be done without compressing the jugular veins (ie, using a tilt table or a foam wedge). The habit of placing a rolled up towel under the neck to elevate the head is potentially dangerous, because compression of the jugular veins has been shown to increase the ICP. Jugular catheters or neck bandages should not be placed in head trauma patients. Any blood needed should be drawn from a peripheral vein or by means of a long saphenous catheter.

In people, measurement of the ICP can be made directly, but this is impractical in most veterinary situations. In adult dogs, the Cushing's reflex can be helpful in gauging increasing ICP. When the ICP increases, the systemic blood pressure rises, and as a response, the heart rate decreases. The appearance of a bradycardic hypertensive head trauma animal is highly suggestive of increased ICP. Unfortunately, this has not been evaluated in neonatal and pediatric patients. Because the autonomic nervous system does not mature until 9 to 10 weeks of age, there is reason to believe that the Cushing's reflex may be unreliable in this age group.

In summary, the magnitude of head trauma can be difficult to assess in neonatal and pediatric patients. Treatment involves optimizing systemic blood pressure using fluids and vasopressors as needed, raising the head 30° without compression of the jugular veins, and optimizing oxygenation and ventilation. The reader is referred to the article on assessment and treatment of CNS abnormalities in the emergency patient for a more in-depth discussion of head trauma.

Summary

The unique anatomic and physiologic characteristics of neonatal and pediatric patients make diagnosis, monitoring, and treatment a challenge. Adult parameters cannot be relied on in these patients, and an awareness of these unique characteristics is essential for any practitioner with a neonatal and pediatric patient base. In addition, many laboratory and pharmacologic data differ dramatically in neonates compared with adults of the same species. Familiarity with these variations is essential in the monitoring and treatment of the neonatal and pediatric illness, such as hypovolemia, shock, and sepsis.

References

[1] Murtaugh R, Kaplan P. Veterinary emergency and critical care medicine. St. Louis: Mosby; 1992.
[2] Hoskins JD. Pediatric health care and management. Vet Clin N Am Small Anim Pract 1999; 29(4):837–52.
[3] Averill DR Jr. The neurologic examination. Vet Clin N Am Small Anim Pract 1981;11(3): 511–21.
[4] Otto C, Kaufman G, Crowe D. Intraosseous infusion of fluids and therapeutics. Compend Contin Educ Pract Vet 1989;11(4):421–30.
[5] Fiser DH. Intraosseous infusion. N Engl J Med 1990;322(22):1579–81.
[6] Boothe DM, Tannert K. Special considerations for drug and fluid therapy in the pediatric patient. Compend Contin Educ Pract Vet 1992;14:313–29.
[7] Levitsky LL, Fisher DE, Paton JB, et al. Fasting plasma levels of glucose, acetoacetate, D-beta-hydroxybutyrate, glycerol, and lactate in the baboon infant: correlation with cerebral uptake of substrates and oxygen. Pediatr Res 1977;11(4):298–302.
[8] Hellmann J, Vannucci RC, Nardis EE. Blood-brain barrier permeability to lactic acid in the newborn dog: lactate as a cerebral metabolic fuel. Pediatr Res 1982;16(1):40–4.
[9] Earl FL, Melveger BE, Wilson RL. The hemogram and bone marrow profile of normal neonatal and weanling beagle dogs. Lab Anim Sci 1973;23(5):690–5.
[10] Meyers-Wallen V. Hematologic values in healthy neonatal, weanling and juvenile kittens. Am J Vet Res 1984;45:1322–7.
[11] Massicotte P, Mitchell L, Andrew M. A comparative study of coagulation systems in newborn animals. Pediatr Res 1986;20(10):961–5.
[12] Center S, Hornbuckle W. Veterinary pediatrics: dogs and cats from birth to six months. Philadelphia: WB Saunders; 1990.
[13] Magrini F. Haemodynamic determinants of the arterial blood pressure rise during growth in conscious puppies. Cardiovasc Res 1978;12(7):422–8.
[14] Partington B. Diagnostic imaging techniques. In: Hoskins JD, editor. Veterinary pediatrics: dogs and cats from birth to six months. Philadelphia: WB Saunders; 1995. p. 7–21.
[15] Boothe DM. Special consideration for drug and fluid therapy in the pediatric patient. Compend Contin Educ Pract Vet 1992;14(3):313–29.
[16] Short CR. Drug disposition in neonatal animals. J Am Vet Med Assoc 1984;184(9):1161–2.
[17] Peters E, Farber T, Heider A. The development of drug metabolizing enzymes in the young dog [abstract 2040]. Fed Proc Am Soc Biol 1971;30:560.
[18] Cowan RH, Jukkola AF, Arant BS Jr. Pathophysiologic evidence of gentamicin nephrotoxicity in neonatal puppies. Pediatr Res 1980;14(11):1204–11.
[19] Plumb D. Veterinary drug handbook. White Bear Lake, MN: Pharma Vet Publishing; 1991.
[20] Driscoll DJ, Gillette PC, Lewis RM, et al. Comparative hemodynamic effects of isopro-terenol, dopamine, and dobutamine in the newborn dog. Pediatr Res 1979;13(9):1006–9.
[21] Mary-Rabine L, Rosen MR. Lidocaine effects on action potentials of Purkinje fibers from neonatal and adult dogs. J Pharmacol Exp Ther 1978;205(1):204–11.
[22] Woods WT, Urthaler F, James TN. Progressive postnatal changes in sinus node response to atropine and propranolol. Am J Physiol 1978;234(4):H412–5.
[23] Textile D, Hoffman JIE. Ventricular function. In: Glickman PD, Heyman MA, editors. Pediatrics and perinatology: the scientific basis. London: Arnold; 1996. p. 737–48.
[24] Bovie KC. Genetic and metabolic diseases of the kidney. In: Canine nephrology. Philadelphia: Harel Publishing; 1984. p. 339–54.
[25] Atkins C. Disorders of glucose homeostasis in neonatal and juvenile dogs: hypoglycemia— part 1. Compend Contin Educ Pract Vet 1984;6(2):197–204.
[26] Textile D, Hoffman JIE. Coronary circulation and myocardial oxygen consumption. In: Glickman PD, Heyman MA, editors. Pediatrics and perinatology: the scientific basis. London: Arnold; 1996. p. 731–6.

[27] Holster M, Keeler BJ. Intracortical distribution of number and volume of glomeruli during postnatal maturation in the dog. J Clin Invest 1971;50:796–800.

[28] Mace SE, Levy MN. Neural control of heart rate: a comparison between puppies and adult animals. Pediatr Res 1983;17:491–5.

[29] Margin F. Hemodynamic determinants of the arterial blood pressure rise during growth in conscious puppies. Cardiol Res 1978;12:422–8.

[30] Kleegman LI, Lube RJ. Factors affecting maturation of the glomerular filtration rate and renal plasma flow in the newborn dog. J Physio 1972;223:395–409.

[31] Fetuin M, Allen T. Development aspects of fluid and electrolyte metabolism and renal function in neonates. Compend Contin Educ Pract Vet 1991;13(4):392–402.

[32] Aporia A. Regulation of water balance. In: Glickman PD, Heyman MA, editors. Pediatrics and perinatology: the scientific basis. London: Arnold; 1996. p. 959–60.

[33] McIntire D. Pediatric intensive care. Vet Clin N Am Small Anim Pract 1999;29:837–52.

[34] Benitz WE, Han MY, Madan A, et al. Serial serum C-reactive protein levels in the diagnosis of neonatal infection [abstract]. Pediatrics 1998;102(4):E41.

[35] Thomas NJ, Carcillo JA. Hypovolemic shock in pediatric patients. New Horiz 1998;6(2): 120–9.

[36] Poffenbarger EM, Olson PN, Chandler ML, et al. Use of adult dog serum as a substitute for colostrum in the neonatal dog. Am J Vet Res 1991;52(8):1221–4.

[37] Levy JK, Crawford PC, Collante WR, et al. Use of adult cat serum to correct failure of passive transfer in kittens. J Am Vet Med Assoc 2001;219(10):1401–5.

[38] Jenkins S. Oxygen toxicity. J Crit Care Med 1988;3:137–52.

[39] Watson RS, Carcillo JA, Linde-Zwirble WT, et al. The epidemiology of severe sepsis in children in the United States. Am J Respir Crit Care Med 2003;167(5):695–701.

[40] Aggarwal R, Paul VK, Deorari AK. Latest guidelines on neonatal resuscitation. Indian J Pediatr 2003;70(1):51–5.

[41] Krauss AN. New methods advance treatment for respiratory distress syndrome. Pediatr Ann 2003;32(9):585–91.

[42] Soifer S. Specific circulations. In: Gluckman P, Heyman MA, editors. Pediatrics and perinatology: the scientific basis. London: Arnold; 1996. p. 749–61.

[43] Wenzel V, Krismer AC, Arntz HR, et al. A comparison of vasopressin and epinephrine for out-of-hospital cardiopulmonary resuscitation. N Engl J Med 2004;350(2):105–13.

[44] Voelckel WG, Wenzel V, Lindner KH. Is one drug enough? Arginine vasopressin in pediatric cardiopulmonary resuscitation. Resuscitation 2002;52(2):157–8.

[45] Stewart JM, Zeballos GA, Woolf PK, et al. Variable arginine vasopressin levels in neonatal congestive heart failure. J Am Coll Cardiol 1988;11(3):645–50.

[46] Rosenzweig EB, Starc TJ, Chen JM, et al. Intravenous arginine-vasopressin in children with vasodilatory shock after cardiac surgery. Circulation 1999;100(19 Suppl):II182–6.

[47] Mann K, Berg RA, Nadkarni V. Beneficial effects of vasopressin in prolonged pediatric cardiac arrest: a case series. Resuscitation 2002;52(2):149–56.

[48] Niermeyer S, Kattwinkel J, Van Reempts P, et al. International Guidelines for Neonatal Resuscitation: An excerpt from the Guidelines 2000 for Cardiopulmonary Resuscitation and Emergency Cardiovascular Care: International Consensus on Science. Contributors and Reviewers for the Neonatal Resuscitation Guidelines [abstract]. Pediatrics 2000;106(3):E29.

[49] Singhi SC, Singh J, Prasad R. Hypocalcaemia in a paediatric intensive care unit. J Trop Pediatr 2003;49(5):298–302.

[50] Mazzola CA, Adelson PD. Critical care management of head trauma in children. Crit Care Med 2002;30(11 Suppl):S393–401.

[51] Adelson PD, Clyde B, Kochanek PM, et al. Cerebrovascular response in infants and young children following severe traumatic brain injury: a preliminary report. Pediatr Neurosurg 1997;26(4):200–7.

[52] Magrini F. Haemodynamic determinants of the arterial blood pressure rise during growth in conscious puppies. Cardiovasc Res 1978;12(7):422–8.

ELSEVIER
SAUNDERS

Vet Clin Small Anim
35 (2005) 435–453

VETERINARY
CLINICS
Small Animal Practice

Anesthetic Protocols for Common Emergencies

Vicki L. Campbell, DVM

James L. Voss Veterinary Teaching Hospital, Colorado State University,
300 West Drake Road, Fort Collins, CO 80523–1620, USA

It is often necessary to perform anesthesia and sedation in the emergency patient to obtain diagnostics or perform minor procedures. In addition, pain control is essential in treating animals with traumatic injuries, painful medical conditions, or surgical disorders. Thorough knowledge and understanding of the drugs used in anesthesia, sedation, and pain management are required to choose a safe yet effective protocol.

Sedating or anesthetizing the emergency patient is a task that should be taken seriously and with precaution. Many animals that are presented to the emergency room are in shock or are on the verge of going into shock. The sympathetic nervous system is stimulated in the emergency situation in an attempt to maintain blood flow and oxygen delivery to the tissues. Almost all anesthetics blunt the response of the sympathetic nervous system. Therefore, the patient that is in compensatory shock may decompensate when given a sedative or anesthetic agent. In addition to interfering with the cardiovascular system, sedatives and anesthetics can compromise the respiratory system, which could be detrimental to a patient that is in respiratory distress.

Pain control in the emergency patient should be a high priority. Pain can adversely affect a patient by causing potentially detrimental sympathetic stimulation. If pain is left uncontrolled for extensive periods, the pain becomes more difficult to treat as the result of a phenomenon called "wind-up" [1]. A painful animal is also more difficult to assess and may put animal handlers at risk for misdirected aggression from the patient.

The goal of this article is to familiarize the reader with the various drugs that are used during sedation, anesthesia, and pain management and to present several common emergency sedation and anesthetic scenarios.

E-mail address: vcampbel@lamar.colostate.edu

Sedation

Sedation is defined as an awake but calm state in which an animal can be aroused [2,3]. The term *sedation* is sometimes used interchangeably with the term *tranquilization* [3]. Sedation is not a form of "light" anesthesia and technically should not be used in this fashion. There are only three classes of true sedatives that are commonly used in small animal veterinary medicine. These include the benzodiazepines, phenothiazines, and α_2-agonists [2,3]. A list of the "pros" and "cons" of each of the aforementioned drug categories is found in Table 1. The butyrophenones are also sedatives but are not currently used commonly in small animal medicine and are not discussed. The opioids are not technically considered sedatives but are commonly used in sedation protocols because they have sedative properties in addition to their ability to control pain.

In the emergency setting, the safest sedatives are cardiopulmonary sparing, titratable, and reversible. Phenothiazines and α_2-agonists can cause significant cardiovascular compromise and hypotension; therefore, these drugs are not recommended for sedation in an unstable or hypotensive critical patient (see Table 1) [2–7]. This is true even though the α_2-agonists are reversible. In addition, acepromazine causes significant splenic sequestration of red blood cells [5] as well as leading to potential platelet dysfunction, and it is not recommended in anemic or bleeding patients [5]. The benzodiazepines are cardiopulmonary sparing and reversible, making a nice addition to emergency sedation (see Table 1) [2–4]. Adding an opioid to a benzodiazepine is probably one of the safest sedative combinations that can be used in an emergency situation. The pros and cons of various opioids are listed in Table 2 [2–4]. Combining an opioid with a sedative or tranquilizer is termed *neuroleptanalgesia* [2,3].

Keep in mind that there is no perfect way to sedate a patient. The availability of the drug, familiarity with the drug, procedure being performed, and ability to monitor the patient for complications all contribute to the relative "safeness" of a drug. Remember the familiar saying by Robert Smith: "There are no safe anesthetic agents; there are no safe anesthetic procedures; there are only safe anesthetists" [3].

General anesthesia

Many veterinarians would prefer general anesthesia as opposed to true sedation in the emergency patient to treat or diagnose the problem. This is because most animals that are truly sedated are still arousable during minor surgical procedures, which may be undesirable. A balanced anesthesia technique that uses several different drug types to reduce the overall amount of anesthetics needed is a safe approach to general anesthesia in the emergency patient. Unfortunately, all general anesthetics have the potential to cause some cardiopulmonary compromise.

Table 1
Pros and cons of common sedatives and tranquilizers

Pros	Cons
Benzodiazepines: diazepam, midazolam	
Cardiopulmonary sparing	May cause excitement in cats/some dogs
Amnestic	Effects may be prolonged with liver disease
Midazolam is water soluble	Diazepam is not water soluble,
(can be given IM or SQ	which may cause unreliable
with reliable absorption)	IM or SQ absorption
Mild tranquilization/anxiolytic	Diazepam is painful on IM injection
Decreases MAC	Diazepam may cause sterile
	abscessation if given IM
Reversible with flumazenil	Midazolam is expensive
Good muscle relaxation	No analgesia
Anticonvulsant	
Phenothiazines: acepromazine	
Good sedative	Not reversible
Lowers threshold for arrhythmias	Hypotension (α-blockade, vasodilation)
Antiemetic (centrally	Platelet aggregation inhibition
antidopaminergic)	Long acting, especially with liver disease
	Mild respiratory depressant
	No analgesia
	Lowers seizure threshold in epileptics
α_2-agonists: xylazine, medetomidine	
Excellent sedation	Hypertension (α_1 and α_2 stimulation,
	vasoconstriction), followed by hypotension
	(central sympathetic blockade resulting
	in decreased cardiac output)
Excellent muscle relaxation	Severe bradycardia (reflex bradycardia
	and central sympathetic blockade)
Mild analgesia (especially GI pain)	May cause emesis
Reversible with yohimbine	First, second, or third degree AV block
or atipamezole	Increased sensitivity to
	catecholamine-induced arrhythmias
	May cause stridor in brachycephalic breeds
	Depresses respiratory center
	Promotes diuresis
	Inhibits insulin, hyperglycemia may result

Abbreviations: AV, atrioventricular; GI, gastrointestinal; IM, intramuscular; MAC, maximum allowable concentration; SQ, subcutaneous.
Data from Refs. [2–7].

General anesthesia is technically defined as loss of consciousness, muscle relaxation, immobility, and analgesia [2,3]. To obtain an anesthetic plane, the addition of an injectable or inhalation anesthetic agent to neuroleptanalgesia is frequently used in the emergency setting. The key term to remember during anesthesia of the emergency patient is *titration*. Allow a little more time than usual for the drug to take effect, because it takes longer for the drug to circulate and reach effective brain concentrations if cardiac output is significantly decreased. Regardless of the drug that is used

Table 2
Pros and cons of common opioids

Pros	Cons
Pure agonists: morphine, hydromorphone, oxymorphone, fentanyl, meperidine, methadone	
Excellent analgesia/euphoria	Dysphoria
Reversible with naloxone, naltrexone	Panting
Mild cardiopulmonary effects (bradycardia and decreased respiratory rate, dose dependent)	Decreased GI motility
Synergistic with tranquilizers/sedatives	Controlled drugs (schedule II)
	Morphine and meperidine can cause histamine release when given IV
	Vomiting
	Excitement/aggression in some cats
Partial agonists and agonist/antagonists: buprenorphine, butorphanol	
Tend to cause less dysphoria than pure agonists	May be less analgesic than pure agonists
Butorphanol can be used in small doses to antagonize dysphoric effects of pure agonists	Butorphanol is short acting (1–2 hours)
Buprenorphine is long lasting (6–8 hours) and can be given orally/buccally to cats	Controlled drugs (schedule III and IV)
Butorphanol is the most potent cough suppressant of all the opioids	
Less likely to cause vomiting than pure opioids	
Good analgesic effect without significant dysphoria in cats	

Abbreviations: GI, gastrointestinal; IV, intravenous.
Data from Refs. [1–4,36–38].

to induce general anesthesia, injectable anesthetics may cause significant cardiopulmonary compromise, even at low doses.

The four most commonly used injectable anesthetics are propofol, thiopental, ketamine, and etomidate (Table 3) [2–4]. A common misconception is that propofol is a safe general anesthetic. Propofol is a useful anesthetic because of its quick redistribution, rapid induction and recovery, and lack of accumulation with repeated doses. If used improperly (ie, too high a dose or given too quickly), however, it can cause apnea and significant hypotension. In fact, propofol (2.5 mg/kg administered intravenously) has been shown to cause longer lasting respiratory depression than thiopental (4.0 mg/kg administered intravenously) in healthy human beings [8]. A study in dogs found that the cardiorespiratory effects of propofol are similar to those of thiopental, with the main advantage of propofol being a rapid smooth recovery [9]. Lastly, one study found that animals given propofol were 3.8 times more likely to develop postoperative

Table 3
Pros and cons of intravenous general anesthetics

Pros	Cons
Propofol	
Rapidly acting general anesthetic	Hypotension (vasodilation)
Rapidly metabolized and redistributed	Respiratory depression/apnea
No cumulative effect with repeat administration	No analgesia
Easily titratable	May cause muscle twitching
	May cause pain on IV injection
	IV route only
	Can cause Heinz body anemia in cats
	May predispose to wound infection
Ketamine	
Water soluble, can be given IM	May cause apneustic breathing pattern
Rapid anesthesia	Causes myocardial depression if animal is catecholamine depleted, which may lead to hypotension
Supports cardiovascular system (direct sympathetic stimulation), may increase blood pressure and heart rate	Increases intracranial pressure
Analgesic	Increases salivary secretions
Good anesthetic in cats	Hallucinatory
	Painful on IM injection
	Metabolized by liver in dogs and excreted unchanged in urine in cats
	Not reversible
Etomidate	
Cardiopulmonary sparing	Expensive
Hypnotic	May cause vomiting
Sparing to brain circulation	May cause twitching
	Suppresses adrenocortical axis
	Propylene glycol base, may cause hemolysis
	IV route only
Barbiturates: thiopental	
Relatively cardiopulmonary sparing	May cause arrhythmias
Maintains cerebral blood vessel response to carbon dioxide	May cause transient apnea
Short acting	Cumulative with repeat doses
Inexpensive	Liver metabolized, recoveries may be prolonged with liver disease
	Causes sloughing if extravasation occurs
	Cumulative with repeat dosing

Abbreviations: IM, intramuscular; IV, intravenous.
Data from Refs. [2–4,8–17].

wound infections compared with animals not receiving propofol for anesthetic induction [10].

Thiopental seems to have experienced a significant reduction in popularity since propofol has become so readily available in veterinary medicine. Recall that thiopental is an ultra–short-acting barbiturate and that its short duration of action is a result of redistribution. If given in repeat boluses, however, it accumulates and leads to a prolonged recovery [2–4]. Thiopental does sensitize the heart to catecholamine-induced arrhythmias [11]. A nice combination is to use a 1:1 combination of propofol and thiopental (17.5-mg/mL solution given intravenously at 1.5-mg/kg boluses to effect), which reduces the amount of both drugs that are given, has similar cardiorespiratory effects compared with propofol or thiopental alone, and leads to smooth induction and recovery [12].

Many veterinarians think that ketamine is a safe anesthetic drug in the emergency setting because it "supports" the cardiovascular system. Ketamine causes direct central nervous system stimulation, leading to increased sympathetic outflow and increased heart rate and blood pressure [13]. In the isolated denervated myocardium, however, it is a direct myocardial depressant [3]. Therefore, in the animal that is already catecholamine depleted, ketamine depresses the cardiovascular system. Experimentally, ketamine has been shown to decrease cardiac output and ventricular contractility in critically ill human patients [14]. In a study in hypovolemic swine, ketamine failed to show any advantage cardiovascularly compared with thiopental [15]. In healthy dogs that received ketamine-diazepam induction, there were no pressor or cardiovascular stimulating effects detected and there were few differences between the ketamine-diazepam induction and thiopentone induction [16]. Ketamine is not reversible and should not be used in animals with cardiac disease. It should be used with caution in critically ill patients, and the veterinarian should be aware of that fact that ketamine does not necessarily support the cardiovascular system.

Etomidate is used infrequently in the private veterinary sector because of its expense. It is probably the most cardiovascularly sparing general anesthetic available but is not without some drawbacks [2,3]. It can lead to rough induction if the animal is not properly premedicated and frequently causes vomiting or retching. Intubation may be difficult, because the airway maintains function and is frequently reactive during intubation. It can cause transient, albeit significant, adrenocortical suppression for several hours after a bolus dose in the dog and cat [17,18]. This adrenocortical suppression could potentially become detrimental in an animal that is catecholamine depleted from Addison's disease or from chronic critical illness.

Inhalation agents are usually quickly titratable and have little systemic metabolism, which may be desirable in the emergency setting. Inhalant anesthetics can cause significant hypotension by decreasing cardiac output and causing peripheral vasodilation, however [2,3]. Therefore, they must be used with caution and with proper patient monitoring.

If general anesthesia is planned, the airway should be controlled via intubation and oxygen provided. Many emergency patients are presented with a full stomach and are at high risk for aspiration if they vomit or regurgitate during a procedure, making airway protection crucial. Monitoring of the anesthetized patient is discussed in further detail elsewhere in this article.

Anticholinergics

The decision to add an anticholinergic to the sedative or anesthetic protocol is controversial. The pros and cons of anticholinergics need to be weighed (Table 4) [2–4]. Procedures that cause significant vagal stimulation should be recognized, and the patient should be preemptively treated with an anticholinergic in these situations. Types of procedures that may stimulate significant vagal reflexes include ocular surgery or manipulation; esophagostomy tube placement; manipulation of the gastrointestinal, urinary, or genital tract; joint capsule manipulation; or chest tube placement. Regardless of the decision about whether to give an anticholinergic, one should always be available and a dose ready to be given intravenously if a problem arises with bradycardia.

Pain management

Pain management in the emergency patient should be the routine standard of care and not an optional treatment. Excessive pain has been shown to be detrimental to animals, leading to the wind-up phenomenon, adverse sympathetic stimulation, and immunosuppression [1]. There are five ways to interrupt the pain pathway. The five components of the pain pathway are transduction (at the receptor level in the periphery), transmission (the afferent nerve going to the spinal cord), modulation (at the level of the spinal cord), projection (to the brain), and assimilation (at the brain and descending pathways) [1]. Nonsteroidal anti-inflammatory drugs (NSAIDS) and local anesthetics prevent transduction. Local anesthetics can prevent transmission. Epidural analgesics can prevent modulation

Table 4
Pros and cons of anticholinergics

Pros	Cons
Atropine and glycopyrrolate	
Increases heart rate	May cause tachycardia and increase myocardial oxygen consumption
Antisialagogue (glyco > atropine)	Decreased GI motility
Glycopyrrolate does not cross BBB or placental barrier	At low doses, may cause AV block
Decreases response to vagal stimulation	Mydriasis
Bronchodilation	

Abbreviations: AV, atrioventricular; BBB, blood-brain barrier; GI, gastrointestinal.
Data from Refs. [2–4].

at the level of the spinal cord. Effective analgesics given epidurally include opioids, local anesthetics, ketamine, and α_2-agonists. Parenteral administration of opioids and low-dose ketamine also helps with modulation. Opioids, α_2-agonists, and ketamine all can effect projection and assimilation in the brain [1].

Opioids are the most effective means of achieving short-term quick analgesia (see Table 2) [1–4]. Constant rate infusions (CRIs) of opioids are a great way to prevent "rollercoaster" analgesia if analgesia is needed long term and allow easy titration for each animal. The addition of ketamine via a low-dose CRI, in conjunction with opioid therapy, helps to prevent the wind-up phenomenon, enhances the analgesic effects of opioids, and is an excellent way to control pain [19,20]. A low dose or analgesic dose of ketamine does not tend to have cardiopulmonary or dissociative side effects [19]. Low-dose intravenous CRIs of lidocaine in conjunction with other analgesics may decrease the pain threshold [21,22]. In addition, local infiltration of local anesthetics is a nice adjunct to pain control. The toxic doses of local anesthetics should be kept in mind when using local anesthetics. Low-dose use of α_2-agonists, such as medetomidine, may aid in pain control [23,24], but the cardiovascular effects of medetomidine still occur even when given in microdoses [25]. NSAIDS are an excellent means of pain control if pain is inflammation mediated (Table 5) [1]. Keep in mind that NSAIDS may interfere with platelet function and may compromise kidney function [1,4]; thus, they should not be given to an actively bleeding animal, an animal in shock, or an animal with renal failure.

Monitoring

Before sedation or anesthesia, it is wise to obtain an extended database on the patient. This would ideally consist of packed cell volume (PCV), total protein, blood glucose, blood urea nitrogen (BUN), electrolytes, lactate, acid-base status, urine specific gravity, ECG, blood pressure, and pulse oximetry. Whenever possible, it is highly recommended to have immediate

Table 5
Pros and cons of nonsteroidal anti-inflammatory drugs

Pros	Cons
Carprofen, aspirin, deracoxib, tepoxalin, meloxicam, ketoprofen	
Anti-inflammatory	GI upset/ulceration
May decrease wind-up phenomenon	Decreased renal blood flow
Good analgesics	Possible liver/kidney damage
	Platelet dysfunction
	Should be avoided if steroids are given

Abbreviation: GI, gastrointestinal.
Data from Refs. [1,4].

intravenous access via a patent intravenous or intraosseous catheter before sedation or anesthesia. If the patient is fractious or is severely distressed by attempts to gain access intravenously, it is reasonable to administer a subcutaneous or intramuscular premedication before intravenous or intraosseous catheter placement. Because of the fragile nature of emergency patients, clients should be properly forewarned about the pros and cons of sedation or anesthesia in their pet.

Regardless of why an emergency patient is being sedated or anesthetized, there are several general principles that should be applied to every patient to ensure safety during the procedure. The safest way to approach emergency sedation or anesthesia is to have a person dedicated to monitoring the animal, because these animals are typically dynamic; therefore, their status can change dramatically from minute to minute. In addition, an anesthetic record should be kept, and at the absolute minimum, the pulse rate, respiration rate, and blood pressure should be recorded every 5 minutes, as outlined in the American College of Veterinary Anesthesiologists (ACVA) guidelines for anesthetic management. Temperature monitoring, eye lubrication, and intravenous fluid therapy should also be standard practice.

Airway management is crucial. All patients should be given supplemental oxygen during the procedure. This maximizes oxygen delivery to the tissues, which is especially important in an already compromised patient. Many of these animals have not been fasted and are prone to vomiting or regurgitation and subsequent aspiration if the airway is not protected. If general anesthetics, such as propofol, are used, the animal should be intubated and the endotracheal cuff inflated. This allows the airway to be protected from aspiration as well providing the opportunity to ventilate the patient if needed.

Cardiovascular monitoring is just as essential as respiratory monitoring. A means of obtaining a true pulse or heart beat should be used. This may consist of a person feeling for a pulse continuously, an audible Doppler pulse, use of a traditional stethoscope on the chest, use of an esophageal stethoscope, or pulse oximetry. ECG monitoring is extremely helpful and can aid in the diagnosis of arrhythmias. It should not be relied on as the sole means of cardiovascular monitoring, however, because electrical activity can continue in a fairly normal fashion for several minutes after mechanical function of the heart has ceased (known as pulseless electrical activity [PEA]).

Blood pressure monitoring via use of indirect measurements is extremely useful in determining if a patient is hypotensive. Doppler blood pressure monitors or the use of an oscillometric blood pressure machine has been validated in small animals and provides tremendous insight into the blood pressure status of an animal [26–32]. Traditionally, oscillometric blood pressure monitors have been unreliable in the cat [30]. In cats, the recently validated Cardell oscillometric blood pressure monitor (Cardell Veterinary Blood Pressure Monitor 9301V, CAS Medical Systems, Inc., Branford, CT) [32] has proven to be extremely useful in the emergency situation, however.

Pulse oximetry is a useful tool in determining hemoglobin saturation, in addition to monitoring pulse rate [33–35]. Pulse oximetry has inherent limitations, and various situations, such as excess ambient light, poor perfusion, or excess motion, may interfere with the reading. The limitations of the pulse oximeter should be known, and if a reading seems to be unacceptable, it should be verified with an arterial blood gas measurement.

Capnography is helpful to use in the intubated patient and can provide insight into the ventilatory status of the patient [35]. In addition, when cardiac output falls dramatically (as seen with cardiac arrest), the end-tidal carbon dioxide concentration drops to less than 10 mm Hg and may be the first clue to the anesthetist that cardiac arrest has occurred or is imminent. As with pulse oximetry, capnography has its limitations, and any aberrant readings should be verified with an arterial blood gas measurement.

Case studies

The following are case studies of common emergencies that may require sedation, anesthesia, or extensive pain management. Keep in mind that there is no set way to approach a specific scenario and that each protocol needs to be tailored to the individual patient. In addition, many drugs have similar actions (eg, various opioids), and choosing one drug over another may be a matter of availability, experience, individual patient needs, and personal preference (Table 6).

Although many emergency situations may require immobilization of a patient to ensure proper treatment, the need to sedate or anesthetize an emergency patient should be seriously reconsidered in patients with head trauma, shock, pulmonary contusions, chest trauma, or a recent meal.

Case 1

A 2-year-old, male, castrated Labrador Retriever named "Buster" is presented to the emergency room 30 minutes after being hit by a car. The owners report that he initially stood up after being hit, ran into yard (but was not using one of the hind limbs), and then collapsed. According to the owners, he has had no previous medical problems; has not urinated since the accident; has had no evidence of vomiting, diarrhea, coughing, or sneezing since the accident; and last ate approximately 6 hours ago.

On physical examination, Buster's heart rate is 180 beats per minute (bpm) with weak pulses, his respiratory rate is 40 breaths per minute with lung sounds present in all fields, and his mucous membranes are pale pink with a capillary refill time of 3 seconds. He has no evidence of abdominal pain on palpation, has a small palpable bladder, and is laterally recumbent.

Table 6
Drug doses

Drug	Dose
Diazepam	0.2–0.5 mg/kg IV bolus
Midazolam	0.2–0.5 mg/kg IV, IM, or SQ
Acepromazine	0.01–0.02 mg/kg IV, IM, or SQ (avoid if possible)
Medetomidine	1–10 µg/kg IV, IM or SQ (avoid if possible)
Xylazine	0.2–0.5 mg/kg IV, IM or SQ (avoid if possible)
Atropine	0.01–0.02 mg/kg IM, SQ, or IV (IV dosing may cause tachycardia)
Glycopyrrolate	0.005–0.01 mg/kg IM, SQ, or IV
Propofol	1-mg/kg IV boluses slowly to effect (watch for apnea and hypotension)
Ketamine	2-mg/kg boluses IV to effect, 4–6 mg/kg IM
Ketamine CRI	0.1-mg/kg IV loading dose, then 2 µg/kg/min (0.1 mg/kg/h) CRI (for pain management)
Etomidate	0.2-mg/kg boluses IV to effect, dilute 50:50 in saline in cats or in animals with renal disease to avoid hemolysis
Thiopental	2–4 mg/kg boluses IV to effect
Morphine	0.2–1 mg/kg IM or SQ (use low dose in cats)
Morphine CRI	0.3-mg/kg IV loading dose (slowly to avoid histamine release), then 0.1 mg/kg/h
Epidural morphine	0.1 mg/kg epidurally with saline or bupivacaine, use preservative-free morphine in epidural space (eg, Duramorph)
Hydromorphone	0.025–0.2 mg/kg (most common range is 0.05–0.1 mg/kg) IV, IM, or SQ (use low dose in cats)
Hydromorphone CRI	0.01–0.04 mg/kg/h CRI (use low dose in cats)
Oxymorphone	0.05–0.1 mg/kg IV, IM, or SQ
Butorphanol	0.2–0.4 mg/kg IV, IM, or SQ
Butorphanol CRI	0.1–0.2 mg/kg/h (excellent in cats)
Buprenorphine	6–10 µg/kg IV, IM, or SQ; can be given orally on buccal membrane surface in cats
Lidocaine CRI	20–30 µg/kg/min CRI (for pain management)
Naloxone	0.01–0.02 mg/kg IV, IM, or SQ
Flumazenil	0.01–0.02 mg/kg IV, IM, or SQ (expensive)

Drug doses are suggestions for sedation, analgesia, and routes of administration in the emergency patient. Cats tend to do better at the low end of the dose range with most of the drugs, especially the benzodiazepines and opioids. If the patient is unstable, start with the lower end of the dose range and titrate to effect.

Abbreviations: CRI, constant rate infusion; IM, intramuscular; IV, intravenous; SQ, subcutaneous.

Data from Refs. [1–4].

His pupillary light reflexes are normal, and he has a normal pupil size. There is evidence of a right tibial fracture on palpation, and he has a 5-cm deep laceration over the right humerus that continues to bleed and is contaminated with gravel.

After two one-quarter shock doses of intravenous crystalloids and flow-by oxygen, the heart rate has decreased to 130 bpm and the respiratory rate is 24 breaths per minute. Because Buster has seemed to respond well to initial stabilization, it is decided that he needs to have a Robert Jones bandage placed for the tibia fracture and that the laceration needs to be aggressively cleaned and the bleeding stopped.

This situation is ideal for the use of neuroleptanalgesia. Intravenous hydromorphone (0.05–0.2 mg/kg) and diazepam (0.2–0.5 mg/kg) can provide excellent sedation and analgesia in this patient. In addition, this combination is cardiopulmonary sparing, which is important in a patient that was recently in hypovolemic shock. It is important to have an anticholinergic, such as atropine (0.02 mg/kg) drawn up in case it is needed quickly. Local block of the laceration with lidocaine at a maximum of dose of 2 mg/kg can help with analgesia during manipulation of the wound over the humerus.

This protocol is likely to allow placement of a Robert Jones bandage and flushing of the wound. If minor surgery is required on the laceration or the broken leg needs to be significantly manipulated, however, general anesthesia may need to be instituted. In this situation, a low dose of propofol (1–2 mg/kg boluses administered intravenously slowly to effect for intubation) could be used for intubation, followed by an inhalational anesthetic, such as isoflurane.

After provision of anesthesia, a one-time dose of an NSAID may help with analgesia (injectable carprofen, 4 mg/kg). The dog should be appropriately volume resuscitated and not have evidence of kidney or liver dysfunction before giving the NSAID. Long-term analgesia for the leg fracture may consist of a low-dose ketamine CRI at a rate of 2 μg/kg/min in conjunction with an opioid CRI of fentanyl or hydromorphone. Alternatively, an intermittent long-acting injectable opioid, such as morphine, could be used subcutaneously or intramuscularly. The addition of a fentanyl patch may aid in analgesia, but keep in mind that this is an adjunctive analgesia therapy and does not take effect for 12 to 24 hours [36]. An epidural injection of preservative-free morphine (given while the dog is under general anesthesia) is another option for pain management of the fractured tibia in this dog.

Case 2

"Tommy," a 3-year-old, male, castrated domestic short hair cat, is presented to the emergency hospital for stranguria for 48 hours. The owners have not seen any urine production for the past 24 hours, and the cat has been lethargic and anorexic for the past day. Tommy has not had a history of urinary problems and was negative for feline leukemia virus (FeLV) and feline immunodeficiency virus (FIV) as a kitten. He is an indoor-only cat and has no other past pertinent medical history.

On physical examination he is estimated to be approximately 5% dehydrated, with tacky mucous membranes, a heart rate of 120 bpm with fair pulses, and a respiratory rate of 30 beats per minute with normal lung sounds. He has a painful abdomen with a large, firm, nonexpressible bladder. His mentation is depressed, but he is arousable.

ECG reveals evidence of spiked T waves, absent P waves, and bradycardia. An extended database reveals the following abnormalities: potassium of 8.0 mEq/L, BUN of 109 mg/dL, PCV of 44%, total protein of 8.0 g/dL, and glucose of 160 mg/dL.

Tommy is diagnosed with a lower urinary obstruction and hyperkalemia-induced bradycardia. Before sedating the cat for urinary catheter placement, it is imperative that the hyperkalemia-induced bradycardia be treated. Therefore, an intravenous catheter is placed, intravenous fluids are started, calcium gluconate is given intravenously slowly to protect the heart, and dextrose/insulin is given to treat the hyperkalemia. Shortly after this treatment, the heart rate is 150 bpm, P waves are present on ECG, and the repeat potassium level is 5.7 mEq/L. The cat now seems to be stable enough for sedation, because, ultimately, the obstruction needs to be repaired to permanently fix his life-threatening hyperkalemia.

This scenario initially requires the use of neuroleptanalgesia. Analgesics in this situation are an absolute must, because urinary obstruction is painful. Cats do not tolerate high doses of pure opioids well because such doses frequently cause excitement and aggression [2–4]. The benzodiazepines are useful because they aid in urethral relaxation [4]. The author's preference is to use butorphanol, an opioid agonist/antagonist, at a dose of 0.2 mg/kg administered intravenously in conjunction with a benzodiazepine, such as midazolam or diazepam (Valium), at a dose 0.2 mg/kg administered intravenously. Keep in mind that benzodiazepines can also cause excitement in cats, [2–4] but that the sedative properties of butorphanol usually mask any excitement seen from the benzodiazepines. The analgesic effects of butorphanol only last approximately 1 to 2 hours, so long-term analgesic management still needs to be considered [23,37].

This neuroleptanalgesia protocol commonly does not provide enough sedation to pass a urinary catheter without pain. Adding a low dose of ketamine at 2 mg/kg administered intravenously frequently allows successful urinary catheterization. The butorphanol or benzodiazepine dose may need to be repeated if the procedure is prolonged. The use of ketamine in urinary-obstructed cats is controversial, because ketamine is excreted unchanged through the kidney in the cat [2]. Therefore, if the cat cannot be successfully unblocked, the ketamine can accumulate in the body. Ketamine is an excellent anesthetic in cats, and these cats can be successfully unblocked most of the time, which makes the use of ketamine in these cats a "nonissue". The author recommends avoiding repeat doses of ketamine in cats that are difficult to unblock, however, and avoids ketamine altogether in cats that have had multiple obstructions in the past because they are more likely to have strictures and may be difficult to unblock. Lastly, it is contraindicated to give ketamine to a cat with cardiac disease.

Therefore, it is always recommended to auscult the heart of the cat before the procedure and to avoid ketamine if a heart murmur is present.

Once the urinary catheter is in place, long-term pain management is indicated. A one-time dose of ketoprofen, meloxicam, or a low-dose steroid helps with inflammation and makes the cat more comfortable. For additional pain control, adding a butorphanol CRI at a rate of 0.1 to 0.2 mg/kg/h or buccal buprenorphine (6–10 μg/kg into the buccal pouch every 6–8 hours) [38] works well in cats.

Case 3

"Isabelle" is a 20-week-old, female, intact Chihuahua that was attacked by a German Shepherd dog 1 hour before presentation to the emergency room. She was normal before the attack but has not been able to walk since the attack. She is up to date on vaccines.

On physical examination, she is in shock with tachycardia, white mucous membranes, and weak pulses. Her respiratory rate is 60 breaths per minute with crackles in the right middle lung lobe, and she has palpable rib fractures on the right side. Her mentation is obtunded, and she has anisocoria (greater in the right pupil than in the left pupil). She has severe bite wounds present over her chest and abdomen.

Flow-by oxygen is immediately instituted. An intraosseous catheter is placed, and two 5-mL/kg boluses of hetastarch are given for volume resuscitation. Maintenance crystalloids are started, and mannitol, 0.5 g/kg, is given intraosseously after the mean arterial pressure is normal. Her head is elevated 30°.

Isabelle responded well to treatment and is more mentally alert. Anisocoria is still present, and she remains tachypneic with focal crackles, leading to a presumptive diagnosis of pulmonary contusions. She is now acting painful from her bite wounds and rib fractures. The abdominal wounds are severe enough that they need to be explored before resolution of the head trauma to ensure that there is no abdominal cavity penetration.

To safely anesthetize Isabelle, she needs to be intubated to allow manual ventilation and maintenance of $Paco_2$ in the low normal range. Elevated carbon dioxide concentrations are dangerous in head trauma patients because they lead to cerebral vasodilation and elevated intracranial pressure. Many of the opioids are respiratory depressants, and ventilation may be necessary to maintain low normal $Paco_2$ if they are used. Intubating and ventilating the dog are not without risk. Intubation can cause transient increases in intracranial pressure. Ventilation has to be performed cautiously to prevent barotrauma and possible pneumothorax, especially because of the suspicion of pulmonary contusions.

The anesthetic induction should consist of drugs that maintain the cerebral vascular response to $Paco_2$ and do not increase the intracranial pressure. A low-dose opioid, such as oxymorphone, 0.05 mg/kg, has excellent analgesic properties and is cardiovascularly sparing. A low-dose benzodiazepine, such as midazolam, 0.2 mg/kg, can lower the amount of other anesthetics used [39,40], is cardiopulmonary sparing, and has excellent muscle relaxation properties. Adding a 2-mg/kg lidocaine bolus administered intravenously can decrease the cough reflex [41] and may reduce the amount of other anesthetics needed to induce general anesthesia. Thiopental given intravenously in 2-mg/kg boluses to effect allows smooth induction. In addition, thiopental significantly reduces the cerebral metabolic oxygen demand [2]. A low dose of atropine (0.01–0.02 mg/kg) should be available. Recall that the blood pressure in puppies and kittens is mostly controlled by heart rate as the result of an underdeveloped sympathetic nervous system [42–44].

Intraoperative anesthesia can be maintained with an inhalation anesthetic that maintains the cerebral vascular response to carbon dioxide, such as isoflurane, sevoflurane, or desflurane. Halothane does not maintain the cerebral vascular response to carbon dioxide [2]. There is controversy as to whether inhalation anesthetics should be used at all if elevated intracranial pressure is a concern. During normocapnia in human beings, isoflurane resulted in much greater cerebral blood volume and flow compared with propofol [44]. Propofol does not seem to maintain the cerebral vascular response to hyperventilation compared with isoflurane, however [44]. A fentanyl CRI during surgery can reduce the amount of inhalation agent that is needed to keep the dog anesthetized and aids in analgesia.

After surgery, the ability of the dog to ventilate and maintain $Paco_2$ needs to be determined. Performing an intercostal nerve block along the fractured ribs before the dog awakens (maximum dose of bupivacaine, 1.5 mg/kg) may significantly improve its ability to ventilate. If the dog is not ventilating adequately, a partial reversal of the pure opioids with a low dose of butorphanol (25–50 µg/kg) or nalbuphine administered intravenously can be attempted. This frequently reverses the respiratory depressant effects of the pure opioids, although maintaining the analgesic effects. For long-term pain management, a respiratory-sparing opioid CRI, such as butorphanol at a rate of 0.2 mg/kg/h, can be tried. Butorphanol can be expensive to use as a CRI in larger dogs and may not provide adequate analgesia for the rib fractures. Another option would be to use a low-dose fentanyl CRI at a rate of 2 to 5 µg/kg/h.

Case 4

"Brutus," a 4-year-old, male, intact Rottweiler is presented for acute onset of vomiting. He has been vomiting for approximately 12 hours after eating a sock 36 hours previously. He has not been to see a veterinarian since he was a puppy because of severe aggression. He is not up to date on vaccines, including rabies.

A physical examination cannot be performed because of profound aggression and lunging. It is decided that Brutus needs to be sedated to place an intravenous catheter, perform a physical examination, obtain blood work samples, and take abdominal radiographs.

Cardiovascularly sparing drugs should be used, because Brutus is likely to be sicker than he is outwardly showing. In addition, his cardiovascular status is not known because of the inability to perform a physical examination. The owner should sign an informed consent indicating that Brutus is a dangerous dog and allowing permission to administer sedation without performing a physical examination. Personnel safety needs to be foremost, and in situations of aggressive animals, sedation protocols may need to include drugs that are not necessarily the most cardiovascularly sparing.

If there is no major concern about heart disease, a high dose of a pure opioid (eg, morphine, 1–2 mg/kg; hydromorphone, 0.2–0.3 mg/kg) with a phenothiazine (acepromazine, 0.03–0.05 mg/kg) and an anticholinergic (atropine, 0.02 mg/kg) can be used intramuscularly. Alternatively, a high dose of a pure opioid (eg, morphine, 1–2 mg/kg; hydromorphone, 0.2–0.3 mg/kg) with an α_2-agonist (medetomidine, 10 μg/kg) and atropine (0.02 mg/kg) can be used intramuscularly.

If there is concern about heart disease, a high-dose opioid (morphine, 2 mg/kg, or hydromorphone, 0.3–0.4 mg/kg) and an anticholinergic (glycopyrrolate, 0.01 mg/kg) can be given intramuscularly. Addition of a water-soluble benzodiazepine (midazolam, 0.25–0.5 mg/kg) can aid in the sedation; however, it is expensive. If midazolam is added to the protocol, the morphine and hydromorphone doses may be able to be reduced slightly.

Case 5

A 14-year-old, female, spayed calico cat is presented to the emergency room with a wound on her back. She got into a fight with a new cat 3 days ago and has a 24-hour history of lethargy and anorexia. Past pertinent medical history includes hypertrophic cardiomyopathy and anorexia. She is currently medicated with diltiazem and methimazole Tapazole.

On physical examination, the cat has a heart rate of 180 bpm with a grade II/VI systolic heart murmur, a palpable thyroid nodule, and a temperature of 104.5°F, and an abscess is present over the dorsum of the back near the right hip.

Because of this cat's heart disease, the heart rate should be kept as normal as possible during anesthesia (ie, avoid tachycardia and bradycardia). Drugs that cause tachycardia (eg, ketamine, atropine); excessive excitement in the cat, which may lead to thyroid storm (eg, pure opioids, high-dose benzodiazepines); and agents that are known to cause severe cardiovascular compromise (α_2-agonists) should be avoided.

Premedication should be administered to decrease the stress of placing an intravenous catheter. Low-dose acepromazine (0.02 mg/kg) with buprenorphine (10 μg/kg) may be used subcutaneously or intramuscularly. A dose of glycopyrrolate (0.01 mg/kg) should be available. After the intravenous catheter is placed, anesthesia induction can occur with etomidate, low-dose propofol, or thiopental administered intravenously to effect for intubation.

Summary

Anesthesia, sedation, and pain management should be taken seriously in the emergency patient. Proper knowledge of the drugs available and their pharmacokinetics and pharmacodynamics are necessary to administer anesthesia safely to critical patients. A proactive approach regarding monitoring, titration of anesthetic drugs, and anticipation of life-threatening complications helps in achieving successful anesthetic outcomes.

References

[1] Muir W, Gaynor J. Handbook of veterinary pain management. St. Louis: Mosby; 2002.
[2] Thurman JC, Tranquilli WJ, Benson GJ. Lumb and Jones' veterinary anesthesia. 3rd edition. Baltimore: Williams & Wilkins; 1996.
[3] Muir WW, Hubbell JAE, Skarda RT, et al. Handbook of veterinary anesthesia. 3rd edition. St. Louis: Mosby; 2000.
[4] Plumb DC. Veterinary drug handbook. 4th edition. Ames (IA): Iowa State University Press; 2002.
[5] Lang SM, Eglen RM, Henry AC. Acetylpromazine administration: its effect on canine hematology. Vet Rec 1979;105:397–8.
[6] Klide AM, Calderwood HW, Soma LR. Cardiopulmonary effects of xylazine in dogs. Am J Vet Res 1975;36(7):931–5.
[7] Pypendop B, Verstegen J. Cardiorespiratory effects of a combination of medetomidine, midazolam, and butorphanol in dogs. Am J Vet Res 1999;60(9):1148–54.
[8] Blouin RT, Conard PF, Gross JB. Time course of ventilatory depression following induction doses of propofol and thiopental. Anesthesiology 1991;75:940–4.
[9] Quandt JE, Robinson EP, Rivers WJ, et al. Cardiorespiratory and anesthetic effects of propofol and thiopental in dogs. Am J Vet Res 1998;59(9):1137–43.
[10] Heldmann E, Brown DC, Shofer F. The association of propofol usage with postoperative wound infection rate in clean wounds: a retrospective study. Vet Surg 1999;28:256–9.
[11] Muir WW. Electrocardiographic interpretation of thiobarbiturate-induced dysrhythmias in dogs. J Am Vet Med Assoc 1977;170:1419–24.
[12] Ko JCH, Golder FJ, Mandsager RE, et al. Anesthetic and cardiorespiratory effects of a 1:1 mixture of propofol and thiopental sodium in dogs. J Am Vet Med Assoc 1999;215(9): 1292–6.
[13] Wong DHW, Jenkins LC. An experimental study of the mechanism of action of ketamine on the central nervous system. Can Anaesth Soc J 1974;21(1):57–67.
[14] Waxman K, Shoemaker WC, Lippmann M. Cardiovascular effects of anesthetic induction with ketamine. Anesth Analg 1980;59(5):355–8.
[15] Weiskopf RB, Bogetz MS, Roizen MF, et al. Cardiovascular and metabolic sequelae of inducing anesthesia with ketamine or thiopental in hypovolemic swine. Anesthesiology 1984; 60:214–9.
[16] White KL, Taylor PM. Comparison of diazepam-ketamine and thiopentone for induction of anaesthesia in healthy dogs. Vet Anaesth Analg 2001;28:42–8.

[17] Dodam JR, Kruse-Elliott KT, Aucoin DP, et al. Duration of etomidate-induced adrenocortical suppression during surgery in dogs. Am J Vet Res 1990;51(5):786–8.

[18] Moon PF. Cortisol suppression in cats after induction of anesthesia with etomidate, compared with ketamine-diazepam combination. Am J Vet Res 1997;58(8):868–71.

[19] Wagner AE, Walton JA, Hellyer PW, et al. Use of low doses of ketamine administered by constant rate infusion as an adjunct for postoperative analgesia in dogs. J Am Vet Med Assoc 2002;221(1):72–5.

[20] Schmid RL, Sandler AN, Katz J. Use and efficacy of low-dose ketamine in the management of acute postoperative pain: a review of current techniques and outcomes. Pain 1999;82: 111–25.

[21] Cassuto J, Wallin G, Hogstrom S, et al. Inhibition of postoperative pain by continuous low-dose intravenous infusion of lidocaine. Anesth Analg 1985;64(10):971–4.

[22] Smith LJ, Bentley E, Shih A, et al. Systemic lidocaine infusion as an analgesic for intraocular surgery in dogs: a pilot study. Vet Anaesth Analg 2004;31(1):53–63.

[23] Grimm KA, Tranquilli WJ, Thurmon JC, et al. Duration of nonresponse to noxious stimulation after intramuscular administration of butorphanol, medetomidine, or a butorphanol-medetomidine combination during isoflurane administration in dogs. Am J Vet Res 2000;61(1):42–7.

[24] Kauppila T, Kemppainen P, Tanila H, et al. Effect of systemic medetomidine, an alpha$_2$ adrenoceptor agonist, on experimental pain in humans. Anesthesiology 1991;74:3–8.

[25] Pypendop BH, Verstegen JP. Hemodynamic effects of medetomidine in the dog: a dose titration study. Vet Surg 1998;27(6):612–22.

[26] Sawyer DC, Guikema AH, Siegel EM. Evaluation of a new oscillometric blood pressure monitor in isoflurane-anesthetized dogs. Vet Anaesth Analg 2004;31:27–39.

[27] Gains MJ, Grodecki KM, Jacobs RM, et al. Comparison of direct and indirect blood pressure measurements in anesthetized dogs. Can J Vet Res 1995;59(3):238–40.

[28] Chalifoux A, Dallaire A, Blais D, et al. Evaluation of the arterial blood pressure of dogs by two noninvasive methods. Can J Comp Med 1985;49(4):419–23.

[29] Caulkett NA, Cantwell SL, Houston DM. A comparison of indirect blood pressure monitoring techniques in the anesthetized cat. Vet Surg 1998;27:370–7.

[30] Binns SH, Sisson DD, Buoscio DA, et al. Doppler ultrasonographic, oscillometric sphygmomanometric, and photoplethysmographic techniques for noninvasive blood pressure measurement in anesthetized cats. J Vet Intern Med 1995;9(6):405–14.

[31] Grandy JL, Dunlop CI, Hodgson DS, et al. Evaluation of the Doppler ultrasonic method of measuring systolic arterial blood pressure in cats. Am J Vet Res 1992;53(7):1166–9.

[32] Pedersen KM, Butler MA, Ersboll AK, et al. Evaluation of an oscillometric blood pressure monitor for use in anesthetized cats. J Am Vet Med Assoc 2002;221(5):646–50.

[33] Fairman NB. Evaluation of pulse oximetry as a continuous monitoring technique in critically ill dogs in the small animal intensive care unit. J Vet Emerg Crit Care 1992;2(2): 50–6.

[34] Barton LJ, Devey JJ, Gorski S, et al. Evaluation of transmittance and reflectance pulse oximetry in a canine model of hypotension and desaturation. J Vet Emerg Crit Care 1996; 6(1):21–8.

[35] Wright B, Hellyer PW. Respiratory monitoring during anesthesia: pulse oximetry and capnography. Compend Contin Educ Pract Vet 1996;18(10):1083–97.

[36] Egger CM, Duke T, Archer J, et al. Comparison of plasma fentanyl concentrations by using three transdermal fentanyl patch sizes in dogs. Vet Surg 1998;27(2):159–66.

[37] Pollet R, Claxton R, Raffe M. Using butorphanol tartrate to manage pain in cats. Vet Med 1998;93(2):146–55.

[38] Robertson SA, Taylor PM, Sear JW. Systemic uptake of buprenorphine by cats after oral mucosal administration. Vet Rec 2003;152:675–8.

[39] Greene SA, Benson GJ, Hartsfield SM. Thiamylal-sparing effect of midazolam for canine endotracheal intubation: a clinical study of 118 dogs. Vet Surg 1993;22(1):69–72.

[40] Hellyer PW, Mama KR, Shafford HL, et al. Effects of diazepam and flumazenil on minimum alveolar concentrations for dogs anesthetized with isoflurane or a combination of isoflurane and fentanyl. Am J Vet Res 2001;62(4):555–60.

[41] Steinhaus JE, Gaskin L. A study of intravenous lidocaine as a suppressant of cough reflex. Anesthesiology 1963;24(3):285–90.

[42] Adelman RD, Wright J. Systolic blood pressure and heart rate in the growing beagle puppy. Dev Pharmacol Ther 1985;8:396–401.

[43] Gauthier P, Nadeau RA, DeChamplain J. The development of sympathetic innervation and the functional state of the cardiovascular system in newborn dogs. Can J Physiol Pharmacol 1975;53:763–76.

[44] Cenic A, Craen RA, Lee T, et al. Cerebral blood volume and blood flow responses to hyperventilation in brain tumors during isoflurane or propofol anesthesia. Anesth Analg 2002;94(3):661–6.

Animals with anterior uveitis, glaucoma, hyphema, and corneal ulcers can all present as an emergency with a history of a "red eye." Sudden blindness may result from retinal separation (detachment), sudden acquired retinal degeneration syndrome (SARDS), fluoroquinolone toxicity, optic neuritis, or central nervous system disease.

This article discusses the clinical signs, diagnosis, and treatment as well as the prognosis of some of the more common ophthalmic emergencies.

Anterior uveitis

Anterior uveitis, inflammation of the iris and ciliary body, is a relatively common emergency (Fig. 1). The animal is usually presented for a painful red eye, with or without vision loss. Clinical signs include conjunctival hyperemia; a protruding third eyelid; an inflamed, reddened, swollen, or "fluffy" iris; iridocyclospasm (miotic pupil); aqueous flare; hypopyon; hyphema; and blepharospasm. The intraocular pressure (IOP) may be decreased to less than 10 mm Hg as a result of decreased aqueous production.

Possible causes of anterior uveitis are listed in Box 1 [1–6]. The diagnostic workup for a dog with uveitis should include a complete blood cell count, serum chemistry panel, urinalysis, specific infectious disease titers, chest radiographs, and, if indicated, abdominal ultrasound. In endemic areas, tickborne diseases, fungal disease, or toxoplasmosis should be considered. In a cat, viral serologic testing for feline leukemia virus, feline immunodeficiency virus, and feline infectious peritonitis is important. If the anterior uveitis is mild, treatment can be considered before a full medical workup is performed. Owners should be warned that neoplasia cannot be ruled out just because there are no other systemic signs (eg, lymphosarcoma, a common cause of anterior uveitis in dogs, can surface many months later).

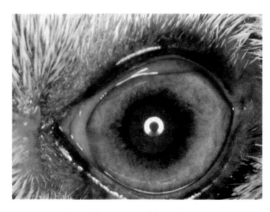

Fig. 1. Anterior uveitis in a dog. The iris is reddened and inflamed and appears "fluffy."

Box 1. Causes of uveitis

Canine
  Trauma
  Infectious
    Tickborne disease
    Fungal disease
    Bacterial disease
      Toxoplasmosis
      Leptospirosis
  Sepsis
  Lens abnormalities
    Cataract or lens luxation
  Immune-mediated disease
    Uveodermatologic syndrome (VKH)
    Pigmentary uveitis in the Golden Retriever
  Neoplasia
  Lymphosarcoma
Feline
  Trauma
  Infectious
    Feline leukemia virus
    Feline immunodeficiency virus
    Feline infectious peritonitis virus
    Toxoplasmosis
    Fungal diseases
    Sepsis
  Lens abnormalities
    Cataract or lens luxation
  Immune-mediated
  Neoplasia
  Lymphosarcoma

Anterior uveitis can result from cataract or injury to the lens. This lens-induced uveitis can be intense and difficult to control. Surgery to remove the lens or lens material may be necessary at the time of injury to control inflammation.

Immune-mediated disease can also lead to uveitis. One example, uveodermatologic syndrome or Voyt-Koyanagi-Harada–like syndrome (VKH) [7], is a disease directed against melanocytes, which can result in a panophthalmitis and skin changes (alopecia, vitiligo, and poliosis). VKH has been documented in a number of breeds, particularly in Japanese breeds, such as the Akita. Immunosuppressive doses of corticosteroids or

(2 mg/kg administered orally) dehydrate the aqueous humor and vitreous body. After intravenous administration of mannitol, a decrease in IOP is evident within 30 minutes and can last for at least 5 hours. Mannitol should be used cautiously in patients that are dehydrated or have preexisting cardiovascular or renal disease. Glycerol can cause vomiting, and the change in IOP is less predictable than with mannitol, but it is also reported to be effective within 1 hour. Food and water should be withheld from the animal for several hours after administration of mannitol. Mannitol depends on an intact blood-aqueous barrier to be effective, so it may be unpredictable in uveitis.

Latanoprost (Xalatan, administered once daily), a prostaglandin analogue, increases drainage of aqueous humor mainly through an alternative outflow route (uveoscleral outflow). It has been reported to rapidly decrease IOP by 40% to 60%. Extreme miosis is documented in most dogs after administration, and the drug should be used with caution in dogs with glaucoma secondary to anterior uveitis. The ocular hypotensive effects of latanoprost are additive to those of other glaucoma drugs.

An oral carbonic anhydrase inhibitor (CAI) should be considered to maximize the reduction in IOP. CAIs (eg, methazolamide [Neptazane] at a dose of 2.5–5 mg/kg) decrease aqueous humor production by the ciliary body. The onset of action is several hours, but the decrease in IOP can be significant. Unfortunately, side effects are common. Gastrointestinal signs, panting, and disorientation are frequently noted because of the presence of carbonic anhydrase in the nephrons of the kidney and in erythrocytes. Topical CAIs (eg, dorzolamide [Trusopt] administered three times daily) have been developed to reduce these adverse side effects [10,11]. Topical β-antagonists (eg, 0.5% timolol [Timoptic]) and epinephrine compounds (eg, dipivefrin) are medications that can be added to reduce IOP further.

After the initial reduction in IOP, vision may or may not improve. The IOP needs to be maintained within normal limits using a combination of topical and oral medications. If the initial glaucoma attack resulted in temporary blindness, it may take days to weeks for limited vision to return. In some dogs, despite aggressive treatment of acute glaucoma, vision never returns.

Systemic corticosteroids at an anti-inflammatory dose have been shown to improve optic nerve head edema in acute glaucoma. The use of calcium channel blockers as neuroprotective agents has also been investigated.

Anterior lens luxation is a frequent cause of secondary glaucoma in dogs. Primary lens luxations occur in many terrier breeds (eg, Jack Russell Terrier) because of an inherited defect in the lens zonular attachment. As well as being a cause of secondary glaucoma, lens luxations can be the result of chronic glaucoma and anterior uveitis. Age-related degeneration of the lens zonules is found in dogs with or without cataract development.

Anterior lens luxations that are determined to be primary in the dog are a surgical emergency. Clinical signs of an anterior lens luxation include anterior uveitis, iridodonesis (movement of the iris), corneal edema, and an increase in the depth of the anterior chamber. The edge of the lens may be visible, especially dorsally (Fig. 3). If IOP is elevated, mannitol should be started as described previously. The lens should be removed as soon as possible if there is to be any chance for regaining vision or controlling IOP. There are inherent risks of intraocular surgery, and owners should be warned that complications, including glaucoma, can occur after surgery.

Subluxation or posterior luxation of the lens is not considered a surgical emergency. These animals should be treated medically, if necessary, for glaucoma and anterior uveitis and referred to an ophthalmologist for follow-up care.

Prognosis

After emergency treatment for acute congestive glaucoma, the dog should be rechecked, preferably by a veterinary ophthalmologist, within a few days. If IOP cannot be controlled medically, a definitive surgical procedure is needed. The amount of time for which IOP can be controlled is variable. Some dogs need immediate definitive treatment, whereas other dogs with glaucoma might have IOP controlled medically for several months.

Laser transscleral cyclophotocoagulation (TSCP) and cyclocryotherapy are relatively noninvasive procedures that destroy the ciliary body and consequently decrease aqueous humor production. A combination of cycloablation and gonioimplantation (shunt to improve aqueous humor outflow) has been successful at maintaining vision in some dogs.

Despite aggressive therapy, the long-term prognosis for a dog with primary glaucoma is poor. Enucleation may be the ultimate outcome. Owners should be educated about the disease and warned that the onset of glaucoma in the unaffected eye can occur within months.

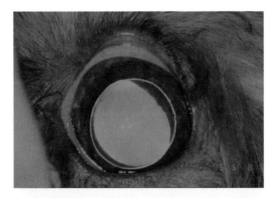

Fig. 3. An anterior lens luxation in a dog. Note the edge of the lens in the dorsal margin. (*From* Mandell DC. Ophthalmological emergencies. In: King L, Hammond R, editors. Manual of canine and feline emergency and critical care. Cheltenham: British Small Animal Veterinary Association; 1999. p. 124; with permission.)

medial rectus muscle frequently ruptures, resulting in a lateral strabismus that may gradually improve over time. Damage to more than three extraocular muscles can lead to phthisis bulbi, because the anterior ciliary arteries enter the eye through these muscles.

Prognosis

The prognosis for saving the eye (but not vision) can be good.

Enucleation

The reader is encouraged to consult a surgery or ophthalmology textbook for techniques of enucleation.

Hyphema

Hyphema, or blood in the anterior chamber, may be the only clinical finding in an animal with a red eye (Fig. 6). There are numerous causes of hyphema (Box 3) [4].

A thorough physical examination should be performed. If no other evidence of hemorrhage or trauma is found, a complete coagulation screen should be submitted and a diagnostic workup for anterior uveitis should be started.

Treatment

Treatment for hyphema involves identifying the underlying cause. If an underlying cause is found, specific treatment should be initiated and the

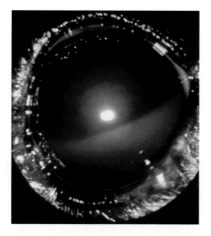

Fig. 6. Hyphema in a dog. Trauma and coagulopathy should be ruled out first. (*From* Mandell DC. Ophthalmic emergencies. Clin Tech Small Anim Pract 2000;15(2):99; with permission.)

Box 3. Causes of hyphema

Trauma
Uveitis
Coagulopathy
  Thrombocytopenia/thrombocytopathia
  Coagulation factor deficiency
  Disseminated intravascular coagulation
Neoplasia
Congenital anomalies
Hyperviscosity syndrome
  Multiple myeloma
Systemic hypertension
Chronic glaucoma
Retinal detachment

---

blood should gradually reabsorb. Atropine (1% administered twice daily) is indicated to minimize the chance of posterior synechiae but only if the IOP can be closely monitored. The use of topical corticosteroids and antibiotics has not been conclusively shown to be of benefit.

Prognosis

The prognosis is dependent on the underlying cause and whether the bleeding can be controlled. In a recent retrospective study, 38 dogs were examined and retinal detachment was found to be the most common cause of hyphema in dogs; the prognosis for vision was found to be poor, but it was better in cases of small hyphema volumes not associated with retinal detachment [13].

Corneal ulcer

An ulcer involves the loss of corneal stroma in addition to loss of corneal epithelium [14]. A variable degree of reflex uveitis can accompany an ulcer. Corneal ulcers are common ocular emergencies. Although usually traumatic in origin, eyelid conformation or an underlying disease process may predispose an animal to develop an ulcer (Box 4). Lagophthalmic breeds are frequently susceptible to central corneal ulcers; ulcers in these breeds can progress and deepen rapidly. A vertical or longitudinal ulceration can be the result of foreign material lodged in the conjunctiva (Fig. 7). Topical anesthesia and a cotton-tipped swab can facilitate examination of the bulbar surface of the nictitating membrane and the palpebral conjunctiva in search of a foreign body. An STT for keratoconjunctivitis sicca (KCS) in the dog

---

Box 4. Causes of corneal ulcers

Trauma
Foreign body
Infection
  Viral
  Bacterial
  Fungal
KCS
Topical irritants
Exposure keratitis (lagophthalmic breeds)
  Facial nerve paralysis
Entropion

(average 19 mm/min) and then fluorescein dye to characterize the ulcer should be performed.

Clinical signs of corneal ulceration include blepharospasm, conjunctival hyperemia, a relatively clear ocular discharge, corneal edema, and miosis (iridocyclospasm). A yellow-white stromal infiltrate usually accompanies infected ulcers. Infected ulcers tend to be deep and can progress quickly if untreated. Gram-positive and gram-negative organisms are capable of infecting the cornea. Gram-negative rods produce proteases (collagenases), which can result in rapid and progressive destruction ("melting") of corneal tissue (Fig. 8).

Superficial corneal ulcers appear as relatively clear defects in the cornea. Some are visible only with the application of fluorescein dye (Fig. 9). Uncomplicated superficial ulcerations should heal by re-epithelialization within 3 to 5 days. Superficial ulcers that do not heal in the expected time frame are referred to as indolent, refractory, or nonhealing ulcers. Indolent ulcers may be the result of an anterior stromal or epithelial basement membrane defect as seen in the Boxer dog. With an indolent ulcer, there is

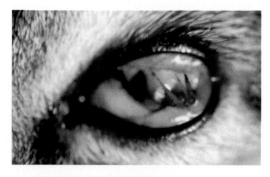

Fig. 7. Foxtails imbedded in the conjunctiva.

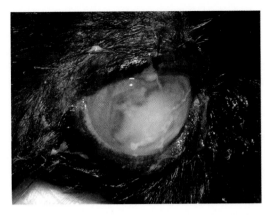

Fig. 8. An infected "melting" ulcer. Notice the white-yellow stromal infiltrate and white thick discharge over the ulcer.

often intense fluorescein dye retention over the area of exposed stroma, surrounded by a ring of less intense dye retention. The lighter staining ring represents the zone in which corneal epithelial cells are present but are not attached to the underlying stroma.

Deep corneal ulcers (stromal ulcers) require vascularization, particularly if they involve more than a third of the corneal thickness. These ulcers can take up to 3 weeks to heal. If the ulcer is deep enough to expose Descemet's membrane, only one cell layer, the endothelium, remains of the original corneal tissue and perforation of the globe is imminent. Descemet's membrane often appears clear or black; fluorescein retention occurs in the surrounding

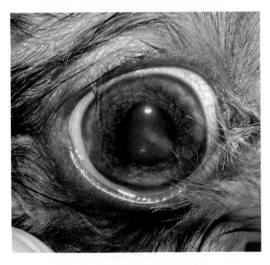

Fig. 9. A superficial corneal ulcer.

exposed stroma, but the membrane itself does not take up stain (Fig. 10). Descemet's membrane is always under some tension and may herniate through the surrounding corneal stroma to bulge anteriorly (descemetocele). Restraint or any pressure on the neck or jugular vein of an animal with a descemetocele can cause IOP to increase and the cornea to rupture.

Treatment

The emergency treatment of corneal ulcers depends on the depth of the ulcer, whether or not infection is present, and the underlying cause. If a topical irritant is suspected, the eye should be irrigated with copious amounts of saline or sterile eyewash.

Referral to an ophthalmologist for corneal surgery, specifically for conjunctival flaps or other grafting procedures, should be considered in animals with the following symptoms:

- Ulcer is deep (>80% stromal loss)
- Ulcer progresses (deepens) in spite of appropriate medical therapy
- Corneal perforation or a descemetocele is present

Although surgery may be indicated, it is not always possible. In these animals, medical therapy should be initiated and the eye rechecked frequently. There is a chance that even a ruptured cornea may heal with medical therapy alone (Fig. 11).

Medical therapy for corneal ulcerations should focus on relief of pain and treatment of infection, if present. Iridocyclospasm (if miosis is present) is treated with 1% atropine (administered two to four times daily). If the pupil

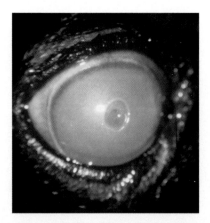

Fig. 10. A corneal ulcer down to Descemet's membrane in a pug. Notice the central clear area. This area does not take up fluorescein stain. These are surgical emergencies. (*From* Mandell DC. Ophthalmological emergencies. In: King L, Hammond R, editors. Manual of canine and feline emergency and critical care. Cheltenham: British Small Animal Veterinary Association; 1999. p. 122; with permission.)

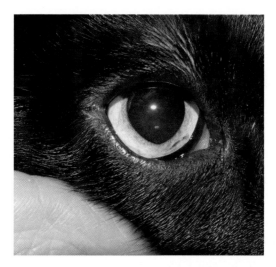

Fig. 11. A corneal perforation in a cat. This healed with medical therapy alone.

is well dilated, there is probably adequate iridocycloplegia. If the cornea is infected, samples for culture/sensitivity and cytologic testing should be submitted. Antibiotic therapy is started and then adjusted depending on the results. Topical corticosteroids are contraindicated in the treatment of corneal ulcers. Topical nonsteroidal anti-inflammatory drugs (NSAIDS) can also delay healing of ulcers but less so than topical steroids. Placement of an Elizabethan collar is essential.

Superficial corneal ulcer

Most superficial ulcerations are not infected, and topical antibiotics are prescribed to help prevent organisms from colonizing the exposed corneal stroma. Neopolybacitracin (Neobacimyx, administered three to four times daily) is a good broad-spectrum antibiotic in dogs. Erythromycin or tetracycline (administered three to four times daily) may be preferred in cats because of their greater sensitivity to the topical allergen, neomycin, which can cause severe chemosis. Anaphylactic reactions to neomycin have been reported in cats [15].

If an indolent or nonhealing ulcer is seen based on the results of fluorescein staining, it can be vigorously debrided with a cotton-tipped swab after application of a topical anesthetic. A grid keratotomy or punctate keratotomy procedure may be performed in dogs after the dry debridement but should be avoided in cats (Fig. 12).

Prognosis

The affected eye should be rechecked and restained with fluorescein dye in 1 week. Most superficial corneal ulcerations heal without complication.

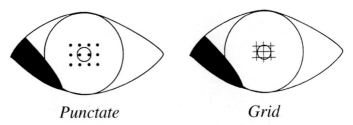

Punctate   Grid

Fig. 12. Punctate and grid keratotomy. After topical anesthetic and debridement with a cotton swab, a 25-gauge needle is used to make punctate or grid marks on (not through) the corneal epithelium. (*From* Mandell DC. Ophthalmological emergencies. In: King L, Hammond R, editors. Manual of canine and feline emergency and critical care. Cheltenham: British Small Animal Veterinary Association; 1999. p. 121; with permission.)

Deep corneal ulcer

If the ulcer spans into the stroma but is not infected, it can be treated like a superficial ulcer but can take up to 3 weeks to heal. Again, if there is greater than 80% stromal loss, a conjunctival flap should be placed.

Infected stromal (deep) ulcer

A white or yellow stromal infiltrate is seen adjacent to the ulcer (Fig. 13). Infected ulcers are potentially serious and need to be treated aggressively. Topical broad-spectrum antibiotics can be initiated (eg, fluoroquinolone [ciprofloxacin (Ciloxan)] administered every 3 hours). Gentamicin or

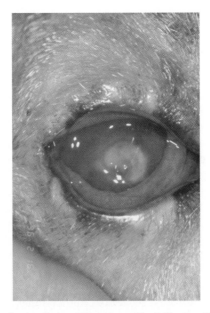

Fig. 13. An infected corneal ulcer. There is a white infiltrate adjacent to the ulcer.

tobramycin (administered every 3 hours) can be added to broaden this spectrum if gram-negative organisms are seen on cytologic examination. Antibiotic therapy may need to be adjusted when culture and sensitivity results are available. Antibiotic solutions or suspensions are preferred over ointments if a corneal perforation is suspected or imminent. Topical atropine (1% administered two to four times daily) should be started to control iridocyclospasm. Collagenase inhibitors, such as autologous serum (one to two drops administered every 2–6 hours) or acetylcysteine, can be considered in a rapidly deepening ulcer.

Prognosis

Infected stromal ulcers can progress quickly to corneal perforation. The eye should be monitored for changes in the shape and color of the cornea and for increasing discomfort. The animal can be hospitalized for the first 24 hours to ensure appropriate treatment, or if the animal is treated at home, the eye should be rechecked frequently. If the corneal ulcer worsens (deepens) despite appropriate medical therapy, surgery is indicated.

Descemetocele

A descemetocele, or an ulcer that exposes Descemet's membrane, is a surgical emergency. Medical therapy similar to that for an infected stromal ulcer can be started before surgery unless the animal struggles or resents restraint. The animal should be handled with extreme care, and any unnecessary pressure on the globe should be avoided. Cage rest must be strictly enforced.

Corneal perforation

A corneal perforation is a surgical emergency. Clinical signs include blepharospasm, pain, corneal edema, a misshapen cornea, and pink or red tissue over the defect (eg, a fibrin clot, Fig. 14), and there may be a change in anterior chamber depth and dyscoria (misshapen pupil). The iris may be adherent to the rent in the cornea or protrude through as a brown or black mass (iris prolapse, Fig. 15). A Seidel test can be performed to check for leakage of aqueous humor. Fluorescein dye is liberally applied to the cornea, and the cornea is gently pressed with a cotton-tipped swab; if corneal integrity is compromised, aqueous humor leaks through the site of perforation and the dye forms rivulets.

Treatment

If surgery is not possible, corneal perforations are treated much like an infected stromal ulcer, with the addition of systemic broad-spectrum antibiotics (amoxicillin-clavulanic acid [Clavamox], 13.75 mg/kg, administered twice a day or enrofloxacin, [Baytril], 10 mg/kg [in the dog], administered once a day) and NSAIDs (carprofen [Rimadyl], 2 mg/kg,

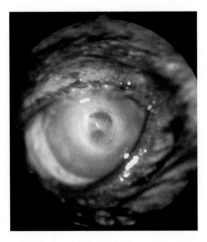

Fig. 14. Corneal rupture in a Shih Tzu. The white and red material over the cornea is the fibrin clot sealing the defect.

administered twice a day). The use of atropine is particularly important, especially if the iris is prolapsed through the wound. The animal should be handled with extreme care, and any unnecessary pressure on the globe should be avoided. Cage rest must be strictly enforced.

Prognosis

The prognosis for a corneal perforation is guarded. Prompt surgical repair of the cornea can save the eye and, possibly, vision. If surgery is not possible and the response to medical therapy is poor, enucleation is appropriate.

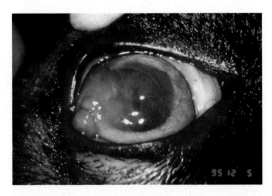

Fig. 15. Iris prolapse. The iris is protruding through the edge of the ulcer. (*From* Mandell DC. Ophthalmological emergencies. In: King L, Hammond R, editors. Manual of canine and feline emergency and critical care. Cheltenham: British Small Animal Veterinary Association; 1999. p. 122; with permission.)

Corneal laceration

The cornea can sustain a laceration secondary to trauma, such as a cat scratch. Corneal edema surrounds the edges of the laceration (Fig. 16). Treatment depends on whether the laceration is partial or full thickness through the cornea and whether the lens is involved. Medical therapy is similar to that for a corneal ulcer as described previously.

Treatment

If a corneal laceration is partial thickness, it may heal with medical therapy alone. If a full-thickness laceration is present, consider referral to an ophthalmologist for direct suturing of the defect.

The close proximity of the lens to the cornea can result in damage to the anterior lens capsule. If the lens capsule has been disturbed, an intense anterior uveitis that is difficult to control may follow. Anti-inflammatory doses of oral corticosteroids should be considered to control the lens-induced uveitis. The clinician should advise owners that the lens material may need to be removed surgically to control the inflammation.

Prognosis

With appropriate treatment, the prognosis for corneal lacerations is good. If the iris is prolapsed through the laceration, the prognosis for retention of vision is guarded, however.

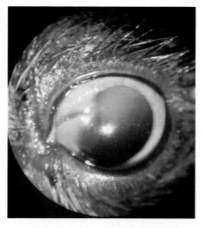

Fig. 16. Corneal laceration in a cat. Notice the corneal edema around the edges of the laceration. All cases should be extensively evaluated for a foreign body. The defect is sutured using 6-0 to 9-0 absorbable suture. (*From* Mandell DC. Ophthalmological emergencies. In: King L, Hammond R, editors. Manual of canine and feline emergency and critical care. Cheltenham: British Small Animal Veterinary Association; 1999. p. 123; with permission.)

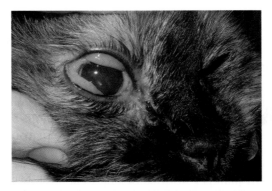

Fig. 19. Conjunctivitis and chemosis in a cat. This was caused by *Chlamydophilia felis* (*Chlamydia psittaci*).

primary conjunctival pathogens. Supportive care and topical antibiotics (erythromycin or oxytetracycline-polymixin [Terramycin] ointment administered three times daily) are preferred in an acute episode of conjunctivitis. Corticosteroids are contraindicated. Antiviral medications are available for use in animals with presumed FHV-1 infection. Topical antivirals (eg, idoxuridine, trifluridine) are virostatic and must be used frequently (five to six times daily) if they are to be effective.

Prognosis

The prognosis is dependent on the underlying cause. Older cats with FHV-1 conjunctivitis are more likely to have recurrences.

Sudden blindness

A thorough history and physical examination are important in all cases of sudden blindness. It is possible that an "acute" blindness has resulted from a slowly progressive insidious disease (eg, progressive retinal atrophy [PRA]). A minimum database (complete blood cell count, serum chemistry panel, urinalysis, and thoracic radiographs) and blood pressure measurement should be acquired to try to establish an underlying cause. Selection of additional diagnostic tests in dogs and cats is based on diseases endemic to a given practice area. Referral to an ophthalmologist for an electroretinogram (ERG) may be necessary for assessment of retinal function.

Retinal separation (Detachment)

Any increase in permeability within the choroidal blood vessels, such as that occurring with systemic hypertension or acute inflammation (choroiditis), results in accumulation of fluid between the retinal pigment epithelium and photoreceptors, creating a serous or exudative retinal separation (Fig. 20) [6,20]. The nature of the subretinal fluid and the magnitude of the separation influence the extent of photoreceptor injury.

Clinical signs include a poor to absent PLR, and the pupils may be dilated in ambient light. When viewed through a dilated pupil with a bright focal light source, a large separation appears as a grayish blue vascularized membrane positioned directly behind the posterior lens capsule and bulging anteriorly. A retinal separation may occupy part of or all the vitreous space. If the fundus is examined with a direct ophthalmoscope or indirect lens, the separated retina can be difficult to see clearly.

Granulomatous meningoencephalitis (GME), trauma, panuveitis (including bacterial, rickettsial, and mycotic infections), immune-mediated disease, and systemic hypertension are possible causes of retinal separation (Box 5).

Treatment

Treatment depends on determination of the underlying cause. Even extensive retinal separations can reattach, with return of vision provided that treatment is started early. Failure to reattach leads to retinal degeneration. Retinal separations that result from GME, immune-mediated disease, or inflammatory disease require high doses of systemic prednisone (1–2 mg/kg administered every 12–24 hours) initially to reattach the retina. If an infectious cause of retinal separation is determined, systemic corticosteroids are contraindicated.

Systemic hypertension (typically >160 mm Hg) is common in older cats [21]. Return of vision after detachment depends on rapid antihypertensive therapy. Amlodipine (Norvasc, 0.625 mg administered once daily) is usually effective at lowering the blood pressure. The rate of retinal reattachment

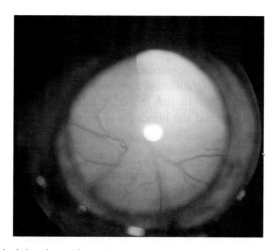

Fig. 20. Retinal detachment in a 15-year-old cat secondary to systemic hypertension.

[12] Mandell DC. Ophthalmological emergencies. In: King L, Hammond R, editors. Manual of canine and feline emergency and critical care. Cheltenham: British Small Animal Veterinary Association; 1999. p. 117–26.

[13] Paul TA, Ward DA. Clinical features, etiologies and outcomes of hyphema in dogs. A retrospective study (1999–2002). In: Proceedings of the American College of Veterinary Opthalmologists 34th Annual Conference. 2003.

[14] Whitley RD, Gilger BC. Diseases of the canine cornea and sclera. In: Gelatt KN, editor. Veterinary ophthalmology. 3rd edition. Baltimore (MD): Lippincott Williams & Wilkins; 1999. p. 635–73.

[15] Plunkett SJ. Anaphylaxis to ophthalmic medication in a cat. J Vet Emerg Crit Care 2000; 10(3):169–71.

[16] Hendrix DVH. Diseases and surgery of the canine conjunctiva. In: Gelatt KN, editor. Veterinary ophthalmology. 3rd edition. Baltimore (MD): Lippincott Williams & Wilkins; 1999. p. 619–34.

[17] Whitley RD, Whitley EM, McLaughlin SA. Diagnosing and treating disorders of the feline conjunctiva and cornea. Vet Med 1993;88:1138–49.

[18] Gionfriddo JR. Identifying and treating conjunctivitis in dogs and cats. Vet Med 1995;90: 242–53.

[19] Wilkie DA. Therapeutics in practice. Management of keratoconjunctivitis sicca in dogs. Compend Contin Educ Pract Vet 1993;15:58–63.

[20] Narfstrom K, Ekesten B. Diseases of canine ocular fundus. In: Gelatt KN, editor. Veterinary ophthalmology. 3rd edition. Baltimore (MD): Lippincott Williams & Wilkins; 1999. p. 869–933.

[21] Komaromy AM, Andrew SE, Denis HM, et al. Hypertensive retinopathy and choroidopathy in a cat. Vet Ophthalmol 2004;7(1):3–9.

ELSEVIER
SAUNDERS

Vet Clin Small Anim
35 (2005) 481–515

VETERINARY
CLINICS
Small Animal Practice

Analgesia and Chemical Restraint for the Emergent Patient

Karol A. Mathews, DVM, DVSc*, Doris H. Dyson, DVM, DVSc

Department of Clinical Studies, Ontario Veterinary College, University of Guelph, Guelph, Ontario, Canada N1G 2W1

Pain level is considered the fifth vital sign in human patients [1], and hospital accreditation may include the institution's approach to pain assessment and management [2]. This assertive approach emphasizes the importance of pain management and has also been included in the American Animal Hospital Association's recommendations. Because animals feel and anticipate pain by similar mechanisms as people [3], this emphasis on pain management should also apply to animals. Continual painful experience in any animal is detrimental to the overall healing process as well as to the general well-being of any animal or person [4–6]. Pain often results in a prolonged hospital stay and increases the potential for secondary problems. Because there may be a link between acute pain and chronic pain in human beings, with the hypothesis that if the acute pain were better controlled, the chronic pain would not develop [7], this is another factor to consider in animals. Although all the negative physiologic effects associated with the experience of pain should be considered, above all, one's actions should be governed by the inhumane aspects of this unnecessary experience. Expected level of pain associated with various emergent conditions is given in Box 1.

Analgesics are frequently withheld in the emergent patient, because a common misconception is that analgesics "mask" physiologic indicators (eg, heart rate, respiratory rate) of patient deterioration (eg, hypotension, hypoxia). This is not the case. Evidence exists in the human literature [8], and has also been an observation in veterinary patients [9], that analgesics do not mask the signs of patient deterioration and should not be withheld for this reason. Even when large doses of opioids are used as a constant rate

---

* Corresponding author.
E-mail address: kmathews@ovc.uoguelph.ca (K.A. Mathews).

0195-5616/05/$ - see front matter © 2005 Elsevier Inc. All rights reserved.
doi:10.1016/j.cvsm.2004.10.012
vetsmall.theclinics.com

Box 1. Expected level of pain associated with various emergent conditions

Severe to excruciating
  Neuropathic pain: nerve entrapment, cervical intervertebral
    disk herniation, inflammation (ie, bacterial, chemical,
    impingement)
  Central nervous system infarction/tumors
  Meningitis
  Inflammation: extensive (ie, peritonitis, fasciitis [especially
    streptococcal], cellulitis)
  Multiple fracture repair when extensive soft tissue injury
    exists
  Necrotizing pancreatitis
  Necrotizing cholecystitis
  Pathologic fractures
  Bone cancer
Moderate to severe and severe (varies with degree of illness or
  injury)
  Osteoarthritis, acute polyarthritis
  Early or resolving stages of soft tissue injuries/inflammation/
    disease
  Peritonitis (ie, bacterial, urine, bile, pancreatic)
  Capsular pain caused by organomegaly (ie, pyelonephritis,
    hepatitis, splenitis, splenic torsion)
  Hollow organ distention
  Mesenteric, gastric, testicular, or other torsion
  Ureteral/urethral/biliary obstruction
  Pleuritis
  Traumatic diaphragmatic hernia repair (associated with
    organ and extensive tissue injury)
  Trauma (ie, orthopedic, extensive soft tissue, head)
  Thoracolumbar disk disease
  Rewarming after accidental hypothermia
  Frostbite
  Cancer pain
  Mucositis after radiation therapy
  Thrombosis/ischemia (arterial or venous), aortic saddle
    thrombosis
  Hypertrophic osteodystrophy
  Panosteitis
  Corneal abrasion/ulceration
  Glaucoma

Uveitis
Whelping/queening
  Mastitis
Moderate
  Diaphragmatic hernia repair (acute, simple with no organ
    injury)
  Soft tissue injuries (ie, less severe than those mentioned
    previously)
  Urethral obstruction
  Early or resolving conditions as mentioned previously
Mild to moderate
  Some dental problems
  Some lacerations
  Cystitis
  Otitis
  Chest drains
  Early or resolving conditions mentioned previously
Mild
  Early, resolving, or simple involvement of conditions
    mentioned previously

This list is far from complete. These examples and their assessed levels of pain are only presumed (see Tables 1 through 8 for suggested analgesic therapy with dose and interval adjustment based on the individual patient response).

infusion (CRI) to treat pain, heart rate is still high in response to hypotension, hypoxia, hypovolemia, or hypercarbia. In fact, when the patient is treated adequately for pain, the potential for the tachycardia being pain related is eliminated and the clinician is alerted to patient deterioration. If analgesics are not used, the tachycardia may be presumed to be caused by pain and other reasons are not considered.

Another major concern with analgesic use expressed by many veterinarians is the potential toxicity or adverse reactions associated with drug administration [10–12]. It is the impression of the authors and others that these adverse effects, primarily those associated with opioid use, are overemphasized. With respect to ventilation, opioid administration after a traumatic incident may improve ventilation rather than impair it. Recent studies confirm that oxymorphone or hydromorphone does not result in deterioration in hemodynamics when administered to dogs with 30% blood loss [13]. This concern for potential adverse effects of various analgesics is also a major reason for less frequent analgesic administration to cats [10,11,14]. Given our current level of understanding of the adverse effects of many analgesics in cats [15], however, there is no longer an overriding reason for withholding them in this species. Throughout the veterinary literature, various analgesic regimens are suggested for many painful states in cats and dogs, and it is recommended that these "tried and true" guidelines be used rather than sticking to "traditional" or outdated single-study dogma.

The use of nonsteroidal anti-inflammatory analgesics (NSAIAs) in the emergent patient may be a concern, and these agents should be withheld until the volume, cardiovascular, and renal status of patients is determined to be within normal limits and with no potential for deterioration [16]. As a guideline, until studies indicate safety in this group of patients, NSAIAs should not be administered to patients with acute renal insufficiency, hepatic insufficiency, dehydration, hypotension, conditions associated with low "effective circulating volume" (eg, congestive heart failure, ascites), coagulopathies (eg, factor deficiencies, thrombocytopenia, von Willebrand disease), or evidence of gastric ulceration or a gastrointestinal disorder of any kind (eg, vomiting with or without the presence of "coffee ground material," melena). Concurrent use of other NSAIAs (eg, aspirin) or corticosteroids is not recommended. NSAIAs are contraindicated in patients with spinal injury (including herniated intervertebral disk) because of the potential for hemorrhage with associated neurologic deterioration if cyclooxygenase (COX)-1 selective NSAIAs are used. COX-2 NSAIAs may not be a problem; however, even minor hemorrhage in the spinal cord may be deleterious. NSAIAs should never be administered to patients in shock, trauma cases on presentation, or patients with evidence of hemorrhage (eg, epistaxis, hemangiosarcoma, head trauma). Patients with severe or poorly controlled asthma or other moderate to severe pulmonary disease may deteriorate with NSAIA administration. Although administration of NSAIAs in head trauma, pulmonary diseases, or thrombocytopenia is generally contraindicated, COX-2 preferential or COX-1–sparing NSAIAs (eg, meloxicam, etodolac, carprofen, tolfenamic acid) may prove to be safe with further study. NSAIAs may have effects on the reproductive tract and fetus [17]; therefore, NSAIAs should not be administered during pregnancy. Because COX-2 induction is necessary for ovulation and subsequent implantation of the embryo [17], NSAIAs should also be avoided in breeding female animals during this stage of the reproductive cycle.

In addition to analgesia for pain, many injured or ill animals require analgesia to facilitate restraint, diagnostic, and emergency procedures. Because each animal is presented with varying levels of injury or illness and is experiencing different degrees of pain, individual drug selection and dosing to effect are essential rather than considering a standard regimen for all patients.

Aggression

It is not uncommon for patients to be aggressive on presentation, preventing even the simplest of assessments or treatments. Cats are likely to be aggressive in a strange environment and after a fearful car trip. Animals may seem to be reasonably stable when acting aggressively on admission, but this assumption should not be made hastily. Endorphin and epinephrine release can mask the seriousness of the patient's clinical condition. In the authors' experience, for example, severely dehydrated cats can be so difficult to handle that a proper assessment is impossible without some chemical restraint (Table 1). These animals should be cautiously assessed from afar and a thorough history taken, before selecting a method of restraint. Chemical restraint rather than force is the humane and often safer way to deal with these animals. Once the reason for the aggression has been decided on, a more direct approach to the problem might be possible. Aggression may be secondary to significant pain and fear in traumatized animals. Respiratory distress may appear as a combination of panic and aggression.

If possible, place an oxygen mask on these animals or provide "flow-by" oxygen for supplementation when stress, poor perfusion, or respiratory compromise could exist. An oxygen mask provides a degree of protection to the handler as a type of muzzle for dogs. The aggressive cat could be allowed to settle down in an induction chamber with oxygen administration. If pain is a component of the aggression, opioid administration is a safe and effective approach to management. Opioids are considered extremely safe from the cardiovascular standpoint, with side effects that are usually easy to treat (administration of anticholinergic agent in the case of bradycardia or titration of naloxone should other unwanted effects occur). Because the intravenous route is often not possible in these animals, drugs that can be administered intramuscularly, absorbed through mucous membranes, or inhaled are considered. The dose of opioid does not need to be reduced because of advanced or young age but, rather, on the basis of clinical condition. When doubt exists as to the origin of the animal's illness, it may be wise to use meperidine initially (eg, mild effect, short duration, minimal respiratory depression or panting that rarely produces nausea and is reversible). Meperidine at a dose of 3 to 10 mg/kg administered intramuscularly is suggested (lower doses for giant breeds and higher doses for cats and small dogs). If this is not effective, a more profound opioid or a mild sedative can be administered. When upper gastrointestinal obstruction or significant central nervous system (CNS) trauma is not present, a profound opioid, such as oxymorphone at a dose of 0.03 to 0.1 mg/kg administered intramuscularly or intravenously, hydromorphone at a dose of 0.05 to 0.2 mg/kg administered intramuscularly or intravenously, or morphine at a dose of 0.5 to 1 mg/kg administered intramuscularly (dogs) or 0.2 mg/kg administered intramuscularly (cats), repeating the dose if needed, should have a more calming effect. Mydriasis is noted in cats as the opioid effects occur. Young healthier animals may require the higher dose, and a sedative is also usually required. When the physiologic status of the patient is not known, the safest supplement to opioid sedation is

Table 1
Commonly used drugs for most trauma patients

Drug	Dose (mg/kg)	Route	Comments
Opioids			
Meperidine	3–10	IM	This is the suggested dose (low doses for giant breeds and high doses for cats and small dogs); if this is not effective, a more profound opioid or a mild sedative can be administered
Oxymorphone or	0.03–0.1	IM, IV	These are preferred when upper gastrointestinal obstruction or
Hydromorphone	0.03–0.15	IM, IV	significant CNS trauma is not present; the younger and healthier an animal is, the higher is the dose required and the less sedative effect these opioids have if given alone; if concerns exist, titrate to effect at low doses initially
Butorphanol	0.1–0.4	IM, IV	If concerns exist, titrate to effect at low doses initially; use of analgesia is necessary in neurologic cases regardless of potential respiratory depression; hand or mechanical positive-pressure ventilation can be instituted if this risk exists
Fentanyl	~4 µg/kg/h		Titrated to effect as a CRI, is recommended for moderate to severe pain; administration can be stopped periodically to allow for neurologic assessment in such cases.
Sedatives			
Midazolam or Diazepam	0.2–0.5	IV recommended	These are the safest supplements to opioid sedation; IM absorption of midazolam is better than that of diazepam because of the solubility characteristics, and it is preferred, if available, when an IM route is chosen
α_2-agonists: Medetomidine	0.01–0.02 (for healthy animals)		The ability to reverse these drugs provides added safety and convenience for outpatients; can also be used at low doses (0.005–0.01 mg/kg) with opioids to provide dependable and profound restraint in healthy animals

Table 1 (*continued*)

Drug	Dose (mg/kg)	Route	Comments
Other drugs			
Ketamine	2–10	Preferably IV	Given by any route (including squirting a dose in the mouth) can easily and effectively restrain aggressive cats
Combinations			
Hydromorphone	0.1–0.2	IM, IV	These can be administered in
or			combination for more sedation
Morphine (dogs only)	0.5–1	IM, SC	and restraint when minor compromise is apparent and
or			advanced age is not a concern;
Butorphanol	0.1–0.4		higher doses can be administered
with			for smaller animals and when
Acepromazine	0.01–0.05		more restraint needed; lower
	0.05–0.15 (cats)		doses are given in older animals (acepromazine) or larger animals
Ketamine (as above)		IV recommended	These should be combined with ketamine in cats when an IM
with			route is possible to produce better
Midazolam/	0.2–0.5		restraint and relaxation with
Diazepam			lower doses of ketamine; avoid
or			ketamine in cats if the possibility
Acepromazine (cats)	0.05–0.15		exists of significant renal compromise because it requires renal excretion for recovery
Medetomidine	0.005–0.01 mg/kg		The ability to reverse these drugs
with	(for healthy		provides added safety and
Opioids (any	animals) (see		convenience for healthy
of the	doses above)		outpatients; may provide more
above)			dependable and profound restraint in healthy animals when combined

Abbreviations: CNS, central nervous system; CRI, constant rate infusion; IM, intramuscular; IV, intravenous; SC, subcutaneous.

From Mathews K, editor. Pain: how to understand, recognize, treat, and stop [12-hour tutorial]. CD-ROM ISBN0-9732655-0-7. Guelph: Jonkar Computer Systems; 2003; with permission.

midazolam or diazepam (0.2–0.5 mg/kg). Absorption of midazolam is better than that of diazepam when given intramuscularly because of solubility characteristics, and midazolam is preferred when an intramuscular route is chosen. Occasionally, the benzodiazepines are unpredictable, and excitement may occur. When minor compromise is apparent and advanced age is not a concern, the aggressive animal can be most effectively and predictably sedated with a profound opioid and acepromazine at a dose of 0.02 to 0.05 mg/kg (dogs) or 0.05 to 0.15 mg/kg (cats). Aggressive cats can be restrained effectively and easily with ketamine (2–10 mg/kg) given by any route, including squirting a dose into the mouth. Midazolam, diazepam, or acepromazine should be combined with ketamine when an intramuscular route is possible so as to produce better restraint and relaxation with a lower dose of ketamine. Avoid ketamine in cats if the possibility of significant renal compromise exists, because it requires renal excretion for recovery [18]. α_2-Agonists can be used at low doses with opioids to provide dependable and profound restraint in healthy animals. It is important to stress "low doses" and "healthy animals," because arrhythmias, cardiac output depression, and mortality have been associated with the use of xylazine in small animals when anesthesia follows [19,20]. Although the newer drugs in this class (eg, medetomidine, romifidine) produce similar cardiac output effects and bradycardia, they may prove useful if used judiciously and combined with opioids to reduce the dose required. Healthy animals can be given xylazine at a dose of 0.05 to 0.2 mg/kg or medetomidine at a dose of 0.005 to 0.02 mg/kg with low to moderate doses of opioids. The ability to reverse these drugs provides added safety and convenience for outpatients. Obtain intravenous access as soon as the animal allows it.

An aggressive animal with unknown health status should not be given intramuscular doses of any drug at levels capable of producing anesthesia even if anesthesia might be required. Attempt mild to moderate restraint with initial drug therapy; if the animal then proves to be sensitive to the drugs, there is less chance of adverse effects or overdose. If you have achieved some restraint, you can then carry out a proper evaluation of the patient, allowing formulation of a safe anesthetic plan if required.

Because of the potential for extremely sick cats to remain aggressive (sometimes in spite of opioid administration), and because restraint for an intramuscular injection may be difficult and stressful, chamber inhalant induction is often required. This is a good choice in aggressive cats with suspected renal failure or older cats with an unknown medical condition. Allow the animal to calm down in the tank before turning on the inhalant. Oxygen should be provided, and, initially, a towel covering the chamber may help to reduce the animal's stress. Observe the animal frequently during this time, and move the tank to assess the level of restraint achieved. Remove the cat and transfer it to a mask as soon as possible to allow better in-depth evaluation. Isoflurane is the drug of choice for induction but should not be administered until the cat's epinephrine release has minimized. Recognize that complete anesthetic induction is not always required for restraint and that sedation alone is possible with isoflurane. If respiratory depression or obstruction occurs with this degree of restraint, complete induction and intubation are required—so be prepared. The patient requires cautious monitoring during this time (whether restraint or anesthesia is provided) while catheter placement, blood sample pro- curement, and other diagnostic assessments may be occurring. An appropriate analgesic can be given after restraint if pain is a component of the problem or diagnostic procedure. The inhalant percentage dialed should be reduced within 5 minutes of administration to avoid a deepened plane.

If anesthetic induction in the cat proceeds more rapidly than expected (2–3 minutes), this implies that significant cardiac output depression may be present; rapid crystalloid (20–30 mL/kg) or synthetic colloid (2–10 mL/kg) therapy given over 20 to 30 minutes with inotropic support with dopamine (10 µg/kg/min more or less to effect) is advised. Suggested analgesics and sedatives are listed in Table 1.

Neurologic compromise

Significant CNS depression can be present in animals admitted for emergency care. It is critical to provide oxygen and determine if positive-pressure ventilation is required. Increased respiratory depression with resultant increased $Paco_2$ from opioid drug therapy can result in a rise in intracranial pressure (ICP), as can nausea and vomiting, and could eventually result in brain herniation if not addressed. Although analgesia may seem to be adequate based on the level of CNS depression caused by head trauma, this must be well assessed, because pain also raises ICP. If analgesia is necessary, it should be administered by titrating, slowly to effect, low doses of an opiate (fentanyl, 2–5 µg/kg, administered every 15–20 minutes preferably), regardless of potentiated respiratory depression; positive-pressure ventilation should be instituted if this risk exists. Vomiting must be avoided. Butorphanol administered intravenously at a dose of 0.1 to 0.4 mg/kg or meperidine administered intramuscularly at a dose of 3 to 5 mg/kg is an alternative. A fentanyl CRI in cats and dogs is recommended for moderate to severe pain. Because fentanyl has a short (~20 minutes) duration of action, administration can be stopped periodically to allow for neurologic assessment. The response to these drugs must be monitored cautiously. When indicated, the use of a lidocaine bolus (2 mg/kg), followed by 1 to 2 mg/kg/h, for analgesia in these dogs may be of value for up to 24 hours. A reduction in ICP may also occur with intravenously administered lidocaine (K.A. Mathews, DVM, DVSc, personal observation 1992–2004) [21–23]. Suggested analgesics are listed in Table 2.

Respiratory compromise

Respiratory compromise is usually apparent directly on admission and is often associated with excitement, panic, or anxiety. If severe, it can progress rapidly to respiratory and cardiac arrest and thus must be dealt with immediately. Calming the animal facilitates therapy in mild situations, but anesthesia may be necessary for immediate treatment in severely distressed patients. In these situations, advanced preparation for intubation and ventilation should be undertaken; equipment and drugs with doses calculated should be made available. Personnel who might be involved should be properly briefed on monitoring these patients and on the need to respond quickly and efficiently if deterioration should occur. Recommendations for analgesia in the respiratory-compromised patient are listed in Table 2.

Table 2
Respiratory compromise

Drug	Dose (mg/kg)	Route	Comments
Upper airway obstruction/trauma			
Acepromazine and/or	0.01–0.05 (adjusted for size and age)		These can be beneficial; IV route for rapid effect; if
Butorphanol	0.05–0.2 (adjusted for size and age)		unsuccessful, anesthetic induction and intubation are necessary
Diazepam/ ketamine or	2.5/50 of mixture @ 0.02 mL/kg	IV	Chosen for the advantage of safe and slow induction to effect; these animals may be
Propofol	1	IV	sensitive to the dose used, especially if hypoxic; titrate to effect using one fourth to one fifth of typical induction doses repeated at 15–20 seconds until intubation is possible
Diazepam	0.2	IV	Can be given to reduce the dose of propofol required and potential adverse cardiovascular effects (hypotension from vasodilation)
Corticosteroid	0.25 mg/kg dexamethasone		Administration is advised to reduce edema
Butorphanol or	0.05–0.2		If not already administered as an antitussive and to assist
Meperidine	2.5	IM	recovery extubation
Placement of nasal cannula			
Generous instillation of an ophthalmic local anesthetic into the nasal meatus			
Chest tube placement (dogs)			
Butorphanol or	0.05–0.2	IM, IV	Infiltration of a local anesthetic should be used in
Oxymorphone or	0.05–0.1	IM, IV	addition
Hydromorphone	0.05–0.1	IM, SC	
Morphine or methadone with or without	0.1–0.3	IV	
Acepromazine or	0.01–0.05 (adjusted for size and age)		
Diazepam	0.2		
Chest tube placement (cats)			
Butorphanol ±	0.1–0.4		Short-term anesthesia may be required for these
Diazepam with	0.2		procedures in cats; titration for induction and
Propofol	1 mg/kg increments	IV	isoflurane maintenance is preferred for such a short procedure as a result of rapid recovery

Table 2 (*continued*)

Drug	Dose (mg/kg)	Route	Comments
Ketamine or	Incremental doses at 2 mg/kg	IV to effect	This is a safe approach in cats with severe respiratory compromise and unknown cardiovascular status; The sympathetic drive and lesser respiratory depression may offer a slight advantage of ketamine over propofol, although either may be used if cautious
Diazepam/ ketamine	Slow titration of 2.5/50 of mixture @ 0.02 mL/kg	IV	
Major chest trauma Butorphanol	0.2–0.4	IM, IV	Doses selected are primarily size related (smaller dose per kilogram for bigger dogs); an increased respiratory rate may be an early sign of a mild overdose and should be stopped; although morphine can be given very slowly IV, the possibility of histamine release can be a significant concern; IM administration is recommended (except if an infusion is used)
or Oxymorphone	0.03–0.1	IM, IV	
or Hydromorphone or Methadone or morphine	0.05–0.2 (titrate IV to effect) 0.3–0.5 (dogs), 0.1–0.2 (cats)	IM, dependent on the degree of pain	
Ketamine	1–2	IV	This can provide a short-term analgesia if morphine is selected for the long-term analgesic
Bupivacaine (for intercostal nerve blocks)	0.2 mL/kg of 0.5%		Divided among 4–6 nerves can provide analgesia for 3–6 hours, repeated as needed, for rib fractures
Epidural analgesia with morphine (see Table 4)			

Abbreviations: IM, intramuscular; IV, intravenous; SC, subcutaneous.

From Mathews K, editor. Pain: how to understand, recognize, treat, and stop [12-hour tutorial]. CD-ROM ISBN0-9732655-0-7. Guelph: Jonkar Computer Systems; 2003; with permission.

Upper airway obstruction

Although pain may not be experienced with most cases of airway obstruction, it is present with trauma to the upper airway. Typical causes of obstruction involve laryngeal paralysis, laryngeal or pharyngeal foreign bodies, tumors, inflammation or edema, brachycephalic syndrome, and collapsing trachea. Rapid intervention is usually necessary to guarantee oxygen delivery. Handling the animal may result in increased stress and anxiety that can worsen the situation. Calm the animal while attempting oxygen delivery by mask or flow-by. A mixture of oxygen and helium (Heliox) may be more effective because of ease of inspiration in the presence of increased airway resistance [24]. Use of a low dose of acepromazine (0.01–0.05 mg/kg) adjusted for size and age combined with butorphanol (0.05–0.2 mg/kg) adjusted for size or oxymorphone or hydromorphone (0.02–0.05 mg/kg) titrated slowly should be of benefit. The intravenous route is preferred for the most rapid effect and ability to titrate, avoiding overdose. Overdose may result in panting or vomiting.

Lower respiratory injury

Chemical restraint and analgesia are required to facilitate placement of a nasal oxygen cannula or for chest tube placement or radiographic examination. The method of restraint selected should be the minimum required for the procedure, with supplemental oxygen provided before, during, and after the procedure. Generous instillation of an ophthalmic local anesthetic into the nasal meatus is adequate for oxygen cannula placement in cats and dogs. Before chest tube placement in dogs, butorphanol, oxymorphone, or hydromorphone administered intravenously, together with low-dose acepromazine or diazepam at doses suggested previously, is usually effective. Incremental doses of ketamine at 2 mg/kg administered intravenously to effect may be added, or slow titration of diazepam (1 mL [5 mg/mL]) or ketamine (1 mL [100 mg/mL]) up to 0.05 to 0.15 mL/kg may be provided. Cats should be anesthetized. Infiltration of a local anesthetic through the skin to the pleura should always be used before chest tube placement in cats and dogs, even when anesthetized. A warmed 1% solution of lidocaine or 0.25% bupivacaine is recommended to avoid the "sting" of the more concentrated solution. Intrapleural and intraperitoneal placement of local anesthetics is a useful adjunct to opioid analgesics for thoracic incisional pain or pleuritis or pain associated with pancreatitis. Instill a mixture of 0.5% bupivacaine (0.2 mL/kg) and sodium bicarbonate (0.01 mEq/kg), dilute with 0.9% saline (3 mL in cats and small dogs and 6–12 mL [relative to size of dog] for larger dogs) into the peritoneal or pleural space via a chest drain for intrapleural analgesia or via a catheter for intraperitoneal analgesia, and be careful to use aseptic technique. Flush with saline (3–12 mL or a volume equal to chest tube volume) to ensure placement into the pleural space. The addition of the sodium bicarbonate reduces the pain associated with local anesthetics at this site by increasing the pH of the solution. Do not add more sodium bicarbonate, because doing so makes the solution too alkaline; **the ratio of bupivacaine and sodium bicarbonate must be adhered to**. Without the sodium bicarbonate, local anesthetic instillation is painful. After intrapleural administration, the animal should be placed with the injured or incision side down for 5 minutes to enhance the effect at the desired site. The patient can also be rolled onto its back to allow the local anesthetic to flow into the paravertebral gutters to block nerves before entering the spinal cord.

If the patient still appears uncomfortable, adjust its position to facilitate redistribution of the local anesthetic. Although the addition of sodium bicarbonate reduces the pain experienced, the positioning required and the local anesthetic itself can cause some pain, so be prepared for this.

Diaphragmatic hernia

Oxygen supplementation is critical to the safe management of an animal with a diaphragmatic hernia. Pleural fluid should be removed before any procedure is undertaken to reduce ventilatory and oxygenation impairment. Significant cardiovascular compromise is also possible in these patients, and replacement of fluid deficits is important. Special concerns related to intestinal incarceration exist. Restraint may be required for radiography or thoracocentesis. Opioid or diazepam sedation is the safest approach when significant respiratory compromise is present.

Major chest trauma

Oxygen supplementation is a vital part of the treatment in these patients. These animals also need analgesia and may require some sedation to reduce movement and subsequent painful stimulation. Depending on the degree of pain associated with the injury, butorphanol (0.2–0.4 mg/kg), oxymorphone (0.03–0.1 mg/kg), or hydromorphone (0.03–0.1 mg/kg) administered intravenously or morphine (0.3–0.5 mg/kg [dogs], 0.1–0.2 mg/kg [cats]) administered intramuscularly can be used. Although morphine can be given slowly intravenously, the possibility of histamine release with hypotension is a concern with the intravenous route of administration [25] and in- tramuscular administration is recommended (except when an infusion is used). Doses selected are primarily size related (smaller dose per kilogram for larger dogs) and slowly titrated to effect when administered in- travenously. An increased respiratory rate may be an early sign of a mild overdose, and administration of the opioid can be stopped before panting occurs. Ketamine at a dose of 1 to 2 mg/kg administered intravenously can provide a short-term solution for analgesia if morphine is selected for the long-term analgesic. Consider the use of local anesthesia to supplement systemic analgesia. Intercostal nerve blocks using 0.5% bupivacaine at a dose of 0.2 mL/kg divided among four to six nerves can provide excellent analgesia for 3 to 6 hours and can be repeated as needed for rib fractures. Epidural analgesia using morphine at a rate of 0.1 to 0.3 mg/kg administered every 8 to 12 hours can impart reasonable analgesia in the thorax with limited adverse systemic effects [26].

Other trauma

Obviously, lacerations and fractures from trauma require analgesia. The drug and dose for initial management are determined by the severity and instability of the injury (Table 3). The fractured limb should be immobilized until definitive repair. Immobilization of fractures reduces pain significantly, and this should be performed as soon as possible whenever possible. Few, if any, analgesics can stop incident pain produced by movement of fractured bones. Initially, opioids (see Table 3) should be administered while determining cardiovascular and volume status. If there are no concerns regarding ongoing hemorrhage and hypovolemia or other contraindications for administration of an NSAIA, meloxicam, carprofen, or tolfenamic acid may be administered parenterally (Table 4).

Traumatic injury frequently results in muscle pain as well. We all have experienced this but tend to forget it in our veterinary patients. Even if lacerations and fractures are not identified, muscular pain can be present. This results from a direct blow to the muscle, resulting in contusion. Hemorrhage or hematomas may compromise neural structures or result in muscle necrosis, which can be painful. Evidence of hemorrhage may be visualized as bruising, but if it is severe, blood seeps through the skin. Delayed-onset muscular pain is common in people and usually starts several hours after injury. Muscle contusions are painful, and activity should be reduced but not ceased, unless there is a fracture present. To reduce swelling, and thus further discomfort, injuries to musculotendinous structures may benefit from local ice pack therapy (not placed directly onto the skin) for the first 24 hours; thereafter, heat application with gentle stretching of injured muscles is advocated [27].

Injuries sustained to the abdomen, pelvis, hind limbs, and soft tissue of the posterior portion of the body may also benefit from epidural analgesia as noted previously. Should parenteral opioids, combined with an NSAIA in the stable patient, be inadequate to control pain until definitive repair, epidural analgesia is recommended. If this is not possible, consider the addition of an adjunct analgesic, such as lidocaine or ketamine (see Table 4; Table 5). A urinary catheter should be placed in these animals.

Cardiovascular compromise

Avoid unnecessary sedation and anesthesia whenever possible, but recognize that excessive manual restraint with accompanying stress can be associated with epinephrine release and potential adverse effects. Drug doses selected should be low in most circumstances, and titration to effect is desirable (intravenous or inhalant administration) (Table 6). Any opioid alone is reasonable for sedation. Diazepam at a dose of 0.2 mg/kg administered intravenously can be added to improve the effect. The adverse effects are usually minimal. If bradycardia results, an anticholinergic glycopyrrolate at a dose of 0.005 to 0.01 mg/kg administered intravenously should be given to maintain cardiac output [28]. Low-dose ketamine (5 mg per cat) with diazepam can be used to sedate cats while conferring some

Table 3
Suggested analgesics for the initial management of acute pain in cats and dogs

Severe to excruciating pain
Requires high-dose opioids and titration to effect is recommended. You must give oxymorphone; at least 0.2 mg/kg (dogs and cats); hydromorphone; 0.2^+ mg/kg; or morphine, 1 mg/kg (dogs), or 0.2 mg/kg (cats, give more if needed, to effect) IV, or IM. Suggest titrating opioids to effect over 3–5 minutes. Use the effective dose divided by 2–4 to establish an hourly SC or IV CRI or fentanyl, 10 to 50 µg/kg IV titrated to effect (cats and dogs), ± NSAIAs when not contraindicated, ketamine, 4 mg/kg, combined with the opioid as a bolus (dogs and cats); lidocaine, 2–4-mg/kg bolus followed by 2–4-mg/kg/h CRI (dogs), 0.25–1-mg/kg bolus, and then 0.5–2 mg/kg/h (cats). This should not be included if local anesthetics have been administered via a different route. Do not overdose with local anesthetic. Tachycardia may persist. It may be impossible to control the pain. Consider combining the above analgesics with epidurally placed analgesics or local blocks, or anesthetize the patient while attempting to find or treat the inciting cause. Remove the inciting cause immediately. This degree of pain can cause death.

Drug	Dose	Duration of action or dosing interval
Moderate to severe pain		
Morphine or methadone: use low end of the dose for moderate pain	Cat: $0.1–0.2^+$ mg/kg IM, SC Dog: $0.5–1^+$ mg/kg IM, SC For IV dosing use half the low end dose, titrate over 3–5 minutes	2–6 h IM, SC 1–4 h IV
Oxymorphone: use low end of the dose for moderate pain	Cat: $0.02–0.1^+$ mg/kg IV, IM Dog: $0.05–0.2^+$ mg/kg IV, IM	2–6 h
Hydromorphone: use low end of the dose for moderate pain	Cat and dog: $0.02–0.1^+$ mg/kg IV, IM, SC	2–6 h
Fentanyl: use low end of the dose for moderate pain	Cat and dog: $0.001–0.01^+$ mg/kg	0.3h
Ketamine: use low end of the dose for moderate pain	Cat and dog: 1–4 mg/kg IV Cat and dog: 2–10 mg/kg PO	Prn (~0.5 h)
Mild to moderate pain		
Opioids listed above for moderate pain	Low end of dose range for cats and dogs Cat and dog: 0.1–0.4 IV	0.25–1 h
Butorphanol: use low end of dose for mild pain	Cat: 0.4–0.8 mg/kg IM, SC Dog: 0.1–0.4 mg/kg IM, SC	2–4 h 1–2 (3) h
Buprenorphine: use low end of dose for mild pain	Cat: 0.005–0.01 mg/kg IV, IM; 0.02 mg/kg sublingual Dog: 0.005–0.02 mg/kg IV, IM	4–8 h 7 h 4–8 h
Meperidine (pethidine)	Cat and dog: 5–10 mg/kg IM, SC	20–30 min

Opioids should be given to effect even beyond dosing and frequency noted if necessary.

Abbreviations: CRI, constant rate infusion; h, hours; IM, intramuscular; IV, intravenous; min, minutes; NSAIA, nonsteroidal anti-inflammatory analgesic; PO, by mouth; Prn, as needed; SC, subcutaneous.

From Mathews K, editor. Pain: how to understand, recognize, treat, and stop [12-hour tutorial]. CD-ROM ISBN0-9732655-0-7. Guelph: Jonkar Computer Systems; 2003; with permission.

Table 4
Suggested analgesia for various levels of ongoing pain

Severe to excruciating pain
  Requires high-dose opioids and titration to effect is recommended. You must give
  oxymorphone at least 0.2 mg/kg (dogs and cats); hydromorphone; 0.2^+ mg/kg; or morphine,
  1 mg/kg (dogs) or 0.2 mg/kg (cats, give more if needed, to effect) IM or SC given to effect.
  Suggest titrating opioids to effect over 3–5 minutes. Use the effective dose divided by 2–4 to
  establish an hourly SC or IV CRI or fentanyl, 10–50 µg/kg/h CRI (cats and dogs), ± NSAIAs
  where not contraindicated; ketamine, 4 mg/kg, combined with the opioid above as a bolus
  and followed with 2–4 mg/kg/h CRI (dogs and cats); lidocaine, 2–4 mg/kg bolus followed by
  2–4 mg/kg/h CRI (dogs) or 0.25–1 mg/kg bolus, and then 0.5–2 mg/kg/h (cats). This should
  not be included if local anesthetics have been administered via a different route. Do not
  overdose with local anesthetic. Tachycardia may persist. It may be impossible to control the
  pain. Consider combining the above analgesics with epidurally placed analgesics or local
  blocks, or anesthetize the patient while attempting to find or treat the inciting cause. Remove
  the inciting cause immediately. This degree of pain can cause death.
  For epidural analgesia/anesthesia, a 1:1 mixture of preservative-free morphine (1 mg/mL)
  and 0.25% bupivacaine is prepared and slowly injected over 5–10 minutes (to avoid vomiting
  and development of a patchy block) at 0.1 mL/kg while the animal is in sternal recumbency;
  follow with a CRI at 0.4–0.8 mL/kg/d. A syringe pump is required to deliver these small
  volumes. If lidocaine is given systemically, eliminate bupivacaine from this mixture to avoid
  overdose of local anesthetic. The beneficial effect of the CRI is related to the proximity of
  catheter tip to nerve roots involved. As an alternative to a CRI, intermittent injections (over
  5–10 minutes) of 0.15–0.2 mL/kg every 6 hours may be administered. If hind limb weakness is
  encountered, the bupivacaine dose should be reduced by one half (0.125%) or one quarter
  (0.0625%) by diluting with sterile saline before mixing with the morphine. Sterility must be
  maintained when withdrawing, diluting, and mixing, because these are not bacteriostatic
  solutions. Prepare a single volume of the mixture for each 24 hours of treatment to avoid
  frequent disconnections of the syringe and contamination.

Drug	Dose	Duration
Moderate to severe pain		
Morphine or methadone	Cat: $0.1–0.2^+$ mg/kg IV, titrate to effect over 3–5 minutes	1–4 h
	0.1–0.5 IM, SC	2–6 h
	Dog: 0.3–1 mg/kg IV, IM, SC	2–4 h
	Administer intermittently or follow with a CRI with effective dose over dosing interval	
Oxymorphone	Cat: $0.02–0.1^+$ mg/kg IV, IM, SC	2–4 h
	Dog: 0.05–0.2 mg/kg IV, IM, SC	2–4 h
	Administer intermittently or follow with a CRI with effective dose over dosing interval	
Hydromorphone	Cat and dog: $0.02–0.1^+$ mg/kg IV, IM, SC	2–6 h
	Administer intermittently or follow with a CRI with effective dose over dosing interval	
Fentanyl	Cat and dog: $0.004–0.01^+$ mg/kg IV bolus	0.3 h
	$0.001–0.010^+$ mg/kg/h	CRI
Fentanyl patch	Cat and dog: <10 kg 25 µg/h	3–5 days

Table 4 (*continued*)

Drug	Dose	Duration
	Dogs: 10–20 kg to 50 µg/h 20–30 kg to 75 µg/h >30 kg–100 µg/h	3 days
Ketamine combined with an opioid or sedative	Cat and dog: 1–4[+] mg/kg/h IV, SC	Bolus
	0.2–4 mg/kg IV	CRI
Ketoprofen[a]	Cat: ≤ 2 mg/kg SC, then ≤ 1 mg/kg	Once, then Every 24 h up to 4 days
	Dog: ≤ 2 mg/kg IV, IM, SC, PO then ≤ 1 mg/kg	Once, then Every 24 h up to 4 days
Meloxicam[a]	Cat: ≤ 0.2 mg/kg SC, PO then ≤ 0.1 mg/kg	Once, then Every 24 h up to 3 days
	Dog: ≤ 0.2 mg/kg IV, SC, PO then ≤ 0.1 mg/kg	Once, then Every 24 h
Carprofen[a]	Cat: ≤ 4 (2 suggested) mg/kg SC	Once
	Dog: ≤ 4 mg/kg SC, IV, PO then ≤ 2.2 mg/kg	Once, then Every 12 h, preferably every 24 h
Flunixin meglumine	Cat and dog: 1 mg/kg SC	Once
Ketorolac tromethamine	Cat: 0.25 mg/kg IM	Repeat once in 8–12 h
	Dog: 0.3–0.5 mg/kg IM, IV	Repeat once in 8–12 h
Etodolac	Dog: ≤10–15 mg/kg PO	Every 24 h
Bupivacaine 0.5%	Intrapleural and peritoneal use: 1 mg/kg (0.2 mL/kg lean weight) + 0.01 mEq/kg sodium bicarbonate diluted to 3, 6, or 12 mL (depending on size of the animal) with saline; for intrapleural, flush this through tube with volume of 0.9% saline equal to volume of chest drain	6 h
Mild to moderate pain		
Opioids above	Low dosages	Titrate down to lowest effective dose
Buprenorphine	Cat: 0.005–0.01 mg/kg IV, IM 0.01–0.002 mg/kg sublingual Dog: 0.005–0.02 mg/kg IV, IM	4–8 h 7 h 4–8 h
NSAIAs above	Low dosages	Titrate down to lowest effective dose
Butorphanol	Cat and dog 0.1–0.4 mg/kg IV, IM, SC Administer intermittently or follow with a CRI with the effective dose over 2-hour dosing interval	2 h

(*continued on next page*)

Table 4 (*continued*)

Drug	Dose	Duration
Meperidine (pethidine)	5–10 mg/kg IM, SC for short-duration analgesia or administered at time of NSAIA injection	20–30 minutes
Morphine syrup	0.5 mg/kg PO titrate to effect	Every 4–6 h
Codeine	0.5–2 mg/kg PO titrate to effect	Every 6–12 h
Bupivacaine 0.5%	6 h	
Sedatives to combine with opioids		
Midazolam	Cat and dog: 0.1–0.5 mg/kg IV, IM	Dog: up to 6 h Cat: can be >6 h
Diazepam	Cat and dog: 0.1–0.5 mg/kg IV	Dog: up to 6 h Cat: can be >6 h
Acepromazine	Cat and dog: 0.01–0.05 mg/kg IV	1–2 h
	Cat and dog: 0.02–0.1 mg/kg IM, SC	2–6 h
Medetomidine	0.002–0.004 mg/kg IM, SC	

Note: Opioids, ketamine, or lidocaine as a CRI can be combined in IV crystalloid fluids (lactated Ringer solution or Ringer solution may not be compatible because of calcium content). I suggest placing the medication in a burette in-line with the maintenance fluid rate. Additional individual drugs can be placed in the burette, or additional fluids can be added to dilute if reduction is required.

Abbreviations: CRI, constant rate infusion; h, hours; IM, intramuscular; IV, intravenous; NSAIA, nonsteroidal anti-inflammatory analgesic; PO, by mouth; SC, subcutaneous.

[a] Dosing based on lean body weight is recommended.

From Mathews K, editor. Pain: how to understand, recognize, treat, and stop [12-hour tutorial]. CD-ROM ISBN0-9732655-0-7. Guelph: Jonkar Computer Systems; 2003; with permission.

analgesia. Propofol should not be used in these animals because of the potential for significant hypotension [29].

Opioids are generally considered the safest analgesic and are most effective in reducing the dose of other agents used for restraint and induction or maintenance of anesthesia should this be required. Oxymorphone, fentanyl, alfentanil, and sufentanil are the drugs most widely accepted as safe in patients with cardiovascular compromise. Butorphanol has not been shown to have significant minimum alveolar concentration (MAC)–sparing effects in dogs [30]. Hydromorphone reduces MAC and is similar to oxymorphone in hypovolemic dogs, suggesting safety with its use. Morphine, although it also reduces MAC, is generally not advised because of its venodilation and potential for histamine release [25]. Recommended analgesic doses for various cardiovascular problems are listed in Table 6.

Shock

Provide oxygen by face mask, nasal cannula, tent, or flow-by while proceeding with assessments and treatment. These animals may be 10% to

Table 5
Adjunctive analgesic suggested dosages

Drug	Species	Dosage (mg/kg)	Route of administration	Duration
Ketamine	Dogs and cats	0.2–4	IV	Bolus for control, followed by CRI depending on severity of pain
		02–4 mg/kg/h	IV	
Lidocaine	Dogs	1–4	IV	Bolus, followed by CRI depending on severity of pain
		1–3 mg/kg/h	IV	CRI
	Cats	0.25–1	IV	
		10–40 µg/kg/min	IV	
Gabapentin	Cats	2.5–5 (10)	PO	q12h
	Dogs	5–10 (25)	PO	q8h for pain
		up to 12	PO	q6h for postseizure or post-CPR vocalization and thrashing; wean off slowly

Abbreviations: CPR, cardiopulmonary resuscitation; CRI, constant rate infusion; h, hours; IV, intravenous; min, minutes; PO, by mouth; q, every.

From Mathews K, editor. Pain: how to understand, recognize, treat, and stop [12-hour tutorial]. CD-ROM ISBN0-9732655-0-7. Guelph: Jonkar Computer Systems; 2003; with permission.

15% dehydrated or may have experienced an intravascular fluid volume loss of 30% to 45%. Fluid resuscitation (with at least 50% of the loss corrected) should be achieved before profound chemical restraint or anesthesia is performed. The CNS depression associated with shock should allow catheter placement without any analgesia. When a venous cutdown is required to place a catheter, subcutaneous infiltration of a small volume (0.5–1 mL) of 1% lidocaine can provide local desensitization. A local anesthetic, such as 1% lidocaine, should be used, if time permits, in any sedated, depressed, or stuporous animal before an emergency procedure (eg, chest drain placement, venous cutdown), because although pain is still perceived, the animal cannot respond. This is also effective for jugular catheter placement in such patients. The crystalloid fluids should then be administered at a rate to restore perfusion as soon as possible (45–90 mL/kg/h is typical). This varies with the individual patient and problem.

Once the animal is starting to respond, consider the need for analgesia (as noted previously). The persistent catecholamine release associated with pain further reduces oxygen delivery to the tissues as well as increasing oxygen demand, and this detrimental effect is of greater concern than any adverse opioid effect. Partial reversal with naloxone (0.4-mg/mL solution at a dose of 0.1–0.25 mL diluted in saline [10 mL] titrated in 1-mL increments to effect) is possible if any problem arises. Analgesia is not be reversed, but the unwanted adverse effects using this technique are eliminated.

Table 6
Cardiovascular compromise: shock and dehydration

Drug	Dose (mg/kg)	Route	Comments
Butorphanol or	0.2–0.4		Doses selected are primarily size related (smaller dose per kilogram for bigger dogs); an increased respiratory rate may be an early sign of a mild overdose and should be stopped
Oxymorphone or	0.03–0.1	IM, IV	
Hydromorphone or	0.05–0.2	Titrate IV to effect	
Methadone or	0.3–0.5 (dogs)	IV, IM	
Morphine	0.1–0.2 (cats)	IM, dependent on the degree of pain	Although morphine can be given slowly IV, the possibility of histamine release can be a significant concern; IM administration is recommended (except if an infusion is used)

Abbreviations: IM, intramuscular; IV, intravenous.
From Mathews K, editor. Pain: how to understand, recognize, treat, and stop [12-hour tutorial]. CD-ROM ISBN0-9732655-0-7. Guelph: Jonkar Computer Systems; 2003; with permission.

Dehydration

If analgesia, restraint, or sedation is required in a dehydrated animal, do not use acepromazine. Start with a low-dose opioid, and slowly increase and add diazepam or midazolam as needed to effect.

Arrhythmias

Some trauma patients or other emergent patients may have premature ventricular contractions (PVCs). Such arrhythmias should be controlled before use of profound chemical restraint or anesthesia if at all possible. Careful titration of an opioid may be required, however, because PVCs may be enhanced or caused by pain. Tachyarrhythmias are also frequently related to insufficient management of pain. Address pain with opioids in these cases, because enhanced vagal tone can also be advantageous. Traumatic myocarditis with associated arrhythmias is not uncommon and may be noted on presentation or within the following 48 hours. Such cases are difficult to treat; therefore, analgesics should not be withheld. The rate of PVCs is not as significant an issue as is the effect of these arrhythmias (ie, poor cardiac output and perfusion). Initially, oxygen should be administered to improve O_2 delivery to the myocardium, especially areas of poor perfusion (traumatized).

When concern persists related to the arrhythmia, a bolus of lidocaine at a dose of 2 mg/kg should be given in an attempt to eliminate the arrhythmia (repeat if needed). This is followed by administration of 50 µg/kg/min in the awake animal, whereas 120 µg/kg/min is recommended in dogs during isoflurane anesthesia to provide therapeutic levels when more guaranteed control is warranted [31]. This higher dose, which is recommended during anesthesia, should be reduced after 1 hour to the lower levels that are typically used for long-term treatment (40–80 µg/kg/min). The advantages of treating PVCs in advance of anesthesia are to know that they are possible to treat, to reduce the chance of a fatal arrhythmia during the stress of anesthetic induction and surgery, and to maximize cardiac output. Mild sedation and a MAC-sparing effect occur with therapeutic levels of lidocaine (advantageous, because the inhalant causes significant cardiovascular depression). Procainamide (6–15 µg/kg intramuscularly or intravenously over 20 minutes) to avoid hypotension may be required if there is no response to lidocaine. Hypokalemia or metabolic acidosis may contribute to ventricular arrhythmias. If opioid use results in significant bradycardia in animals without cardiovascular compromise, atropine or glycopyrrolate can be used to treat the bradycardia. Glycopyrrolate is commonly chosen over atropine because of the increased duration of effect and slightly lower incidence of tachycardia and arrhythmias. It can take as long as 3 minutes to see the full effect of glycopyrrolate. Atropine has a more rapid onset of action than glycopyrrolate and is selected when a significant bradycardia is immediately life threatening. If the patient is hypovolemic, treat the hypovolemia before treating opioid-induced bradycardia.

Gastrointestinal or visceral pain

α_2-Agonists, hydromorphone, and morphine have an increased incidence of vomiting when used for premedication or analgesia in the awake animal. These drugs should be avoided in cases in which a foreign body or other obstruction is suspected to avoid vomiting and subsequent worsening of the pain or when the potential for gastrointestinal rupture occurs. Oxymorphone is commonly chosen, but if it is not available, meperidine (3–5 mg/kg administered intramuscularly) can be used for premedication or mild sedation for procedures like radiography or reducing stress and pain as well as for reducing the dose of drugs used for induction. The more profound opioid that is available can be given after induction and stabilization when the vomiting center is less receptive to opioids as a result of the depressant effects of general anesthesia at this site. Analgesic recommendations for the various gastrointestinal problems are listed in Table 7.

Gastric or dilation volvulus

Cardiovascular compromise can present as a primary problem in these cases if shock, dehydration, or arrhythmias are present (refer to the previous

Table 7
Gastrointestinal compromise

Opioid agonists (narcotics)	Dose (mg/kg)	Route of administration	Interval (hours)
Morphine	Dog		
	0.1–0.5	IV, slowly	1–4
	0.1–0.5	IV, over 1 hour	CRI
	0.5–1	IM, SC	1–4 (6)
	0.1–0.3	Epidural	4–8 (12)
	0.5–2	PO, titrate to effect	4–6
	Cat		
	0.05–0.2	IV, slowly IM, SC	2–6
	0.5–1	PO, titrate to effect	8–12
Oxymorphone	Dog		
	0.03–0.1	IV	2–4
	0.05–0.2	IM, SC	2–4 (6)
	0.05–0.3	Epidural	4–6
	Cat		
	0.02–0.1	IV	2–4
	0.05–0.1	IM, SC	2–4
Hydromorphone	Dog		
	0.03–0.1	IV	2–4
	0.1–0.2	IM, SC	2–4 (6)
	Cat		
	0.04–0.20	IV	2–4
	0.10–0.20	IM, SC	2–4 (6)
Methadone	Dog and cat		
	0.1–0.5	IV, IM, SC	2–4
Fentanyl	Cat and dog		
	0.001–0.005[+]	IV loading	0.5–1
	0.001–0.005	IV, 20–60 min	CRI
	0.05 anesthesia	IV, 60 min	CRI
Gastric/dilation volvulus			
Oxymorphone or hydromorphone or	0.03–0.04 0.05–0.2	IV (with or without diazepam)	
Methadone	0.3–0.5	IV The dose for each drug can be diluted in saline and slowly given over 5 min until the desired effect is reached; analgesia can produce an antiarrhythmic benefit	

Abbreviations: CRI, constant rate infusion; IM, intramuscular; IV, intravenous; min, minutes; PO, by mouth; SC, subcutaneous.

From Mathews K, editor. Pain: how to understand, recognize, treat, and stop [12-hour tutorial]. CD-ROM ISBN0-9732655-0-7. Guelph: Jonkar Computer Systems; 2003; with permission.

recommendations for cardiac compromise). Acid-base disorders (metabolic acidosis) and electrolyte disturbances (low potassium) may also be present. Occasionally, respiratory compromise may coexist because of abdominal enlargement and pressure on the diaphragm. Oxymorphone (with or without diazepam) is a popular choice for analgesia. Many of these dogs are large (eg, Great Danes); therefore, the effective dose is lower than the dose typically used (0.03–0.04 mg/kg administered intravenously), especially if cardiovascular compromise exists. The dose can be diluted in saline and slowly given over 5 minutes until the desired effect is reached.

Pancreatitis and peritonitis

Pancreatitis is a not an uncommon primary problem in dogs and cats, causing moderate to excruciating pain. Pancreatitis should be considered in patients presented with abdominal pain and in those recovering from a hypotensive event. Mild to moderate pain can be managed with butorphanol at a dose of 0.4 mg/kg administered every 2 to 3 hours or an hourly CRI at a dose equal to the bolus dose that was effective in relieving pain, divided by 2 or 3. Monitoring the patient dictates whether an increase or decrease is required. For patients with pancreatitis, the question is often raised regarding the opioid effects on sphincter tone. Morphine, fentanyl, and oxymorphone, in decreasing order, increase intracommon biliary ductal pressure in human beings, which has been extrapolated to a similar potential effect on pancreatic ductal pressure in dogs; however, because moderate to severe pancreatitis is extremely painful, opioids are required to control this pain. In one of the authors' (K.A. Mathews) experience in managing pain associated with pancreatitis, the opioids have worked well with no apparent adverse effects. Buprenorphine (0.005–0.02 mg/kg [dogs] and 0.005–0.01 mg/kg [cats] administered every 8 hours) has less effect on intraductal pressure in people and may be the drug of choice in mild to moderate pain associated with pancreatitis. For more severe pancreatitis or pain associated with peritonitis caused by abdominal wall–penetrating injuries, gastrointestinal perforation, biliary rupture, or urinary tract injury, oxymorphone, hydromorphone, or fentanyl can be administered in the same fashion as butorphanol, with the exception of the oxymorphone and hydromorphone dose being divided by 4 for an hourly rate and fentanyl being administered at the effective bolus dose per hour. Again, monitoring the patient should indicate whether the dose should be changed. Lidocaine or ketamine may also be added as a CRI (see Tables 4 and 5). Epidural analgesia via an epidural catheter is also an excellent method of controlling severe pain (see Table 4) [32]. A 1:1 mixture of preservative-free morphine (1 mg/mL) and 0.25% bupivacaine is prepared and slowly injected over 5 to 10 minutes (to avoid vomiting and development of a patchy block) at rate of 0.1 mL/kg while the animal is in sternal recumbency, followed by a CRI at a rate of 0.4 to 0.8 mL/kg/d. A syringe pump is required to deliver these small volumes. If lidocaine is given systemically, bupivacaine should be eliminated from this mixture to avoid overdose. The beneficial effect of continuous local anesthetic infusions is related to the proximity of catheter tip to nerve roots involved. As an alternative to a CRI, intermittent injections (over 5–10 minutes) of 0.15 to 0.2 mL/kg administered every 6 hours may be administered. If hind limb weakness is encountered, the bupivacaine dose should be reduced by one half (0.125%) or one quarter (0.0625%) by diluting with sterile saline before mixing with the morphine. Absolute sterility must be maintained when diluting and mixing. It is advised to prepare a single volume of the mixture for each 24 hours of treatment so as to avoid frequent disconnections of the syringe. Be reminded that the morphine is preservative-free; therefore, strict aseptic technique must be observed when withdrawing and mixing.

Intra-arterial or intravenous catheter placement

Most of the time, percutaneous catheter placement is a fast procedure with minimal discomfort; however, in difficult patients, when time permits, a eutectic mixture of local anesthetic (EMLA Cream 2.5% lidocaine and 2.5% prilocaine combined with thickening agents to form an emulsion, AstraZeneca, Wilmington, DE) cream placed over the previously cleansed arterial or venipuncture site eliminates the pain of catheter placement. Dosing is calculated in a manner similar to that of the injectable formulation. Local anesthetic concentrations are described as weight by volume (grams per 100 mL); therefore, the 2% solution is 2000 mg per 100 mL (2g per 100 mL), or 20 mg/mL, which applies to the creams and gels. This product is not sterile and should be used only on intact skin to provide anesthesia for intravenous (peripheral and central) catheter placement, blood collection, lumbar puncture, and other minor superficial procedures. EMLA cream should be covered with an occlusive dressing for at least 20 minutes, and preferably longer, for optimum effect.

Urinary catheter placement

It is frequently necessary to place a urinary catheter in traumatized patients. This procedure rarely requires more than manual restraint in male animals; however, it is more difficult to carry out in female animals. Unless a male dog is struggling excessively or is small, chemical restraint is rarely needed. Female dogs and cats should receive an analgesic. Because the trauma patient is receiving analgesics as a result of pain from other injuries, no additional restraint is required; however, the authors always apply a local anesthetic to female patients and all cats. A sterile 2% lidocaine gel in a tapered-end cartridge (Astra) can be introduced into the vaginal vault or the penile urethra 5 minutes before catheter placement.

Analgesia for nursing mothers

Occasionally, nursing mothers sustain injuries that are painful and require analgesic therapy. In addition to the humane aspect of treating the mother, analgesia is important because a litter of pups or kittens may aggravate the painful state, potentially triggering aggression in the mother toward the pups or kittens. Clearly, analgesics must be administered; however, there is a lack of information regarding the detrimental effects on the pups or kittens of analgesic administration to lactating dogs or cats. There may be a difference in effect based on age; neonates would potentially be more susceptible because of the immaturity of metabolizing functions. The two classes of analgesics commonly used in veterinary patients are opioids and NSAIAs. These drugs are excreted in the milk; however, the quantity is small in people. This information is not available for the dog and cat.

The lipid solubility of the opioid influences its appearance in the milk; therefore, a more hydrophilic opioid, such as morphine, may appear in smaller amounts than a more lipid-soluble opioid, such as oxymorphone or meperidine. In people, a single dose of meperidine or morphine administered to nursing mothers did not seem to cause any risk to the suckling infant; however, repeated administration of meperidine, in contrast to morphine, had a negative impact on the infant [33,34]. Short-term use of codeine in nursing mothers was also noted to be safe; however, infant plasma samples taken 1 to 4 hours after feeding (20–240 minutes after administration to the mother) showed codeine levels to be higher than those of morphine [35]. A 15-day study of human mothers on a methadone maintenance program (40–105 mg/d) concluded that methadone is "safe" to use in breastfeeding mothers [36]. One of the authors (KAM) has used oxymorphone in lactating mothers after trauma for a minimum of 3 days, during which time puppies were vigorous and playful. The mothers were attentive with apparent normal maternal behavior.

Rather than withhold opioid analgesic therapy because of potential concern for the puppies and kittens, administration with observation of behavior is suggested. To avoid the potential for drug side effects, avoid nursing during peak drug levels; when possible, time nursing immediately before the next dose and avoid sedatives with long half-lives [37]. Short-term pain management using a fentanyl patch may be useful in certain cases. Caution is required because of the risk of the puppies or kittens chewing on the patch; thus, a fentanyl patch is not recommended. One drop of naloxone (0.4 mg/mL) from a 1-mL syringe can be administered (sublingually) to puppies and kittens if depression is noted. With this in mind, opioid drugs and doses are listed in Tables 1 through 4. COX-2 is important in nephron maturation [38]. Because NSAIAs may not be lipid soluble, are highly protein bound to plasma proteins, and may be present (to a great degree) in an ionized form in the plasma, theoretically, only a small amount may appear in breast milk and thus be safe to use. It has been suggested that single-time use of an NSAIA is safe in nursing human mothers [33]. A single dose of a COX-2 preferential NSAIA (eg, carprofen, meloxicam; see Table 4) is commonly used for postoperative pain after cesarean section in cats and dogs. No studies have been conducted investigating the prolonged administration of commonly used NSAIAs in cats and dogs, however; until studies indicate that NSAIAs present in the milk of lactating mothers have no affect on renal maturation and function in the puppy or kitten at maturity, it is difficult to know whether long-term use of NSAIAs in the lactating mother have any deleterious affects on the young.

Doses recommended for these animals are given here as a guide and should be those required to relieve pain. As a result, titration to effect would be the most prudent method of dosing.

Analgesia for neonates, infants, weanlings, and pediatric patients

There tends to be apprehension in administering analgesic drugs, especially opioids, to young animals because of the often-cited "decreased drug metabolism and high risk of overdose." Although this may be true in the neonate, it is not necessarily so through all stages of maturation. Based on the human literature, the analgesic requirement may be higher than in the adult at a certain stage of development, especially in the pediatric human patient [39]. Personal experience with intensive monitoring of the rare young (4–6-month-old) animal that inadvertently received 10 times the recommended opioid dose revealed no adverse effects; on the contrary, these animals seemed to be quite comfortable. This is not to suggest that the opioid dose should be increased but to emphasize that administering the analgesic to effect rather than giving a predetermined dose is the most important method by which to manage pain. Opioids can be reversed with naloxone should there be clinical evidence of the need for this (depending on the size of the animal, 0.05–0.1 mL [0.4 mg/mL solution] diluted in saline [5 mL] administered at a rate of 0.5 mL/min and titrated to effect; Table 8). CNS depression associated with respiratory depression, bradycardia, and hypotension rarely occurs when the animal is in pain. Because the effects of the opioid occur quite rapidly after administration, it is wise to monitor for potential adverse effects rather than ignoring appropriate analgesia for a "potential" problem that may not happen.

Neonates, and potentially infants, need to be considered separately from the weanling or juvenile patient when administering analgesics. Neonates do feel pain; however, because of the immaturity of the nervous system, various drugs and dosages require special consideration [40]. Because the N-methyl-D-aspartate (NMDA) system seems to be underdeveloped in the neonate, ketamine may not be effective. Lower doses of fentanyl or morphine are required for analgesia in the neonate when compared with the 5-week-old puppy. Puppies are also more sensitive to the sedative and respiratory depressant affects of morphine, and it is recommended that fentanyl may be a more suitable opioid in the extremely young, especially the neonate. In addition to the nervous system, the hepatorenal system continues to develop until 3 to 6 weeks of age; this may result in reduced metabolism and excretion, altering dosing and dosing intervals [41]. The presence of milk in the stomach and absorption of medication from the gastrointestinal tract are also altered, potentially resulting in lower blood levels. Suggested drugs and doses are listed in Table 8.

Several studies in neonates and infants have revealed that when pain was experienced and not managed at this young age, an increased sensitivity to pain developed; stress disorders, increased anxiety, and attention-deficit hyperactivity disorders, leading to impaired social skills and patterns of self-destruction behavior, also occurred. This has also been shown in laboratory animals [42], and there is no reason to believe this to be any different in cats and dogs.

Local anesthetics are frequently recommended to prevent pain during various emergency procedures. Infiltration of lidocaine is extremely painful even with 27- to 30-gauge needles, especially in the neonate or pediatric patient [43]. To reduce pain, buffering (as previously described), warming (37°C–42°C), and slow administration are recommended. It might be advisable to use a maximum dose of lidocaine administered to kittens at a rate of 3 mg/kg in the neonate to 6 mg/kg to the older pediatric cat and 6 mg/kg in the neonatal pup to 10 mg/kg in the older pediatric dog. The lower dose is required because of the immaturity of the nerves and not because the younger animals are at any greater risk of toxic side effects. This dose should be diluted in 0.9% saline for accurate dosing, ease of administration, and distribution over the site. Bupivacaine may also be used with a 2-mg/kg maximum dose in the older kitten and puppy, with half of this dose advised for the neonate and weanling. Buffering and warming should be performed as described for lidocaine.

The most frequently used topical cream local anesthetic at our institution is EMLA cream (Astra). In children, the peak effect is at 2 hours; however, our experience in animals is that 30 minutes facilitates procedures like jugular catheter placement using the Seldinger technique. A longer dwell time might be necessary in the more active animal, however. The advantage with this product is that no injection is required. The site should be covered after application for approximately 20 minutes.

Sedatives

Sedatives should be used with caution in young animals, especially those less than 12 weeks of age [44]. The phenothiazine tranquilizers (ie, acepromazine) undergo minimal hepatic biotransformation and may cause prolonged CNS depression. These agents are not analgesic; in fact, they may increase the level of pain if analgesics are not coadministered. These drugs

Table 8
Drug dosages for pediatric patients

Drug	Species	Dose (mg/kg) (lower dosages less than 4 weeks of age)	Route of administration (SC suggested for less than 4 weeks of age)	Interval (hours)
Mild to moderate pain				
Opioid agonists				
Morphine	Dog	0.1–0.5	IM, SC, IV slowly	1–4
		0.05[+]	IV, SC over 1 hour	CRI
		0.25[+]	PO, titrate to effect	4–6 (8)
	Cat	0.05–0.1	IM, SC	1–4
		0.025[+]	IV, SC over 1 hour	CRI
		0.25[+]	PO, titrate to effect	4–6 (8)
Methadone	Dog and cat	0.1–0.5	IV, IM, SC	1–4
Oxymorphone	Dog and cat	0.02–0.05	IV, IM, SC	2–4
Hydromorphone	Dog and cat	0.02	IV, IM, SC	2–4 (6)
Fentanyl	Dog and cat	0.002–0.010	IV loading	0.5–1
		0.001–0.005	IV over 20–60 min	CRI
Meperidine	Dog and cat	2–5	IM	0.5–1
Opioid agonist-antagonists				
Butorphanol	Dog	0.1–0.2	IV, IM, SC	1–4
	Cat	0.1–0.2 (or to effect)	IV, IM, SC	1–4
	Dog and cat	0.05–0.01[+]	IV, SC over 1 hour	CRI
Opioid partial agonists				
Buprenorphine		5–10 μg/kg	SC	~6
Moderate to severe pain				
Opioid agonists				
Morphine	Dog and cat	0.5–1[+]	IM, SC, IV slowly	1–4
		0.05[+]	IV, SC over 1 hour	CRI
		0.5[+]	PO, titrate to effect	4–6 (8)
	Cat	0.1–1	IM, SC	1–4
		0.05[+]	IV, SC over 1 hour	CRI
		0.5[+]	PO, titrate to effect	4–6 (8)
Methadone	Dog	0.5–1[+]	IM, SC, IV	1–4
Oxymorphone	Dog and cat	0.05–0.1[+]	IV, IM, SC	2–4
Hydromorphone	Dog and cat	0.05–0.1[+]	IV, IM, SC	2–4 (6)
Fentanyl	Dog and cat	0.005–0.010[+]	IV loading	0.5–1
		0.001–0.005	IV over 20–60 min	CRI
Meperidine	Dog and cat	2–5	IM	0.5–1
Opioid agonist-antagonists				
Butorphanol	Cat	0.3–0.8 (or to effect)	IV, IM, SC	1–4 (6)
		0.2–0.4	IV over 1 hour	CRI
	Dog	0.1–0.4	IV, IM, SC	1–2

Table 8 (*continued*)

Drug	Species	Dose (mg/kg) (lower dosages less than 4 weeks of age)	Route of administration (SC suggested for less than 4 weeks of age)	Interval (hours)
Naloxone: opioid antagonist				

Naloxone should always be available when opioids are used. The dose depends on the administered opioid, dose, and duration. Start by slowly titrating naloxone IV in 0.004–0.04 mg/kg (0.01–0.1 mL of 0.4 mg/mL solution) increments until desired clinical response is achieved. For easy titration, combine naloxone, 0.05–0.1 mL with 0.9% saline 5 or 10 mL. You may have to redose at varying intervals, because duration of opioid action is longer than that of naloxone.

Sedatives				
Midazolam	Cat and dog	0.05–0.1	IV, IM	Dog up to 6 hours Cat can be >6 hours
Diazepam	Cat and dog	0.05–0.1	IV	Dog up to 6 hours Cat can be >6 hours
Acepromazine	Cat and dog	0.01–0.025	IM, SC	2–6

Abbreviations: CRI, constant rate infusion; h, hour; IM, intramuscular; IV, intravenous; min, minutes; PO, by mouth; SC, subcutaneous.

From Mathews K, editor. Pain: how to understand, recognize, treat, and stop [12-hour tutorial]. CD-ROM ISBN0-9732655-0-7. Guelph: Jonkar Computer Systems; 2003; with permission.

induce peripheral vasodilation, and hypotension and hypothermia may result. If these drugs are required, reduce the dose (eg, acepromazine 0.005–0.025 mg/kg administered intramuscularly or subcutaneously). It is advised that the 10-mg/mL concentration of the commercial product be diluted to 1 mg/mL before withdrawing for administration to facilitate accurate dosing. Opioids have sedating effects, especially in young animals; therefore, if these drugs are required, the addition of a sedative may not be necessary in animals younger than 4 months of age. Should sedatives be required, suggested drugs and doses are listed in Table 8.

Opioids

In veterinary patients, it has been recommended to administer half of the usual adult dose of opioids to puppies and kittens. Based on human pediatric studies, this depends on the degree of pain and the phase of maturation. Standard doses can be used if sedation and restraint are also desired (eg, premedication). Starting at lower doses and increasing to effect is recommended for analgesia. Reversal of any adverse effects may be titrated using naloxone as described previously. The dosing recommendations in Table 8 are ranges published for dogs and cats. Fentanyl transdermal patches and fentanyl "lollipops" (transmucosal) are administered to children [45]. No veterinary studies are available in this young group of patients assessing these routes of administration.

Nonsteroidal anti-inflammatory analgesics

These agents are not recommended for animals less than 6 weeks of age based on the developing hepatorenal system. Potential concerns for the administration of NSAIAs immediately after a traumatic event have been previously described.

Analgesia for pregnant dogs and cats

Pregnant animals may suffer injury requiring management with analgesics. The nonsteroidal analgesics must be avoided in these animals because of several potential problems. NSAIAs may have adverse effects on the reproductive tract and fetus because they block prostaglandin activity, resulting in cessation of labor, premature closure of the ductus arteriosus in the fetus, and disruption of fetal circulation [46]. In addition, adverse effects in the fetus similar to those occurring in the adult may occur because of potential placental transfer, and arrest of nephrogenesis may occur because of the importance of COX-2 for maturation of the embryologic kidney [38]. A single injection after a cesarean section is acceptable. Currently, opioids are the analgesic of choice. A review of the addiction medicine literature with experience gained from pregnant women seeking recovery from opioid addiction concluded that methadone, buprenorphine, and morphine seemed safe for the treatment of pain during pregnancy [47,48].

When opioid analgesia is required, dose to effect and treat the underlying problem. Ensure that there are no other stresses and that the animal has a comfortable and clean environment with normal ambient temperature.

The doses in Tables 3 and 4 are those recommended for nonpregnant cat or dog and are given here as a guide. The dose used in the pregnant animal should be titrated according to lean (nonpregnant) weight. Because the goal is to relieve pain, titration to effect would be the most prudent method of dosing.

Adjuvant analgesic drugs

Adjuvant analgesic drugs, such as lidocaine, ketamine, and tricyclic antidepressants, are not generally considered to be primary or first-choice analgesics. In fact, some of these drugs may have weak or nonexistent analgesic effects when used alone. Adjuvant analgesics are typically used in combination with other known analgesic drugs in acute pain states to manage severe pain, where they seem to enhance their analgesic action, or to reduce the dose of the primary analgesic [49]. Suggested dosing regimens for these drugs are listed in Table 5.

Lidocaine

In addition to its local anesthetic effects, lidocaine has been shown to alleviate neuropathic pain and hyperalgesia and to reduce opioid require-ments after surgery when administered as a CRI [50]. Although not necessarily used as an adjunctive analgesic, lidocaine may be useful in managing head trauma patients during periods of increasing ICP, such as occurs during vomiting or "gagging." Lidocaine has been reported to lower ICP during a period of increasing ICP [51–53]. Head trauma patients experience pain, and in some instances, the use of opioids may increase ICP if vomiting is induced or as a result of mild respiratory depression. The degree and significance of respiratory depression caused by opioids may be exaggerated in the head trauma patient. One of the authors (KAM) has used lidocaine in these cases (1 mg/kg bolus) to treat impending tentorial herniation and suggests a CRI in some cases to reduce the opioid requirement in this acute setting for the ensuing 24 hours only.

Ketamine

Ketamine is an NMDA antagonist, blocking the NMDA receptor wind-up and subsequent sensitization of dorsal horn neurons. Ketamine may also abolish established central sensitization. Ketamine should not be used alone for pain management, because there are no veterinary studies assessing efficacy and adverse effects when ketamine is used as a sole analgesic agent in this setting. Ketamine via CRI is used as an adjunctive analgesic in severe pain states in combination with an opioid to enhance analgesia or to reduce opioid requirements [54]. The infusion should be tapered down before being discontinued so as to prevent potential hyperalgesia. The hourly dose varies considerably and is dependent on the pain experienced. The doses in Table 5 are those recommended; however, one of the authors (K.A.M.) has used a dose as high as 4 mg/kg/h in dogs, in addition to high doses of opioid (fentanyl or morphine), to achieve a level of comfort (light plane of anesthesia) facilitating sleep in patients with severe to excruciating pain. At the lower doses required to relieve pain, the patient is alert and comfortable. Ketamine is excreted via the kidney in cats and metabolized by the liver in dogs. It is essential that these organs are functioning normally before administration of ketamine.

Gabapentin

Gabapentin is used in human patients for management of neuropathic pain associated with diabetes, cancer, or primary nerve compression [55].

One of the classic features of this type of pain is the presence of abnormal pain induced by a nonnoxious stimulus (allodynia). Frequently, conventional analgesics, such as opioids and NSAIAs, show limited value in treating this type of pain. In dogs and cats suffering from neuropathic pain secondary to cervical or thoracolumbar intervertebral disk disease or pelvic trauma, gabapentin has reduced the pain in these severe pain states. In the cases in which one of the authors (KAM) treated neuropathic pain with gabapentin, it seemed that gabapentin contributed greatly to the analgesia these animals were experiencing. Frequently, animals requiring this drug need several weeks to months for resolution, if ever, of their pain. Gabapentin is also useful in treating animals that are extremely restless, disoriented, vocalizing, or manic after cardiopulmonary arrest or seizures. Again, dosing to effect and resolution of these signs are the goals. Sedation is appropriate in this instance. There is an extremely wide dose range for gabapentin, and it should be given to effect. The dose-limiting effect generally observed is sedation. Careful lowering of the drug dose is recommended. Gabapentin is an antiepileptic agent; recent studies have shown that gabapentin interacts specifically with the $\alpha_2\delta$ subunits of voltage-dependent calcium channels, and it is suggested that the antiallodynic actions of gabapentin involve a central mechanism of action. It has been reported that gabapentin binds with the high-affinity $\alpha_2\delta$ subunits of voltage-dependent calcium channels, blocking calcium currents in isolated cortical neurons and blocking maintenance of spinal cord central sensitization.

Gabapentin is excreted by the kidneys; animals with renal insufficiency may require less frequent dosing as a result of slower elimination. Because dosing to effect is the method by which the appropriate dose is selected, once this effect is reached, treatment twice a day rather than three times a day may suffice. Nephrotoxicity is not an issue. Signs of overdose are reduced activity and excessive sleepiness progressing to depression. Tapering the dose down is important, because stopping the drug abruptly may lead to rebound pain, which may be severe.

Nursing care

Because a cold, damp, dirty, or noisy environment contributes to stress and anxiety, which, in turn, lowers the threshold to pain sensation, it is important that the patient be made comfortable, clean, warm, and dry. Stabilization of fractures and primary treatment of wounds and burns also reduce pain. Tender loving care is of utmost importance.

References

[1] McCaffrey M. Pain ratings: the fifth vital sign. Am J Nurs 1997;97:15–6.
[2] Staats P. Pain: assessment and approach to practical pain management in the ICU. Presented at the Society of Critical Care Medicine 29th Educational and Scientific Symposium. Orlando, February 11–15, 2000.

[3] Vierck CJ. Extrapolation from the pain research literature to problems of adequate veterinary care. J Am Vet Med Assoc 1976;168:510–4.

[4] Benson GJ, Wheaton LG, Thurmon JC, et al. Postoperative catecholamine response to onychectomy in isoflurane-anesthetized cats: effect of analgesics. Vet Surg 1991;20(3):222–5.

[5] Morton DB, Griffiths PHM. Guidelines on the recognition of pain, distress and discomfort in experimental animals and an hypothesis for assessment. Vet Rec 1985;116:431–3.

[6] Smith JD, Allen SW, Quandt JE, et al. Indicators of postoperative pain in cats and correlation with clinical criteria. Am J Vet Res 1996;209:1674–8.

[7] Katz J, Jackson M, Kavanagh B, et al. Acute pain after thoracic surgery predicts long-term post-thoracotomy pain. Clin J Pain 1996;12:50–5.

[8] Attard AR, Corlett MJ, Kidner NJ, et al. Safety of early pain relief for acute abdominal pain. BMJ 1992;305:554–6.

[9] Brock N. Treating moderate and severe pain in small animals. Can Vet J 1995;36:658–60.

[10] Dohoo SE, Dohoo IR. Factors influencing the postoperative use of analgesics in dogs and cats by Canadian veterinarians. Can Vet J 1996;37:552–6.

[11] Lascelles BD, Capner CA, Waterman-Pearson AE. Current British veterinary attitudes to perioperative analgesia for cats and small mammals. Vet Rec 1999;145:601–4.

[12] Watson ADJ, Nicholson A, Church DB, et al. Use of anti-inflammatory and analgesic drugs in dogs and cats. Aust Vet J 1996;74:203–10.

[13] Machado CEG. Comparison of oxymorphone and hydromorphone in dogs: impact on isoflurane MAC and induction of anesthesia during hypovolemia [DVSc thesis]. Guelph: University of Guelph; 2002.

[14] Lascelles BDX, Waterman A. Analgesia in cats. In Pract 1997;19(4):203–13.

[15] Wilcke JR. Idiosyncrasies of drug metabolism in cats: effects on pharmacotherapeutics in feline practice. Vet Clin N Am Small Anim Pract 1984;14(6):1345–54.

[16] Mathews KA. Non-steroidal anti-inflammatory analgesics: a review of current practice. J Vet Emerg Crit Care 2002;12(2):89–97.

[17] Clutton RE. Cardiopulmonary disease. In: Seymour C, Gleed R, editors. Manual of small animal anaesthesia and analgesia. Cheltenham: British Small Animal Veterinary Association; 1999. p. 169.

[18] Waterman AE. Influence of premedication with xylazine on the distribution and metabolism of intramuscularly administered ketamine in cats. Res Vet Sci 1983;35:285–90.

[19] Clarke KW, Hall LW. A survey of anaesthesia in small animal practice: Association of Veterinary Anaesthesiology/British Small Animal Veterinary Association Report. J Assoc Vet Anaesthesiol 1990;17:4–10.

[20] Dyson DH, Maxie MG, Schnurr D. Morbidity and mortality associated with anesthetic management in small animal veterinary practice in Ontario. J Am Anim Hosp Assoc 1998; 34:325–35.

[21] Hamill JF, Bedofrd RF, Weaver DC, et al. Lidocaine before endotracheal intubation: intravenous or laryngotracheal? Anesthesiology 1981;55(5):578–81.

[22] Sakabe T, Maekawa T, Ishikawa T. The effects of lidocaine on canine cerebral metabolism and circulation related to the electroencephalogram. Anesthesiology 1974;40:433–41.

[23] White PF, Schlobohm RM, Pitts LH, et al. A randomized study of drugs for preventing increases in intracranial pressure during endotracheal suctioning. Anesthesiology 1982;57: 242–4.

[24] Milner QJ, Abdy S, Allen JG. Management of severe tracheal obstruction with helium/ oxygen and a laryngeal mask airway. Anaesthesia 1997;52:1087–9.

[25] Robinson EP, Fagella AM, Russell WL. Comparison of histamine release induced by morphine and oxymorphone administration in dogs. Am J Vet Res 1988;49:1699–701.

[26] Torske KE, Dyson DH. Epidural analgesia and anesthesia. Vet Clin N Am Small Anim Pract 2000;30(4):859–74.

[27] Wheeler AH, Aaron GW. Muscle pain due to injury. Curr Pain Headache Rep 2001;4: 441–6.

[28] Torske KE, Dyson DH, Conlon PD. Cardiovascular effects of epidurally administered oxymorphone and an oxymorphone-bupivacaine combination in halothane-anesthetized dogs. Am J Vet Res 1999;60:194–200.

[29] Rouby JJ, Andreev A, Leger P, et al. Peripheral vascular effects of thiopental and propofol in humans with artificial hearts. Anesthesiology 1991;75:32–42.

[30] Quandt JE, Rafee MR, Robinson EP. Butorphanol does not reduce the minimum alveolar concentration of halothane in dogs. Vet Surg 1994;23:156–9.

[31] Nunes de Moraes A, Dyson DH, O'Grady MR, et al. Plasma concentrations and cardiovascular influence of lidocaine infusions during isoflurane anesthesia in healthy dogs and dogs with subaortic stenosis. Vet Surg 1998;27:486–97.

[32] Hansen BD. Epidural catheter analgesia in dogs and cats: technique and review of 182 cases (1991–1999). J Vet Emerg Crit Care 2001;11(2):95–103.

[33] Spigset O, Hagg S. Analgesics and breast-feeding: safety considerations. Paediatr Drugs 2000;2(3):223–38.

[34] Wittels B, Scott DT, Sinatra RS. Exogenous opioids in human breast milk and acute neonatal neurobehavior: a preliminary study. Anesthesiology 1990;73:864–9.

[35] Meny RG, Naumburg EG, Alger LS, et al. Codeine and the breastfed neonate. J Hum Lact 1993;4:237–40.

[36] Begg EJ, Malpas TJ, Hackett LP, et al. Distribution of R- and S-methadone into human milk during multiple, medium to high oral dosing. Br J Clin Pharmacol 2001;52(6):681–8.

[37] Bond GM, Holloway AM. Anesthesia and breast-feeding—the effect on mother and infant. Anaesth Intensive Care 1992;20(4):426–30.

[38] Harris RC. Cyclooxygenase-2 in the kidney. Am Soc Nephrol 2000;11:2387–94.

[39] Collins JJ. Palliative care and the child with cancer. Hematol Oncol Clin N Am 2002;16: 657–70.

[40] Pascoe PJ. Perioperative pain management. Vet Clin N Am Small Anim Pract 2000;30: 917–32.

[41] Boothe DM, Bucheler J. Drug and blood component therapy and neonatal isoerythrolysis. In: Hospkins J, editor. Veterinary pediatrics: dogs and cats from birth to six months. Philadelphia: WB Saunders; 2001. p. 35–56.

[42] Lee BH. Managing pain in human neonates—application for animals. J Am Vet Med Assoc 2002;221(2):233–7.

[43] Rodriguez E, Jordan R. Contemporary trends in pediatric sedation and analgesia. Emerg Med Clin N Am 2002;20(1):199–222.

[44] Hosgood G. Surgical and anesthetic management of puppies and kittens. Compend Contin Educ Pract Vet 1992;14(5):345–57.

[45] Ball A, Ferguson S. Analgesia and analgesic drugs in paediatrics. Br J Hosp Med 1996;55(9): 586–90.

[46] Dubois RN, Abramson SB, Crofford L, et al. Cyclooxygenase in biology and disease. FASEB J 1998;12:1063–73.

[47] Nanovskaya T, Deshmukh S, Brooks M, et al. Transplacental transfer and metabolism of buprenorphine. J Pharmacol Exp Ther 2002;300(1):26–33.

[48] Wunsch MJ, Stanard V, Schnoll SH. Treatment of pain in pregnancy. Clin J Pain 2003;19(3): 148–55.

[49] Lamont LA, Tranquilli WJ, Mathews KA. Adjunctive analgesic therapy. Vet Clin N Am Small Anim Pract 2000;30(4):805–13.

[50] Groudine SC, Fisher SAG, Kaufman RP, et al. Intravenous lidocaine speeds the return of bowel function, decreases postoperative pain and shortens hospital stay in patients undergoing radical retropubic prostatectomy. Anesth Analg 1998;86:235–9.

[51] Hamill JF, Bedord RF, Weaver DC, et al. Lidocaine before endotracheal intubation: intravenous or laryngotracheal? Anesthesiology 1981;55:578–81.

[52] Sakabe T, Maekawa T, Ishikawa T. The effects of lidocaine on canine cerebral metabolism and circulation related to the electroencephalogram. Anesthesiology 1974;40:433–41.

[53] White PF, Schlobohm RM, Pitts LH, et al. A randomized study of drugs for preventing increases in intracranial pressure during endotracheal suctioning. Anesthesiology 1982;57: 242–4.

[54] Muir WW III. Drugs used to treat pain. In: Handbook of veterinary pain management. St. Louis: Mosby; 2002. p. 142–63.

[55] Field MJ, McLeary S, Hughes J. Gabapentin and pregabalin, but not morphine and amitriptyline, block both static and dynamic components of mechanical allodynia induced by streptozocin in the rat. Pain 1999;80:391–8.

ELSEVIER
SAUNDERS

Vet Clin Small Anim
35 (2005) 517–525

VETERINARY
CLINICS
Small Animal Practice

Practical Considerations in Emergency Drug Therapy

Tim B. Hackett, DVM, MS[a],*,
Tracy L. Lehman, DVM[b]

[a]Department of Clinical Sciences and Critical Care Unit, Veterinary Teaching Hospital,
Colorado State University, Fort Collins, CO 80523, USA
[b]Department of Microbiology, Immunology, and Pathology, Colorado State University,
Fort Collins, Colorado

"If all the drugs were thrown into the ocean, it would be all the worse for the fishes and all the better for mankind."

—Oliver Wendell Holmes

Drug therapy is an integral part of emergency and critical care medicine. Even the simple act of administering intravenous fluids is a drug therapy. Unfortunately, errors in drug therapy are a documented source of thousands of deaths each year in the human medical arena and likely occur in veterinary medicine as well [1]. Because our most critical patients receive fluids and a multitude of other drugs, clinicians need to be constantly aware of the drugs they are administering and the interactions that can occur when multiple drugs are used. Knowledge of the drugs used in critically ill patients is particularly important, because drug decisions often have to be made rapidly and in patients that may lack normal organ function.

When prescribing drugs for a desired therapeutic outcome, the clinician needs to understand the appropriate dose, frequency, route, and patient factors that may influence drug delivery. The purpose of this article is to review common drug therapies in the emergency setting, routes and dosing concerns, common drug-drug interactions (DDIs), and patient factors influencing drug dosages.

Routes of administration

Although intravenous drug administration is the preferred method in most emergency and critical care cases, other routes are often necessary.

---

* Corresponding author.
E-mail address: Tim.Hackett@ColoState.edu (T.B. Hackett).

0195-5616/05/$ - see front matter © 2005 Elsevier Inc. All rights reserved.
doi:10.1016/j.cvsm.2004.11.003

Intravenous access may not be possible in volume-contracted small animals. Venous cutdowns can be performed but may take precious time. Some medications should not be given intravenously or through the same line as other drugs. Several alternative methods of drug administration exist, including sublingual, intratracheal, intraosseous, intraperitoneal, intracardiac, gingival, and per rectum. Clinicians practicing emergency and critical care medicine should be proficient at all methods of drug administration and understand the indications and dosages used for each method.

Intravenous administration is usually the most ideal means of providing drug therapy in the emergency setting. The cephalic, jugular, medial saphenous (cats), and lateral saphenous (dogs) veins are the most common sites for catheter placement. Emergency clinicians should practice jugular venous cutdowns on cadavers to familiarize themselves with the technique. Knowing the locations of the veins helps to direct the skin incision when blood pressure is low and venous palpation is not reliable. A full description of techniques for venous access can be found elsewhere [2].

When there is no venous access or time for a vascular cutdown, drugs can be given via the sublingual route. The injection is made into the ventral meaty part of the tongue and is rapidly absorbed because of the preferential circulation to the head and brain during shock situations. The sublingual vein can sometimes also be a route of drug administration in sedated or nonresponsive animals.

Drugs like epinephrine, atropine, lidocaine, and dexamethasone can be administered by the intratracheal route in intubated animals. Twice the intravenous dosage is diluted with sterile saline at a rate of 5 to 10 mL and is injected into the endotracheal tube through a long catheter. After infusion of the drug, several deep assisted breaths can help to move the drugs to the pulmonary tissues for absorption. Drugs are then absorbed into the pulmonary circulation and taken to the left side of the heart, where they can reach coronary and systemic circulation.

The intraosseous route can be useful in neonatal and small animals, such as birds and rodents. A spinal needle or bone marrow needle with an inner stylet can be placed through the trochanteric fossa to the medullary cavity of the femur in dogs, cats, and small rodents. The ulna or proximal tibia should be used in birds, because these are nonpneumatic bones [3]. All drugs, including shock dose fluids or blood products, can be administered via this route. Intraosseous catheter use should be limited to 24 hours or less because these catheters are uncomfortable and difficult to cover. Administration of fluids through an intraosseous catheter should improve the circulating volume of the patient so that intravenous catheterization, if necessary, can be performed later.

Appropriate only in cardiac arrest situations, intracardiac injections are generally not recommended if any other method of drug administration can be used successfully. Complications associated with intracardiac injections include lung and coronary vessel lacerations and refractory ventricular fibrillation resulting from intramuscular injection into the myocardium. Intracardiac injection also necessitates cessation of cardiac compressions and respiratory support. Intracardiac injections are most effective and less likely to cause additional problems when performed during internal cardiac massage, because the likelihood of coronary vessel or lung damage is greatly reduced with direct visualization of the heart.

Intraperitoneal, oral, and per rectum dosing are other available routes for drug administration in specific instances. Rectal administration of drugs like diazepam and potassium bromide can be an effective method of seizure control. Lactulose and fluids can also be administered per rectum. Dextrose can be administered orally for the treatment of hypoglycemia. Warm fluids, dialysates, and some analgesics can be administered intraperitoneally through a sterile catheter.

Drug dosages

"Drugs have taught an entire generation of American kids the metric system."
                                                                —P.J. O'Rourke

In a review of human studies published from 1994 to 2001, the most common cause of preventable adverse drug events occurred by prescribing an inappropriate dose of medication [4]. The charged environment of emergency medicine is the last place clinicians should be performing complicated calculations. Dosage charts and prepared calculation programs can be invaluable resources during an emergency, such as cardiopulmonary arrest. Veterinarians and veterinary technicians should double-check dose and volume with one another before administering a new drug to a patient.

Dosage charts based on the drug concentrations available in each hospital should be prepared in the most user-friendly manner possible. This includes dosages for fluids and drugs, such as epinephrine, atropine, lidocaine, magnesium, sodium bicarbonate, dextrose, and calcium gluconate. Examples of emergency drug dosage charts and treatment algorithms are available at the Veterinary Emergency and Critical Care Society's web site (http://veccs.org/public/shopping/posters.html). The charts should be positioned where they can be seen when directing cardiopulmonary resuscitation. The print should be large enough to be easily read from where the clinician(s) and support staff are standing. Appropriate and rapid drug administration can be further encouraged when drugs are kept close to the arrest location and in consistent and labeled compartments. All staff likely to be involved in an arrest situation should be familiar with the location of the drugs and associated materials. To be most effective, cardiopulmonary resuscitation drills should be practiced with the entire staff, including basic and advanced life support techniques.

For more complicated drug dosing, such as continuous rate infusions (CRIs), precalculated charts and computer spreadsheets can help with appropriate dosing. Calculators or computers should be readily available so that such calculations can be performed when necessary. It is advisable to secure inexpensive calculators to walls surrounding emergency treatment areas. This is particularly important, because inappropriate administration of many of the drugs used as CRIs (eg, dopamine, dobutamine, sodium nitroprusside) can lead to life-threatening complications.

Drug references should be readily available for determining drug interactions, dosage calculations, and appropriate suspending agents for commonly used combinations. The ultimate responsibility always belongs to the clinician ordering the drug therapy. Although computer programs and other references can make drug references and complicated calculations easy to perform, they are only as good as the persons who create and use them. Such programs and references must be constantly cross-referenced, updated, and assessed for errors [5].

In addition to checking the calculation of CRIs, support staff must be proficient at administering the CRIs. Properly programmed and functioning infusion pumps are the most reliable way to administer CRIs. Appropriate monitoring of the pumps should maximize the safety of drug infusions.

Finally, no matter what method of calculation is used for drug therapy, clinicians must be aware of the patient factors and drug interactions that can change the dosing of many drugs.

General guidelines

Avoiding drug problems sounds simple: use as few drugs as possible, and know as much as you can about the drugs you do use. The continued production of new drugs and the complications associated with advanced medical care make such principles difficult to follow, however. A mnemonic has been developed to help remind physicians to use drug therapy more appropriately [6]. The mnemonic "SAIL," which stands for Simplify, Adverse effects of drugs, Indications, and List all drugs, has been developed to encourage physicians to consider multiple drug therapy carefully. "Simplify" is a reminder that almost all drugs can be stopped and should be stopped if there are suspected complications. Making changes one at a time helps to define the cause of the problem more clearly. "Adverse effects of drugs" reminds the clinician that all drugs can have reactions even if they are not documented. Even drugs that are used to treat other drug reactions can cause reactions themselves in some patients. "Indications" reminds clinicians that there should be a measurable and measured goal, because all drugs should be given to improve patient health. Finally, "List all drugs" denotes one of the easiest ways to avoid problems: take an accurate drug history and keep accurate and current records of all drugs used. Research each drug, with an emphasis on patient factors and concomitant drug administration that may cause problems. The process is easier and the risk of complications is lower when fewer drugs are used.

Commonly used drugs and their interactions

Any drug can cause problems in individual patients. Polypharmacy, or the use of more than one drug in a patient at a time, increases the risk of complications from the drugs and the administration of them. Unfortunately, research is lacking on the interactions of multidrug administration [7]. Consequently, clinicians should exhaust available resources, use careful patient monitoring, and work to keep drug use to a minimum to avoid iatrogenic drug complications. This article cannot list all the drugs used in emergency and critical care medicine and their known interactions. A few drugs and mechanisms of interaction are discussed below as examples.

Fluids, probably the most commonly administered emergency drug, can have several complications and interactions depending on the route of administration and type of fluid chosen. Lactated Ringer's solution contains calcium and may lead to problems when administered concurrently with other drugs and blood products. Blood products not only interact with other solutions but can cause life-threatening interactions with the patient's immune system. Using type-specific blood, cross-matching, and administering small test doses help to decrease the risk of complications. Use of lipid-containing fluids and parenteral nutrition formulas necessitates separate lines for other fluids and drugs, because the opacity of the solution makes it difficult to see drug precipitation. Ideally, fluids should be discontinued and lines flushed with saline before and after administering any additional drugs. This should help to avoid adverse interactions when using a single line.

Many drugs affect the hepatic cytochrome p450 enzyme system. Administration of multiple drugs having the same metabolic pathways can interfere with function and increase toxicity of one or more of the medications. For example, the H_2 blockers ranitidine and cimetidine inhibit the hepatic cytochrome p450 enzyme system, and concurrent use of drugs like diazepam, theophylline, and procainamide can lead to complications if the dosages are not adjusted. Famotidine, however, does not seem to affect the cytochrome p450 enzyme systems and would potentially be a better choice if an H_2 blocker was necessary in a patient requiring additional drug therapy [8].

H_2 blockers are only one category of drugs known to interact with the cytochrome p450 enzyme system. As more drugs are developed that involve these pathways, clinicians may see treatment failures and unreported DDIs. It is estimated that 50% or more of all drugs interact with the cytochrome p450 pathways. Antifungals (eg, ketoconazole), benzodiazepines, chemotherapeutics, immunosuppressives (eg, tacrolimus, cyclosporine), proton pump inhibitors (eg, omeprazole), warfarin compounds, antivirals, fluoroquinolones, and even antiemetics interact with the cytochrome p450 enzymes. Even herbal supplements like St. John's wort have been found to affect the p450 pathways and may interfere with other drug therapies [9,10]. Awareness of these complications helps to emphasize the importance of

DDIs and can help the clinician to make appropriate drug and monitoring choices.

Patient factors

Several patient factors can dramatically affect the distribution and metabolism of drugs. These factors need to be noted and dosages adjusted to avoid complications.

Age is an important factor to consider when making drug choices. Neonates have immature renal function and should not receive nonsteroidal anti-inflammatory drugs (NSAIDS), aminoglycosides, or angiotensin-converting enzyme (ACE) inhibitors. Dosages of highly protein-bound drugs and anesthetics should be reduced in young animals to prevent prolonged drug effects caused by physiologic hypoalbuminemia and an immature blood-brain barrier. Fluoroquinolones should be avoided in growing animals because they can interfere with cartilage growth [8,11]. These problems are magnified during the perinatal period; thus, pregnant and nursing animals must be treated cautiously to avoid complications in their offspring. Geriatric patients also need careful assessment because they are more likely to have organ dysfunction and altered drug metabolism [12].

Body condition can affect drug dosing. Obese animals often need to be dosed at the ideal body weight, especially when using drugs that can be sequestered in adipose tissue, such as thiobarbiturates. Administration of subcutaneous or intramuscular medications can be more difficult in obese and extremely thin animals. Additionally, animals with an abnormal body condition often have underlying medical problems that should affect drug choices. Every effort should be made to identify the cause for the abnormal body condition before initiating drug therapies.

Hepatic and renal dysfunction is extremely important to drug therapy, because the liver and kidney are involved in the function, breakdown, and clearance of most drugs. The liver manufactures plasma proteins affecting the available concentration of protein-bound drugs, such as furosemide and propofol. Hypoalbuminemia increases the toxicity of these drugs. The liver is also the site of the cytochrome P450 system, which is involved in the action of many commonly used drugs. Liver disease may affect the function of these pathways. Renal disease can decrease the kidney's ability to filter and excrete drugs, leading to extended periods of drug and drug metabolite presence in the body. Aminoglycosides are eliminated primarily by renal mechanisms and should be used with caution and monitoring even in animals with normal renal function [13]. Even the use of potassium-containing fluids can lead to life-threatening serum potassium levels in animals with impaired renal function [14]. Most animals with hepatic and renal disease require lower doses and less frequent administration of most drugs. Cardiovascular disease requires adjustments in fluid type and infusion rates. These patients are often on multiple therapies commonly associated with DDI issues. Dehydration interferes with the absorption of subcutaneous drug administration.

Most patients requiring emergency or critical care medical support have factors that affect drug delivery and metabolism. Care should be taken to provide thorough and repeated assessments to identify such factors and respond to complications rapidly.

Monitoring recommendations

> "I've never had a problem with drugs. I've had problems with the police."
> —Keith Richards

All animals receiving emergency medical care should be monitored closely. This is especially important in those animals receiving multiple drug therapy. In a recent literature review, patient monitoring was one of the two most frequently identified causes of preventable adverse drug events in human medicine, second only to dosage errors [4].

Evaluating and recording vital signs, such as temperature, heart rate and rhythm, pulse rate, respiratory rate, mucous membrane color, and attitude, should be routine in patients on multiple drug therapy. Changes in patient condition should be evaluated for possible drug complications or interactions. Records of type, time, amount, and method of drugs administered should be accurate and current. Proper chronologic records can minimize confusion about drug administration between shifts. Continuous infusions of fluids and CRI medications should be checked often for accuracy so as to avoid complications from overdosing or underdosing. These basic monitoring techniques can help to avoid most major complications and help to initiate early and appropriate responses to problems.

More invasive and specific monitoring is recommended for certain drug therapies. Safe and effective administration of positive inotropes is accomplished with continuous blood pressure monitoring. Continuous electrocardiographic monitoring may be necessary with drugs that affect cardiac function. Examples include intravenous fluids, calcium, epinephrine, dopamine, lidocaine, and procainamide. Blood gas monitoring is recommended to guide bicarbonate therapy. Daily red blood cell counts as well as total protein and electrolyte levels are ideal when patients are receiving fluid and nutritional support. The clinician should be familiar with the complications associated with all drugs being administered and choose the most appropriate monitoring techniques. Animals receiving multiple drugs should have additional preventative monitoring for signs of possible drug interactions. References should be readily available to help the clinician avoid and respond to complications from drug administration.

Plasma drug concentrations should be considered in critical care patients with specific complications or failure to respond to appropriate therapy.

Monitoring plasma concentrations of drugs is necessary when using drugs with a narrow therapeutic spectrum. Examples include warfarin, phenobarbital, and digoxin.

Resources

Books, handheld computer software, and Internet resources are available for assistance in drug use in emergency and critical care practice. Books focused on drug interactions have sections to help clinicians with drug choices. Plumb's *Veterinary Drug Handbook* [8], for example, has sections on drug interactions, adverse effects, and contraindications. The *Physician's Desk Reference* has similar information. The clinician should use several of the available resources in their most current format and cross-reference when possible to avoid printing errors and discrepancies. Unfortunately, complete information on drug interactions is not available, and clinicians need to monitor for complications in all patients receiving drug therapy.

Finally, clinicians should not forget the role of the pharmacist when confronted with multiple drug therapy questions or adverse drug reactions. Pharmacists can provide information on drug choices, interactions, and pharmacokinetics to assist in clinical cases. Pharmacists are also excellent sources of information on new drug information. Involvement of pharmacists in drug therapy for human emergency and critical care patients has been shown to reduce drug errors and adverse drug events and to decrease morbidity, mortality, and the costs of health care [15].

References

[1] Phillips DP, Christenfeld N, Glynn LM. Increase in US medication-error deaths between 1983 and 1993. Lancet 1998;351:643–4.
[2] Wingfield SGB. Emergency vascular access and intravenous catheterization. In: Wingfield WE, Raffe MR, editors. The veterinary ICU book. Jackson, WY: Teton New Media; 2002. p. 58–67.
[3] Quesenberry KE, Hillyer EV. Supportive care and emergency therapy. In: Ritchie BW, Harrison GJ, Harrison LR, editors. Avian medicine: principles and applications. Lake Worth, FL: Wingers Publishing; 1994. p. 382–433.
[4] Kanjanarat P, Winterstein AG, Johns TE, et al. Nature of preventable adverse drug events in hospitals: a literature review. Am J Health Syst Pharm 2003;60:1750–9.
[5] Kraft KE, Dore FH. Computerized drug interaction programs: how reliable [letter]? JAMA 1996;275:1087.
[6] Meador CK. Polypharmacy—old bad habits. J Am Board Fam Pract 1998;11(2):166–7.
[7] Lee RD. Polypharmacy: a case report and new protocol for management. J Am Board Fam Pract 1998;11(2):140–4.
[8] Plumb DC. Veterinary drug handbook. 3rd edition. Ames, IA: Iowa State University Press; 1999.
[9] Jang EH, Park YC, Chung WG. Effects of dietary supplements on induction and inhibition of cytochrome p450s protein expression in rats. Food Chem Toxicol 2004;42(11):1749–56.
[10] Butterweck V, Derendorf H, Gaus W, et al. Pharmacokinetic herb-drug interactions: are preventative screenings necessary and appropriate? Planta Med 2004;70:784–91.

[11] Egerbacker M, Edinger J, Tschulenk W. Effects of enrofloxacin and ciprofloxacin hydrochloride on canine and equine chondrocytes in cultures. Am J Vet Res 2001;62(5):704–8.

[12] Booth DM. Principles of drug therapy. In: Small animal clinical pharmacology and therapeutics. Philadelphia: WB Saunders; 2001. p. 3–17.

[13] Nagai J, Takano M. Molecular aspects of renal handling of aminoglycosides and strategies for preventing the nephrotoxicity. Drug Metab Pharmacokinet 2004;19(3):159–70.

[14] Ross LA. Fluid therapy for acute and chronic renal failure. Vet Clin N Am Small Anim Pract 1989;19(2):343–59.

[15] Papadopoulos J, Rebuck JA, Lober C, et al. The critical care pharmacist: an essential intensive care practitioner. Pharmacotherapy 2002;22:1484–8.

ELSEVIER
SAUNDERS

Vet Clin Small Anim
35 (2005) 527–535

VETERINARY
CLINICS
Small Animal Practice

Index

Note: Page numbers of article titles are in **boldface** type.

0195-5616/05/$ - see front matter © 2005 Elsevier Inc. All rights reserved.
doi:10.1016/S0195-5616(05)00002-1   *vetsmall.theclinics.com*

Changing Your Address?

Make sure your subscription changes too! When you notify us of your new address, you can help make our job easier by including an exact copy of your Clinics label number with your old address (see illustration below.) This number identifies you to our computer system and will speed the processing of your address change. Please be sure this label number accompanies your old address and your corrected address—you can send an old Clinics label with your number on it or just copy it exactly and send it to the address listed below.

We appreciate your help in our attempt to give you continuous coverage. Thank you.

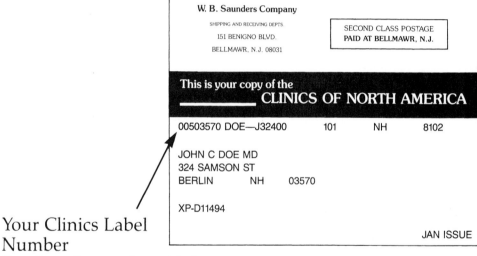

W. B. Saunders Company

SHIPPING AND RECEIVING DEPTS.

151 BENIGNO BLVD.

BELLMAWR, N.J. 08031

SECOND CLASS POSTAGE
PAID AT BELLMAWR, N.J.

This is your copy of the
CLINICS OF NORTH AMERICA

00503570 DOE—J32400   101   NH   8102

JOHN C DOE MD
324 SAMSON ST
BERLIN   NH   03570

XP-D11494

JAN ISSUE

Your Clinics Label Number
Copy it exactly or send your label
along with your address to:
W.B. Saunders Company, Customer Service
Orlando, FL 32887-4800
Call Toll Free 1-800-654-2452

Please allow four to six weeks for delivery of new subscriptions and for processing address changes.